Prentice Hall Health's

high yield facts

of Dental Hygiene

Demetra Daskalos Logothetis, RDH, MS
Director and Associate Professor
University of New Mexico
Health Sciences Center
Division of Dental Hygiene
Albuquerque, New Mexico

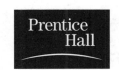

Prentice
Hall

Upper Saddle River, New Jersey 07458

Library of Congress Cataloging-in-Publication Data
Logothetis, Demetra Daskalos.
   High yield facts of dental hygiene/Demetra Daskalos
Logothetis.
      p. ; cm. -- (Success across the boards) (Prentice Hall
Health review series)
Includes bibliographical references.
   ISBN 0-13-089307-2
   1. Dental hygiene--Examinations, questions, etc. 2. Dental
Hygienists--Examinations, questions, etc. 3. Oral medicine--
Examinations, questions, etc.
   [DNLM: 1. Dental Prophylaxis--Examination Questions. 2.
Dental Hygienists--Examination Questions. 3. Dental Polish-
ing--Examination Questions. WU 18.2 :832h 2003] I. Title: II.
Series. III. Series: Prentice Hall Health review series
   RK60.5 .L635 2003
   617.6'01'076--dc21

                                              2002009510

Publisher: Julie Levin Alexander
Assistant to Publisher: Regina Bruno
Senior Acquisitions Editor: Mark Cohen
Assistant Editor: Melissa Kerian
Editorial Assistant: Mary Ellen Ruitenberg
Senior Marketing Manager: Nicole Benson
Marketing Assistant: Janet Ryerson
Product Information Manager: Rachele Strober
Director of Production and Manufacturing:
   Bruce Johnson
Production Managing Editor: Patrick Walsh
Production Liaison: Alexander Ivchenko

Production Editor: Jessica Balch, Pine Tree Composition
Manufacturing Manager: Ilene Sanford
Manufacturing Buyer: Pat Brown
Design Director: Cheryl Asherman
Senior Design Coordinator: Maria Guglielmo Walsh
Cover and Interior Designer: Janice Bielawa
Manager of Media Production: Amy Peltier
New Media Project Manager: Stephen Hartner
Composition: Pine Tree Composition
Printing and Binding: Banta Harrisonburg
Cover Printer: Phoenix Color

Pearson Education, Ltd., *London*
Pearson Education Australia Pty. Limited, *Sydney*
Pearson Education Singapore Pte. Ltd.
Pearson Education North Asia Ltd., *Hong Kong*
Pearson Education Canada, Ltd., *Toronto*
Pearson Educación de Mexico, S.A. de C.V.
Pearson Education—Japan, *Tokyo*
Pearson Education Malaysia, Pte. Ltd.
Pearson Education, *Upper Saddle River, New Jersey*

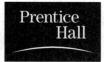

10 9 8 7 6 5 4 3 2 1
ISBN 0-13-089307-2

I dedicate this book to my parents,
Pete and Soula Daskalos, who through their
example have taught me about hard work, diligence, and
perseverance and who devoted themselves to their children
in order to give us a better life. For their love and
support, which has allowed me to make all things possible.

To my husband, Nick, for his endless love and support.
For his ability to make me laugh and feel good
when things get too stressful, and for his encouragement
and understanding on a daily basis.

To my children, Stacy and Costa, who make everything worthwhile.
For their love and understanding.

And in loving memory of my grandparents, Nick and Olga Tzouvaras,
and my dear friend Karen Finley who passed away during the creation
of this text. May the memory of them be eternal.

Contents

Preface

This dental hygiene review textbook is designed to assist the dental hygiene student in preparing for the National Dental Hygiene Board Examination by offering an easy flash card format to study. This book is also an excellent tool for preparing students to take state or regional board examinations. It offers a comprehensive section on local anesthesia and pain control for students who must take a local anesthesia examination to become licensed to administer local anesthesia.

The textbook is designed to provide the most important information needed to take any dental hygiene board examination, and is organized based upon the National Dental Hygiene Board Specifications with the intent to help students prepare for the exam, and understand the breakdown of the exam's contents. The textbook is divided into three sections according to the examination format. Section I, Scientific Basis for Dental Hygiene Practice, encompasses all the basic science coursework. This is an important section for students to review since most students have taken some of these courses as prerequisites and will need to refresh or relearn some information. Section II, Provision of Clinical Dental Hygiene Services, includes information on assessing patient characteristics through comprehensive material on medical history review; head and neck examination; periodontal, oral, and occlusal evaluation; and clinical testing. It includes a complete radiology section along with x-rays to complement the flash cards. Information on infection control, dental emergencies, patient education, pain control, and management of the medically compromised patient can be found in this section under planning and managing dental hygiene care. Section II also includes material on performing periodontal procedures, reassessment and maintenance, preventive agents, and dental materials. Section III, Community Health and Research Principles, includes coursework related to community dental health and research methods.

High Yield Facts of Dental Hygiene is in flash card format for easy reading and memorization. Key concepts (☞) are provided throughout the text to assist the student in retaining important information necessary to be successful at passing the examination.

This textbook is excellent for refreshing student's memories prior to board examinations on information they have already learned in an easy-to-use "dental hygiene in a nutshell" format. However, I also encourage students to use this textbook at the beginning of their dental hygiene education to help study for exams and provide a continuous review of essential material leading up to the national, regional, or state board examinations.

I encourage students to begin studying early, and to continuously review the information provided in this text throughout their dental hygiene education. I sincerely hope that this textbook benefits its readers in a positive way to successfully complete your education and licensure, which you have worked so hard to earn. Best of luck.

Demetra Daskalos Logothetis

Acknowledgments

I would like to thank the contributors of this textbook for their hard work, perseverance, and attention to detail. A special thank you to Mark Cohen, Senior Acquisitions Editor for Prentice Hall, who came up with the idea for this text, for all his support and encouragement. Also, to Melissa Kerian, Assistant Editor Health Professions, Prentice Hall, for all her help and support, and to Martha Currise, freelance developmental editor, for helping me keep on track and for always getting back to me so quickly whenever I had questions.

A special thank you to Christine Nathe who was always willing to help with the Division's administrative work so that I could spend quality time working on this text. Thank you to Charlie Tatlock, DDS, Assistant Professor Clinician Education for UNM Dental Services; Robert Supple, DDS; and Jacqueline Plemons, DDS, Associate Clinical Professor, Department of Periodontics, TAMUS BCOD, for allowing me to use their pathology slides in this text. Thank you to Kirstin Peterson who spent so much of her time helping me collect x-rays for this text. A special thank you to all my students who helped me find x-rays for this book, and especially to April Navalesi who worked so hard at organizing the x-rays. I would also like to thank all the reviewers for offering wonderful feedback and advice.

Reviewers

Eugenia Bearden, RDH, ME
Associate Professor
Dental Hygiene
Clayton College and State University
Morrow, Georgia

Marsha E. Bower, CDA, RDH, MA
Assistant Professor
Dental Studies
Monroe Community College
Rochester, New York

Nancy Cuttic, RDH, BSDH, MEd
Associate Professor
Dental Hygiene Program
Harcum College
Bryn Mawr, Pennsylvania

Rita Hallock, RDH, BA
Assistant Professor
Dental Hygiene Program
Brevard Community College
Cocoa, Florida

Denise Muesch Helm, RDH, MA
Assistant Professor
Northern Arizona University
Department of Dental Hygiene
Flagstaff, Arizona

Carol C. Johnson, RDH, MSHA
Program Director
Dental Hygiene
West Central Technical College
Douglasville, Georgia

C. Merry LeBlond, RDH, MS
Assistant Professor and Coordinator
Dental Hygiene Program
Middlesex County College
Edison, New Jersey

Contributors

Joe R. Anderson, PharmD, BCPS
Assistant Professor
University of New Mexico
College of Pharmacy
Albuquerque, New Mexico

Carla Loiacono, RDH, MS
Associate Professor
University of New Mexico
Division of Dental Hygiene
Albuquerque, New Mexico

Christine Nathe, RDH, MS
Associate Professor
University of New Mexico
Division of Dental Hygiene
Albuquerque, New Mexico

Sandy Roe, RDH, MS
Administrative Director
Participa! Inc. Dental Services
Adjunct Assistant Professor
University of New Mexico
Division of Dental Hygiene
Albuquerque, New Mexico

Catherine Bosiljevac Sovereign, MS, RDH, RD
Adjunct Assistant Professor
University of New Mexico
Division of Dental Hygiene
Albuquerque, New Mexico

Tammy Teague, RDH, BS
Adjunct Assistant Professor
University of New Mexico
Division of Dental Hygiene
Albuquerque, New Mexico

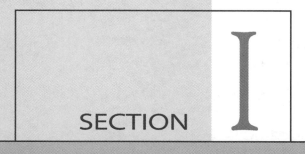

SECTION I

Scientific Basis for Dental Hygiene Practice

➤ Anatomical Science

➤ Physiology

➤ Biochemistry and Nutrition

➤ Microbiology and Immunology

➤ Pathology

➤ Pharmacology

CHAPTER

1 Anatomical Science

Demetra Daskalos Logothetis,
  RDH, MS
Sandy Roe, RDH, MS

➤ HEAD AND NECK ANATOMY

Osseous Anatomy—Skull

ANATOMIC TERMINOLOGY	
DORSAL SIDE	Backbone side ☞ Also called posterior
VENTRAL SIDE	Belly side ☞ Also called anterior
SUPERIOR	Describes something that is on top
INFERIOR	Describes something that is below
MIDLINE	Vertical line dividing the center of the body
MEDIAL	Toward the midline
LATERAL	Away from the midline
FRONTAL SECTION	Slices through the frontal view of the head and neck **Figure 1-1**
SAGITTAL SECTION	Slices through the sagittal view of the head and neck **Figure 1-2**
TRANSVERSE OR CROSS SECTION	Through the head **Figure 1-3**

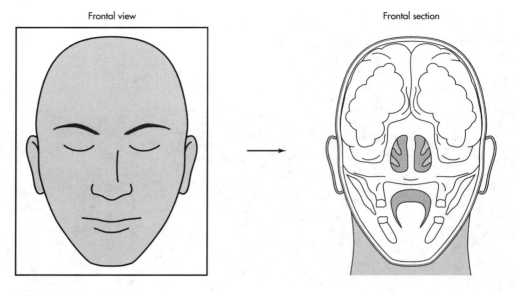

Frontal view   Frontal section

FIGURE 1-1. Frontal Section

CRANIAL	Pertaining to the head
CERVICAL	Pertaining to the neck
SUPERFICIAL	Topmost layer
DEEP	Below it
INTERNAL	Inside
EXTERNAL	Outside
JOINT	Joining of two bones
LIGAMENTS	Strong connective tissue; hold bones together

SKULL There are two portions of the skull	
CRANIUM	Primarily involved in housing and protecting the brain
VISCERAL STRUCTURES	Related to the face

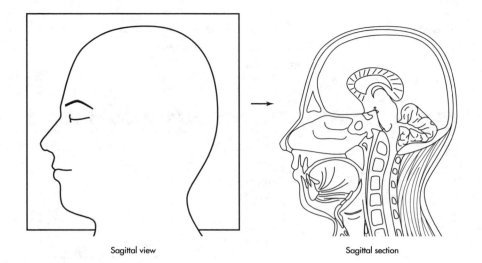

Sagittal view   Sagittal section

FIGURE 1-2. Sagittal Section

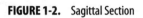

BONES OF THE NECK

CERVICAL VERTEBRAE	Provide strong support for the neck and protective tunnel for important nerves and blood vessels There are seven cervical vertebrae named by number: • C-1—"Atlas"; holds up the cranium • C-2—"Axis"; medial protuberance allows rotation around it • C-3 • C-4 • C-5 • C-6 • C-7

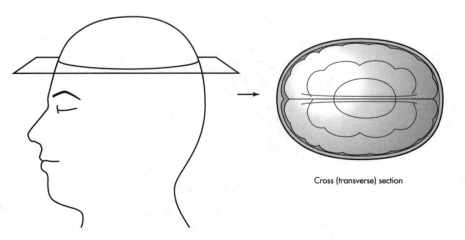

Cross (transverse) section

FIGURE 1-3. Transverse or Cross Section

HYOID BONE	Bone of the neck that is attached to several muscles but to no other bone **Figure 1-4**

BONES OF THE CRANIUM	
SINGLE	• Occipital • Frontal • Sphenoid • Ethmoid
PAIRED	• Parietal • Temporal

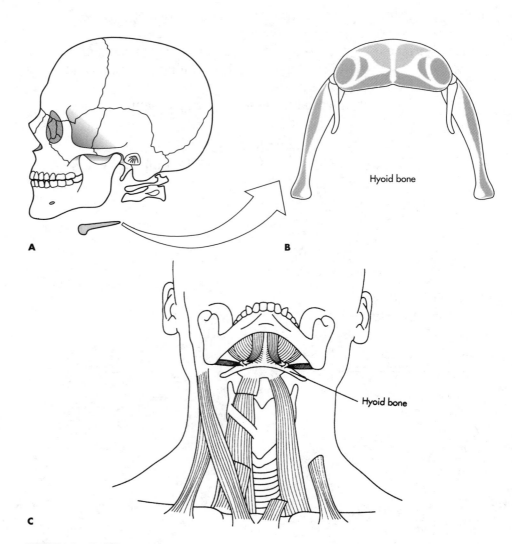

A

B

Hyoid bone

C

Hyoid bone

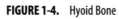

FIGURE 1-4. Hyoid Bone

BONES OF THE FACE

SINGLE	Vomer
PAIRED	• Maxilla • Zygomatic • Nasal • Lacrimal • Palatine

SUPERIOR ASPECT OF THE SKULL Figure 1-5

BONES	• Frontal (single) • Occipital (single) • Parietal (paired)
SUTURES	• Coronal—extends transversely between the frontal and parietal bone • Sagittal—joins the parietal bones • Lambdoidal—lies between the occipital and the two parietal bones • Squamosal—temporal and parietal bones • Temporozygomatic—zygomatic and temporal bones • Median palatine—palatine bones • Tranverse palatine—maxilla and palatine bones

ANTERIOR ASPECT OF THE SKULL
Major bones Figure 1-6

LEFT	• Parietal • Greater wing of sphenoid • Temporal • Sphenoid • Lacrimal ethmoid • Nasal septum—ethmoid vomer • Zygomatic
RIGHT	• Nasal bones • Parietal • Greater wing of sphenoid • Temporal • Zygomatic • Lacrimal • Inferior nasal concha • Mandible

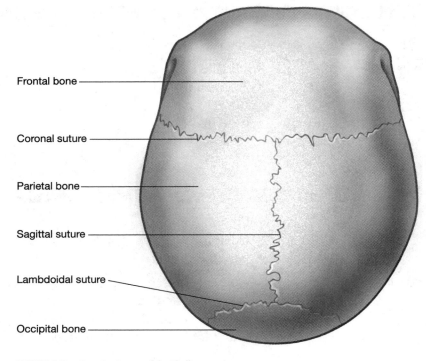

Frontal bone

Coronal suture

Parietal bone

Sagittal suture

Lambdoidal suture

Occipital bone

FIGURE 1-5. Superior Aspect of the Skull

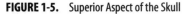

FRONTAL BONE

- Forehead and eyebrow area of the face
- Extends into the eye sockets or orbits

Figure 1-7

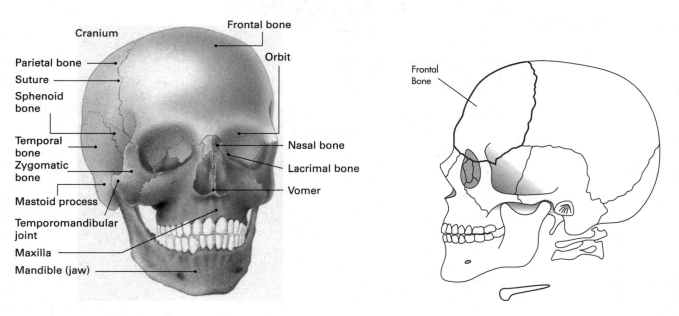

Cranium

Frontal bone

Parietal bone

Orbit

Suture

Sphenoid bone

Temporal bone

Zygomatic bone

Mastoid process

Temporomandibular joint

Maxilla

Mandible (jaw)

Nasal bone

Lacrimal bone

Vomer

Frontal Bone

FIGURE 1-6. Anterior Aspect of the Skull

FIGURE 1-7. Frontal Bone

ANTERIOR CRANIAL FOSSA

Lies in middle of frontal bone and resembles a walnut; comes together with sphenoid bone to form a "shelf" where the cerebrum rests

Figure 1-8

PARIETAL BONES

Constitutes most of the top and sides of the cranium

Figure 1-9

OCCIPITAL BONE

Contains singularly large foramen from interior view—foramen magnum that provides passage for the large spinal cord as it exits the brain; hypoglossal canals transmit cranial nerve (CN) XII

Figure 1-10

Osseous Anatomy—Maxilla

BODY

Orbital, nasal, infratemporal, and facial surfaces

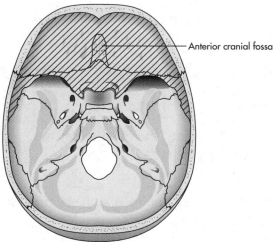

FIGURE 1-8. Anterior Cranial Fossa

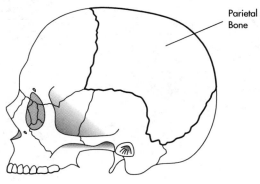

FIGURE 1-9. Parietal Bone

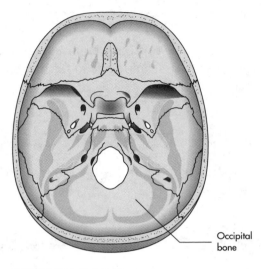

Occipital
bone

FIGURE 1-10. Occipital Bone

MAXILLARY PROCESSES

FRONTAL	• Forms medial orbital rim with the lacrimal bone • Orbital surface is separated from the sphenoid bone by inferior orbital fissure
ZYGOMATIC	Articulates with the zygomatic bone laterally, forming the infraorbital rim
PALATINE	• Two palatine processes articulate to form the hard palate • Suture between two processes is the median palatine suture
ALVEOLAR	Supports the roots of the maxillary teeth ☛ Bone is more porous than mandible ☛ Can use infiltration anesthesia

BONES OF THE MAXILLA

FRONTAL PROCESS	Articulates with frontal bone
NASAL SEPTUM	Vertical midline structure divides the nasal cavity in half **Figure 1-11**
ANTERIOR NASAL SPINE	Small projection of bone at the beginning of nasal septum ☛ May appear in periapical films of maxillary anterior teeth

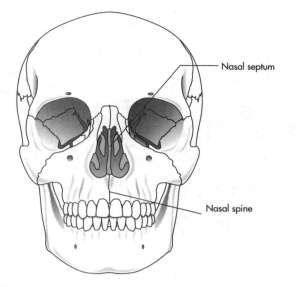

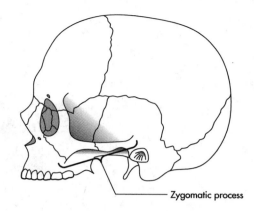
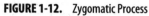

FIGURE 1-12. Zygomatic Process

FIGURE 1-11. Nasal Septum and Nasal Spine

CANINE EMINENCE	Prominence of canine root ☛ Landmark for ASA injection
ZYGOMATIC PROCESS	Composed of portions of the temporal bone, the zygoma bone, and the maxillary bone ☛ Articulates with zygoma to form the cheek ☛ Landmark for PSA, MSA injections **Figure 1-12**
MAXILLARY TUBEROSITY	Bone directly distal to last molar ☛ Posterior superior alveolar nerve
PALATINE PROCESS	Forms anterior portion of hard palate
ALVEOLAR PROCESS	Maxillary bone that surrounds and supports the teeth

MAXILLARY SINUSES

- Part of paranasal sinuses
- Pyramid-shaped spaces in close proximity to roots of posterior maxillary teeth
- ☛ Can be seen on posterior periapical films
Figure 1-13

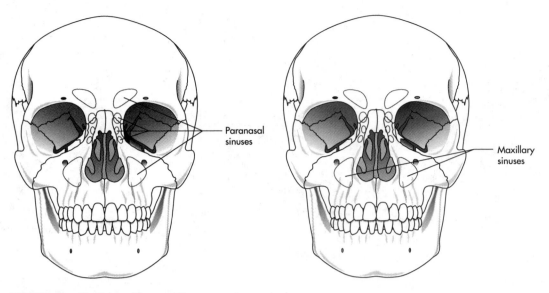

FIGURE 1-13. Maxillary and Paranasal Sinuses

FORAMEN Figures 1-14 and 1-15	
INCISIVE FORAMEN	Behind the central incisors ☞ Nasopalatine nerve—injection site for nasopalatine injection

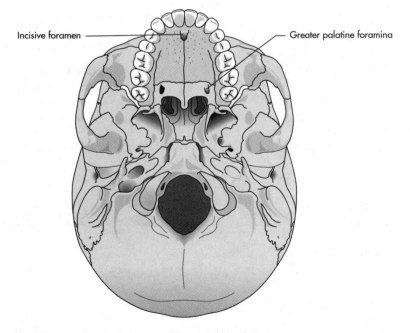

FIGURE 1-14. Incisive Foramen and Greater Palatine Foramina

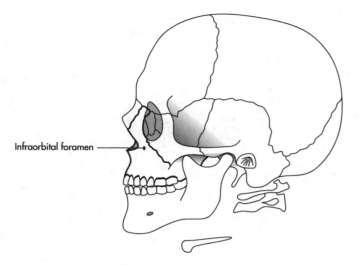

Infraorbital foramen

FIGURE 1-15. Infraorbital Foramen

GREATER PALATINE FORAMEN	Two foramen found on back of palate on either side of palate opposite last molars ☞ Greater palatine nerve—injection site for greater palatine injection ☞ Not part of the maxillary bone
INFRAORBITAL FORAMEN	Provides exit for the infraorbital nerve that innervates the skin of middle of face ☞ Landmark for infraorbital (IO) injection

PALATINE BONE

GREATER (MAJOR) PALATINE FORAMEN	Also called anterior palatine foramen; opening of pterygopalatine canal; greater palatine nerve
MIDDLE AND POSTERIOR PALATINE FORAMEN	Palatine nerves to soft palate and tonsils
MIDPALATINE SUTURE	Suture dividing the palate in half

VOMER BONE

Seen in posterior view of nasal cavity and palate and forms part of the nasal septum

Figure 1-16

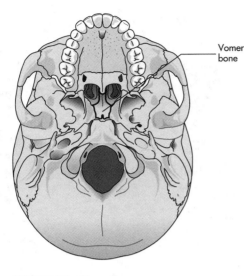

FIGURE 1-16. Vomer Bone

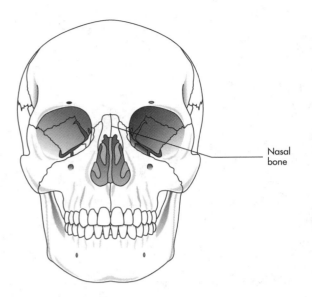
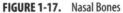

FIGURE 1-17. Nasal Bones

NASAL BONES

Two small bones on bridge of the nasal orifice
❖ Forms bridge of nose
Figure 1-17

ETHMOID BONE

- Interior view—walnut-shaped bone in frontal bone
- Single bone forming posterior portion of nasal cavity
- Contains many sinuses or air cells
- Cribriform plate—perforated with holes; sensory nerves from nose ascend to olfactory bulbs of CNI

LACRIMAL BONES

Two bones—lacrimal glands rest on their fossae; adjacent to naso-lacrimal duct
❖ Smallest bones of cranium

Sphenoid Bone

- Single butterfly-shaped cranial bone
- Supports the base of the brain
- Several foramina through which major nerves exit the brain
Figure 1-18

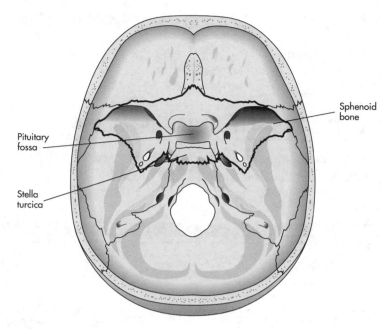

Sphenoid bone

Pituitary fossa

Stella turcica

FIGURE 1-18. Sphenoid Bone

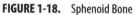

FORAMEN OVALE

Mandibular nerve (V₃) exits
☛ Part of greater wings that form lateral wall of skull
Figure 1-19

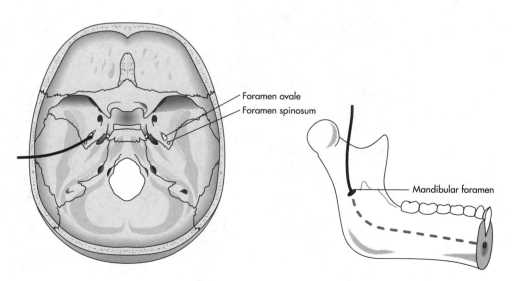

Foramen ovale
Foramen spinosum

Mandibular foramen

FIGURE 1-19. Foramen Ovale, where Mandibular Neve (V₃) Exits onto the Mandible

FORAMEN ROTUNDUM

Maxillary nerve (V_2) exits

Figure 1-20

FORAMEN SPINOSUM

Middle menigeal artery branch of maxillary artery exits
☛ Part of greater wings that form lateral wall of skull

FORAMEN LACERIUM

Internal carotid artery

SUPERIOR ORBITAL FISSURE

- Large fissures rather than foramina
- Nerves and veins to muscles of the eye
- ☛ CNs III, IV, VI, and Ophthalmic (V_1) exit

Figure 1-21

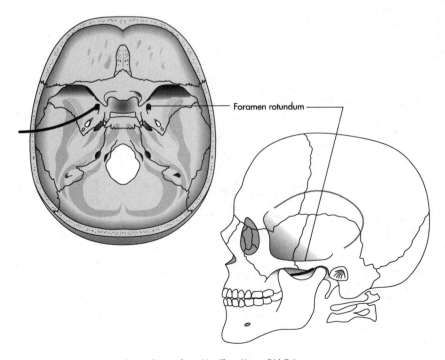

Foramen rotundum

FIGURE 1-20. Foramen Rotundum, where Maxillary Nerve (V_2) Exits

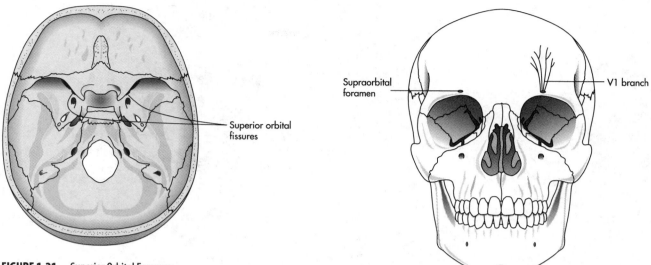

FIGURE 1-21. Superior Orbital Foramen

FIGURE 1-22. Supraorbital Foramen, where Ophthalmic Nerve (V₁) Exits

SUPRAORBITAL FORAMEN

Branch V_1 exits on to the frontal bone
Figure 1-22

INFRAORBITAL FORAMEN

Infraorbital nerve and artery

OPTIC FORAMEN

- Foramina close to each other and close to the stella turcica
- Houses the optic nerve from the eye

ANGULAR SPINE

Sphenomandibular ligament

PTERYGOID PLATES

Four thin "wings" of bone inferior and lateral to the palate
☛ Attachment sites for muscles
Figure 1-23

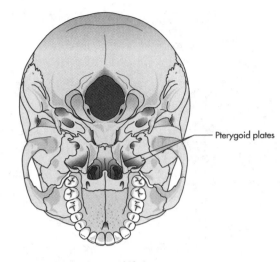

FIGURE 1-23. Pterygoid Plates

PTERYGOID FOSSA

Also called scaphoid fossa

PTERYGOID HAMULI (SINGULAR: HAMULUS)

• Two tiny hooks important to muscles that pass around them
• Pterygomandibular raphe

Figure 1-24

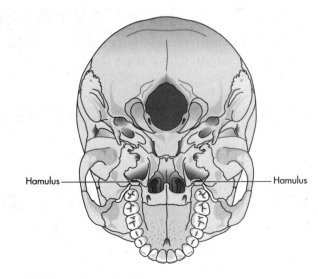

FIGURE 1-24. Pterygoid Hamuli

STELLA TURCICA

- Middle of the sphenoid bone
- Pituitary fossa—pituitary gland rests in the fossa and is attached to the base of the brain

See Figure 1-18

Temporal Bone

Houses the structures of the ear

Figure 1-25

EXTERNAL AUDITORY MEATUS

Bony canal that leads the outer ear into the middle ear and then the inner ear

ARTICULAR FOSSA

- Condyle of the mandible fits into this fossa
- Also called glenoid fossa

MASTOID PROCESS

- Provides muscle attachment
- Large bump directly posterior to the ear
- ☞ Digastric muscle

Figure 1-26

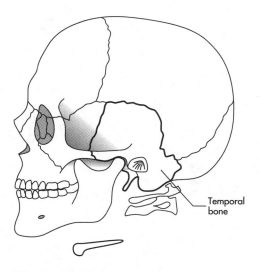

FIGURE 1-25. Temporal Bone

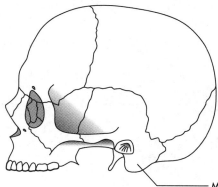

FIGURE 1-26. Mastoid Process

MASTOID NOTCH

- Directly posterior to ear; forms a large bump
- Provides muscle attachment
- ⚿ Stylomandibular ligament

STYLOID PROCESS

- Sagittal view
- Site of muscle and ligament attachment

Figure 1-27

FRONTAL BONE

Supraorbital notch

TEMPOROMANDIBULAR

Creates temporomandibular joint by articulating with the mandible

TEMPOROMANDIBULAR JOINT (TMJ) Movable joint allowing hinge-type movement and gliding-type movement between temporal bone and mandible	
JOINT	Two bones joined together by connective tissue
TMJ	Where the mandible articulates with the cranium within the temporal bone ⚿ "Jaw joint"

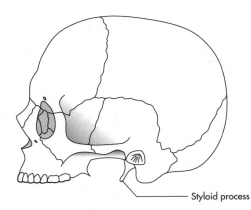

Styloid process

FIGURE 1-27. Styloid Process

ARTICULATIONS	• Condyle of mandible—egg-shaped bone that articulates against the articular eminence • Mandibular fossa • Articular eminence of temporal bone ☛ Condyle and the eminence are covered with fibrous connective tissue and no blood vessels, which makes the TMJ different from all other joints ☛ Most frequently used joint in the body
MENISCUS	• Biconcave disk between the condyle and the eminence • Acts as a cushion ☛ Composed of fibrous connective tissue
TEMPOROMANDIBULAR CAPSULE	Attaches the condyle to the temporal bone by a connective tissue band encircling the joint
LIGAMENTS	• Stylomandibular ligament—connects styloid process of temporal bone to posterior border of ramus of the mandible • Temporomandibular joint ligament—prevents excessive retraction of joint • Sphenomandibular ligament—provides support and connects angular spine of sphenoid bone with lingula of mandible
SYNOVIAL MEMBRANE	• Innermost aspect of the joint capsule lined with thin epithelial membrane • Produces lubricating synovial fluid used to protect and cushion the joint
MOVEMENTS OF TMJ	• Hinge movements—occurs in the inferior joint cavity • Gliding movements—occurs in the superior joint cavity ☛ Combination of two movements allows for chewing and mastication
ASSOCIATE MUSCLES	• Lateral pterygoid—protrusion and lateral deviation of mandible • Posterior portion of temporalis—retraction of mandible • Suprahyoids—opening jaw • Masseter, temporalis, and medial pterygoid—closing jaw

Osseous Anatomy—Mandible

MANDIBLE

☞ Single facial bone
☞ Only freely movable bone of the skull
☞ Largest and strongest facial bone

Figure 1-28

BODY	Horizontal portion, which bears the teeth
RAMUS	On either side of mandible rising vertically ☞ Masseter muscle ☞ Temporalis mscle ☞ Internal pterygoid muscle, stylo-mandibular ligament
ANGLE	☞ Masseter muscle ☞ Internal pterygoid muscle
CONDYLE	• Egg-shaped process • Rests in mandibular fossa • Involved in temporal mandibular joint
PTERYGOID FOSSA OF THE CONDYLE	• Also called fovea of condyle or external • External pterygoid mscle
CORONOID PROCESS	Provides attachment of: • Masseter muscle • Temporal muscle
MANDIBULAR NOTCH	• Also called semiluner or sigmoid • Curved area between coronoid process and condyle

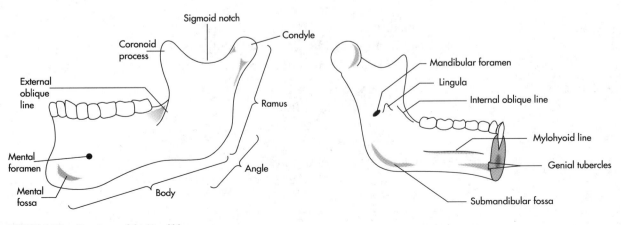

FIGURE 1-28. Structures of the Mandible

EXTERNAL OBLIQUE RIDGE	• Attachment site for muscle of the cheek (the buccinator) • Crest where the ramus joins the body of the mandible ☞ Landmark for inferior alveolar, lingual, and long buccal injections ☞ Visible on posterior radiographs
CORONOID NOTCH	Concave curve of the anterior border of the ramus ☞ Landmark for inferior alveolar block
INTERNAL OBLIQUE RIDGE	• Interior of mandible parallel to external oblique line • Attachment for portion of constrictor muscle ☞ Visible on posterior radiographs ☞ Landmark for inferior alveolar block
RETROMOLAR FOSSA	☞ Landmark for inferior alveolar block and pterygomandibular raphe
ALVEOLAR PROCESS	Contains roots of the mandibular teeth ☞ Alveolar process of posterior teeth is more dense than the mandibular incisors (allowing infiltration of incisors)
MENTAL FOSSA	Near chin depression, where mentalis muscle attaches
MENTAL FORAMEN	Typically between the apices of the first and second mandibular premolars ☞ Mental nerve ☞ Landmark mental nerve block
MENTAL PROTUBERANCE	Bony prominence of the chin ☞ Also called symphysis
GENIAL TUBERCLES	Small projection on the internal surface near midline of mandible ☞ Also called mental spines ☞ Muscle attachment area for geniohyoid and genioglossus muscle
SUBLINGUAL FOSSA	Superior to the anterior portion of the mylohyoid line ☞ Sublingual salivary gland

SUBMANDIBULAR FOSSA	Deep depression below the posterior mandibular teeth ☛ Submandibular salivary gland
MYLOHYOID RIDGE OR LINE	Horizontal line on interior body of mandible ☛ Attachment of mylohyoid muscle that forms the floor of the mouth
MYLOHYOID GROOVE	Mylohyoid nerve
LINGULA	Bony spine that overhangs mandibular foramen ☛ Attachment for sphenomandibular ligament associate with temporomandibular joint ☛ Protects nerves and vessels entering mandibular foramen
MANDIBULAR FORAMEN	Internal surface of the ramus ☛ Where inferior alveolar nerve exits mandible
MANDIBULAR CANAL	Inferior alveolar nerve travels along canal after exiting mandibular foramen

Cranial Nerves

AFFERENT COMPONENT (GENERAL SOMATIC AFFERENT)

- Sensory perception
- Proprioception
- Pain, touch, temperature, and pressure
- Sense of movement
- Skeletal muscle, skin, oral mucosa, alveolar bone, teeth, and TMJ

EFFERENT COMPONENT (SPECIAL VISCERAL EFFERENT)

Provides function of the muscles of mastication

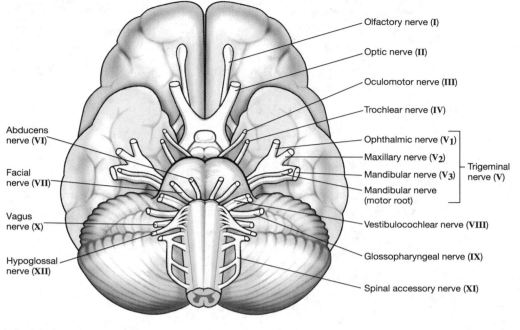

FIGURE 1-29. Twelve Cranial Nerves

Cranial Nerves

Nerve	CN	Function	Type	Mnemonic
Olfactory	I	Smell	Sensory	Some
Optic	II	Sight	Sensory	Say
Oculomotor	III	Eye movement, pupil constriction, accommodation, eyelid opening	Motor	Marry
Trochlear	IV	Eye movement	Motor	Money
Trigeminal	V	Mastication, facial sensation	Both	But
Abducens	VI	Eye movement	Motor	My
Facial	VII	Facial movement, anterior 2/3 taste, lacrimation, salivation (submaxillary and submandibular salivary glands)	Both	Brother
Vestibulocochlear	VIII	Hearing, balance	Sensory	Says
Glossopharyngeal	IX	Posterior 1/3 taste, swallowing, salivation (parotid gland), monitoring carotid body and sinus	Both	Big
Vagus	X	Taste, swallowing, palate elevation, talking, thoracoabdominal viscera	Both	Brains
Accessory	XI	Head turning, shoulder shrugging	Motor	Matter
Hypoglossal	XII	Tongue movements	Motor	Most

Figure 1-29

CRANIAL NERVES AND PASSAGEWAYS	
NERVES	I II III, IV, VI V1 V2 V3 VII, VIII IX, X, XI XII
PASSAGEWAYS	Cribriform plate Optic canal Superior orbital fissure Foramen rotundum Foramen ovale Internal auditory meatus Jugular foramen Hypoglossal canal

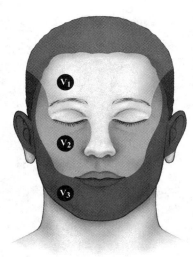

FIGURE 1-30. Divisions of the Trigeminal Nerve

Fifth Cranial Nerve—Trigeminal Nerve

Predominantly sensory; largest cranial nerve of the superficial and deep face; mainly sensory but has a motor and autonomic component

Three major divisions:
- Opthalmic—V1
- Maxillary—V2
- Mandibular—V3

Figure 1-30

Ophthalmic Nerve (V1)

- Purely sensory
- Smallest of the three major divisions of the trigeminal nerve
- Exits from the middle cranial fossa by way of the superior orbital fissure
- Three branches: lacrimal, frontal, and nasociliary

Figure 1-31

LACRIMAL	
SUPPLIES	• Lacrimal gland • Adjacent conjunctiva skin of the lateral angle of the upper eyelid

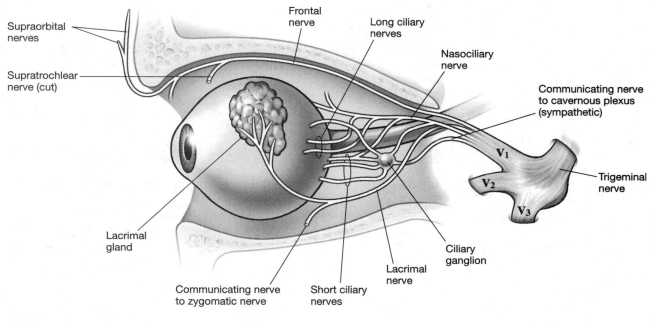

FIGURE 1-31. Divisions of the Ophthalmic Nerve (V1)

FRONTAL	
SUPRAORBITAL	Supplies skin of upper eyelid and scalp
SUPRATROCHELAR	Supplies skin of medial portion of upper eyelid and adjacent forehead

NASOCILIARY	
LONG CILARY	Supplies eyeball
POSTERIOR ETHMOIDAL	Supplies mucous membrane of posterior ethmoidal air cells and sphenoid sinus
INFRATROCHLEAR	Supplies • Skin of eyelids • Lacrimal caruncle • Lacrimal sac • Adjacent conjunctiva • Side of nose
ANTERIOR ETHMOIDAL	Supplies • Anterior ethmoidal air cells • Mucosa of anterior portion of septum • Lateral nasal

Maxillary Nerve (V2)

- Purely sensory
- Passes through the foramen rotundum to reach the pterygopalatine fossa, where it gives off a number of branches: zygomatic, pterygopalatine, posterior superior alveolar, and infraorbital

Figure 1-32

ZYGOMATIC

Enters orbital cavity via the inferior orbital fissure; runs along the lateral wall of the orbital cavity and divides into two branches

ZYGOMATICO-TEMPORAL	Communicates with lacrimal nerve to supply parasympathetic fibers to lacrimal gland then emerges through zygomaticorbital foramen to supply skin of anterior temporal region
ZYGOMATICOFACIAL	Emerges from zygomaticofacial foramen; supplies the skin over prominence of cheek

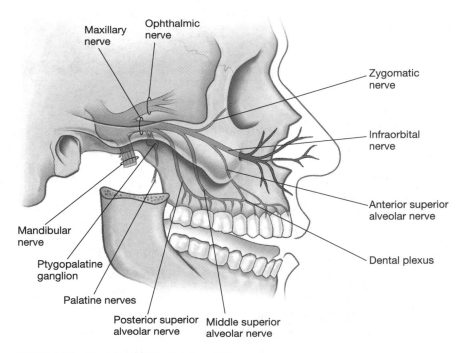

FIGURE 1-32. Divisions of the Maxillary Nerve (V2)

PTERYGOPALATINE NERVES Figure 1-33

Two short trunks of the pterygopalatine nerve leave the main trunk of the maxillary nerve and descend vertically, merging with the pterygopalatine ganglion

ORBITAL	• Transverses inferior orbital fissure • Supplies periosteum of the orbit, mucous membrane of posterior ethmoid and sphenoid sinus
GREATER PALATINE	• (Anterior palatine)—descends through greater palatine canal and exits at greater palatine foramen • Supplies mucous membrane of hard palate to canine area • Gives off posterior inferior lateral nasal branch, which • Supplies middle and inferior meatuses and inferior concha
MIDDLE AND POSTERIOR PALATINE	• Emerge at lesser palatine foramen • Supply palatine tonsil and soft palate
POSTERIOR SUPERIOR LATERAL NASAL BRANCH	• Transverses sphenopalatine foramen • Supplies superior and middle concha, posterior ethmoidal air cells, posterior part of septum • A large branch of this nerve is the nasopalatine

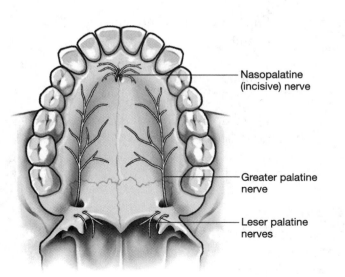

Nasopalatine (incisive) nerve

Greater palatine nerve

Leser palatine nerves

FIGURE 1-33. Pterygoid Palatine Nerves

NASOPALATINE	• Exits via incisive foramen • Supplies septum, anterior palate where it communicates with greater palatine nerve at the canine palatal tissue
PHARYNGEAL	• Runs in pharyngeal canal • Supplies sphenoid sinus, nasopharynx behind the auditory tube

POSTERIOR SUPERIOR ALVEOLAR

• Separates from the main maxillary trunk and courses inferiorly from the pterygopalatine fossa
• Supplies three molar teeth (except mesial buccal root of first molar), adjacent buccal mucoperiosteum (gingiva, bone, and mucous membrane), maxillary sinus

INFRAORBITAL

MIDDLE SUPERIOR ALVEOLAR	• Supplies maxillary premolars, mesial buccal root of maxillary first molar, and adjacent buccal mucoperiosteum (gingivae/bone), maxillary sinus • Enters orbit via inferior orbital fissure, exits at infraorbital foramen
ANTERIOR SUPERIOR ALVEOLAR	• Supplies anterior teeth and adjacent facial mucoperiosteum (gingivae/bone), maxillary sinus, inferior meatus, and floor of nose
TERMINAL BRANCHES OF INFRAORBITAL NERVE— INFERIOR PALPEBRAL	• Supplies skin and conjunctiva of lower eyelid
EXTERNAL NASAL	• Supplies skin of the sides of the nose
SUPERIOR LABIAL	• Supplies skin and mucous membrane of upper lip (anastomose with buccal branches of VII to form infraorbital plexus)

Mandibular Nerve (V3)

• The largest of the three divisions of the trigeminal nerve and the only one that carries both sensory and motor fibers; exits via oval foramen (foramen ovale)

- Divides into an anterior division (mainly motor) and a posterior division (mainly sensory); gives off two branches: meningeal and medial pterygoid

  Figure 1-34

MENINGEAL

- Returns to the cranium via the spinous foramen accompanying the middle meningeal artery
- Supplies dura mater, mastoid air cells

MEDIAL PTERYGOID

- Motor component of the mandibular nerve
- Supplies medial pterygoid muscle, tensor veli palatini muscle, tensor tympani muscle

ANTERIOR DIVISION—MOTOR AND SENSORY

MASSETERIC	• Supplies masseter muscle, temporo-mandibular joint, sensory

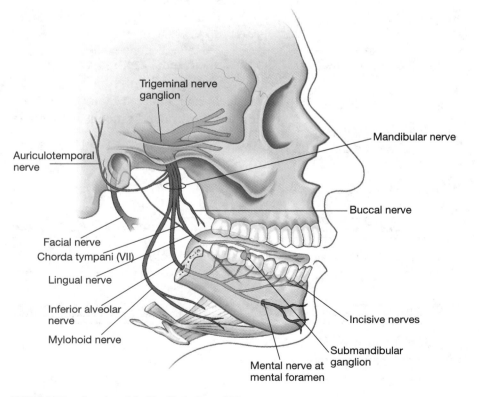

FIGURE 1-34. Branches of the Mandibular Nerve (V3)

DEEP TEMPORAL NERVE	• Usually divides into 2 or 3 branches • Supplies temporal muscle
LATERAL PTERYGOID	• Supplies lateral pterygoid muscle
BUCCAL	• Sensory only • Supplies skin and facia of cheek, mucosa and gingivae distal to the mental foramen

POSTERIOR DIVISION—SENSORY EXCEPT FOR MYLOHYOID BRANCH

AURICULOTEMPORAL	Supplies temporomandibular joint, anterior and superior part of ear, external acoustic meatus, tympanic membrane, skin of temporal region, parotid gland (communicates with optic ganglion, from lesser petrosal nerve, IX, parasympathic fibers)
LINGUAL	Supplies anterior 2/3 of tongue, mucous membrane of floor of mouth, lingual of lower gingivae, joined by chorda tympani with parasympathetic fibers to submandibular and sublingual salivary glands (via VII)
INFERIOR ALVEOLAR	Supplies mandibular teeth; divides into: • Incisive—to mandibular incisor and canine teeth and adjacent facial gingivae • Mental—to skin and mucous membrane of lower lip

Arteries of the Head and Neck

CAROTID ARTERIES

Paired; run along sternocleidomastoid muscle

COMMON CAROTID Figure 1-35

Largest carotid artery
Divides below mandible into:

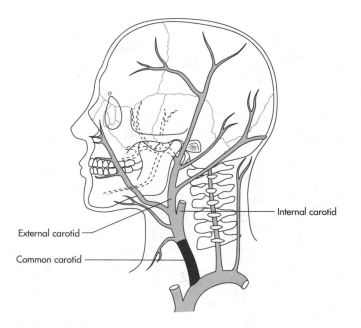

FIGURE 1-35. Common Carotid Artery

EXTERNAL CAROTID	Supplies face and head
INTERNAL CAROTID	Supplies brain

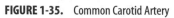

BRANCHES OF EXTERNAL CAROTID ARTERY Figure 1-36

THYROID ARTERY	Paired; supplies thyroid gland
LINGUAL ARTERY	Right and left sides of head; pass under mandible to supply the tongue
FACIAL ARTERY	Passes over inferior boarder of mandible; supplies face
OCCIPITAL ARTERY	Supplies back of skull
POSTAURICULAR	Supplies ear region
SUPERFICIAL TEMPORAL ARTERY	Large branch spreading over temporal and parietal bones
MAXILLARY ARTERY	Travels internally—supplies maxilla, mandible, nasal cavity ☛ Major branch of external carotid

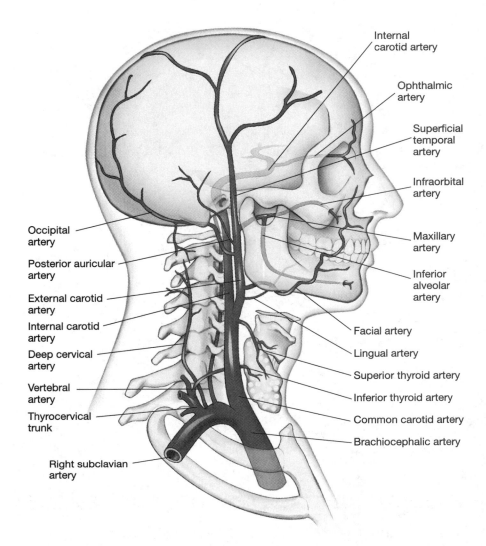

FIGURE 1-36. Anterior Supply of the Head and Neck

MAXILLARY ARTERY BRANCHES Travels behind the neck of the condyle within the infratemporal fossa Figure 1-37	
MIDDLE MENIGEAL ARTERY	Meninges
INFERIOR ALVEOLAR ARTERY	Enters in mandibular canal with inferior alveolar nerve; travels along mandibular canal; supplies mandible and mandibular teeth
DEEP TEMPORAL ARTERY	Branches to the muscles of mastication; supplies temporalis, masseter, buccinator, and pterygoid muscles

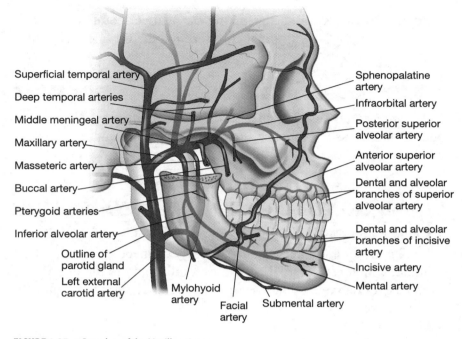

FIGURE 1-37. Branches of the Maxillary Artery

SPHENOPALATINE ARTERY	Supplies the anterior palate and sphenoid sinus
POSTERIOR SUPERIOR ALVEOLAR	Posterior maxillary teeth and maxillary sinus
INFRAORBITAL	Orbital region, face, and anterior max teeth
GREATER PALATINE	Hard and soft palate
BUCCAL ARTERY	Long branch along inner surface of cheek and supplies cheek mucosa

ARTERIES OF THE BRAIN

INTERNAL CAROTID ARTERY	• Middle cerebral artery—supplies large areas of the temporal and pariental regions of the cerebrum • Anterior cerebral artery—supplies the anterior of the cerebrum • Posterior cerebral artery—supplies occipital region

VERTEBRAL ARTERIES	Runs up the cervical vertebral along the spinal cord through the foramen magnum

BASILAR ARTERY

Vertebral arteries fuse together at top of the brainstem and form on vessel; branches supply the brainstem and cerebellum

CIRCLE OF WILLIS

- Connects two sources of blood supply to brain
- Basilar artery and internal carotid artery connect around pituitary gland, which is a safety device for blood supply to the brain
- ⚷ In case of damage to one vessel, blood can be rerouted around the blockage

Veins of the Head and Neck

Carry metabolic waste products and CO_2 down the neck, back to the heart
Figure 1-38

JUGULAR VEINS

Large veins that drain the head and neck

EXTERNAL JUGULAR	• Smaller than internal jugular • Receives outflow from retromandibular vein • Drains extracranial tissues
INTERNAL JUGULAR	Largest of jugular veins and travels to inside of cranium and drains brain and most tissue of the head and neck
ANTERIOR JUGULAR	Blends together with external jugular and subclavian veins to drain anterior portion of neck

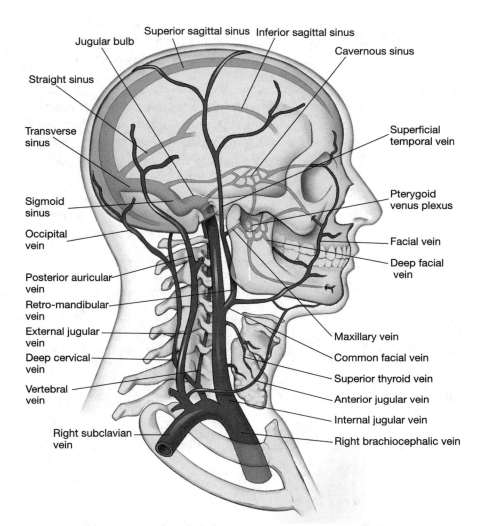

FIGURE 1-38. Venous Drainage of the Head and Neck

BRANCHES OF EXTERNAL JUGULAR VEIN

- Retromandibular vein
- Occipital
- Retroauricular branch
- Superficial temporal vein

BRANCHES OF INTERNAL JUGULAR VEIN

FACIAL VEIN	Drains the face
LINGUAL VEIN	Drains the tongue
THYROID VEIN	Drains the thyroid gland

MAXILLARY VEIN	Branch of both external and internal jugular veins; rapidly becomes pterygoid plexus
PTERYGOID PLEXUS	In infratemporal fossa next to maxillary artery and is a network of veins draining maxilla and nasopalatine; protects the maxillary artery from being compressed during mastication ☛ Area of administration of PSA injection; must avoid penetrating plexus by using a short needle and always aspirate
PSA	Drains maxillary posterior teeth
MSA	Drains maxillary premolars
ASA	Drains maxillary anterior teeth
INFERIOR ALVEOLAR VEIN	Drains mandibular teeth and periodontium
VERTEBRAL	Does not go to the brain; connects with the occipital veins
OCCIPITAL	Connects with the vertebral vein

Lymph Nodes

CERVICAL LYMPH NODES

Run along sternocleidomastoid muscle; drain the tissue fluids of the head down the neck and act as filters
- Cervical deep group
- Cervical superficial group

LYMPH NODES OF THE HEAD Figure 1-39

OCCIPITAL	Drains lymph fluid from base of skull
RETROAURICULAR	Drains lymph fluid from posterior scalp and external ear
PAROTID	Drains lymph fluid from parotid gland and adjacent tissues
ANTERIOR AURICULAR	Drains lymph fluid from anterior to external ear

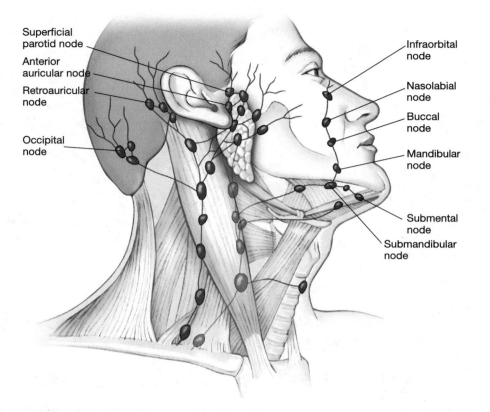

Superficial parotid node
Anterior auricular node
Retroauricular node
Occipital node
Infraorbital node
Nasolabial node
Buccal node
Mandibular node
Submental node
Submandibular node

FIGURE 1-39. Lymph Nodes

FACIAL	Drains lymph from face into submandibular lymph nodes
SUBMANDIBULAR	Located on inferior boarder of mandible; drains most of maxilla and mandible ☞ Infection in maxillary dentition or mandibular posterior teeth causes swelling in the node
SUBMENTAL	Located on mylohyoid muscle and drains lower anterior mandible

JUGULODIGASTRIC

Large nodes that can be felt by palpating along the anterior edge of the sternocleidomastoid muscle

Figure 1-40

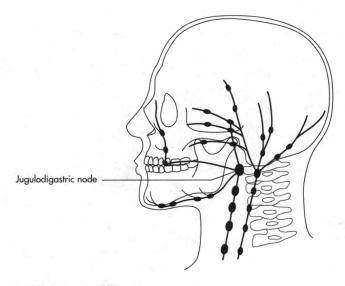

Jugulodigastric node ————

FIGURE 1-40. Jugulodigastric

➤ MUSCLES OF THE HEAD AND NECK

DEFINITIONS	
TENDONS	Connective tissue that attaches muscles to bones
ORIGIN	Stationary attachment of muscle
INSERTION	Attachment that moves
LIGAMENT	Dense regular connective that attaches bone to bone
JOINT	Where two bones come together

MUSCLES OF FACIAL EXPRESSION All innervated by CN VII—facial nerve Figure 1-41	
FRONTALIS	Paired; muscle of forehead and eyebrows
OBICULARIS OCULI	Closes the eye
LEVATOR LABII SUPERIORIS	Elevates upper lip
LEVATOR LABII SUPERIORIS ALAEQUE NASI	• Elevates upper lip • Wiggles or flares nose
OBICULARIS ORIS	Circular muscle around lips, purses lips

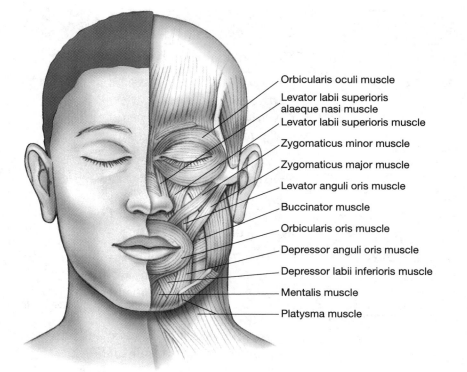

Orbicularis oculi muscle
Levator labii superioris alaeque nasi muscle
Levator labii superioris muscle
Zygomaticus minor muscle
Zygomaticus major muscle
Levator anguli oris muscle
Buccinator muscle
Orbicularis oris muscle
Depressor anguli oris muscle
Depressor labii inferioris muscle
Mentalis muscle
Platysma muscle

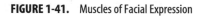

FIGURE 1-41. Muscles of Facial Expression

LEVATOR ANGULI ORIS	• Raises angle of lips • Smiles
DEPRESSOR ANGULI ORIS	Depresses corner of mouth
DEPRESSOR LABII INFERIORIS	Depresses lower lip
METALIS	Pouts, puckers
PLATYSMA	Pulls down corners of mouth
BUCCINATOR	Cheek—chews, swallows
ZYGOMATICUS MAJOR	• Elevates angle of mouth • Smiles
ZYGOMATICUS MINOR	Elevates upper lip
PLATYSMA	• Raises skin of neck • Pulls down corner of mouth

MUSCLES OF MASTICATION Figure 1-42
Elevation and lateral movement of mandible

Four pairs innervated by CN V trigeminal nerve division V3

TEMPORALIS	• *Origin*—temporal fossa • *Insertion*—coronoid process • *Action*—elevation of mandible ⚷ Called closing the mandible
MASSETER	• *Origin*—zygomatic process • *Insertion*—lower border and angle of mandible • *Action*—elevation of mandible ⚷ Called clenching muscle
MEDIAL PTERYGOID	• *Origin*—pterygoid plates • *Insertion*—angle of the mandible • *Action*—elevation of mandible
LATERAL PTERYGOIDS	• *Origin*—pterygoid plates • *Insertion*—neck of condyle and temporomandibular capsule and disk • *Action*—protrusion of mandible

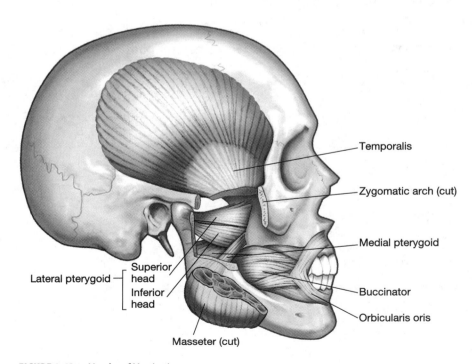

FIGURE 1-42. Muscles of Mastication

POSTERIOR NECK MUSCLES	Figure 1-43
TRAPEZIUS	• *Action*—supporting the head • *Innervation*—CN XI ☛ Runs from head to shoulders and down back in a continuous sheet
STERNOCLEIDO-MASTOID	• *Action*—turning and supporting the head • *Innervation*—CN XI spinal accessory nerve ☛ Paired muscles—runs from the mastoid process inferiorly and anteriorly until it inserts on the sternum and clavicle

Anterior Neck Muscles

SUPRAHYOID MUSCLES	Figure 1-44
DIGASTRIC	• *Origin*—mastoid process • *Insertion*—digastric fossa • *Action*—act as pulley opening or depressing the mandible

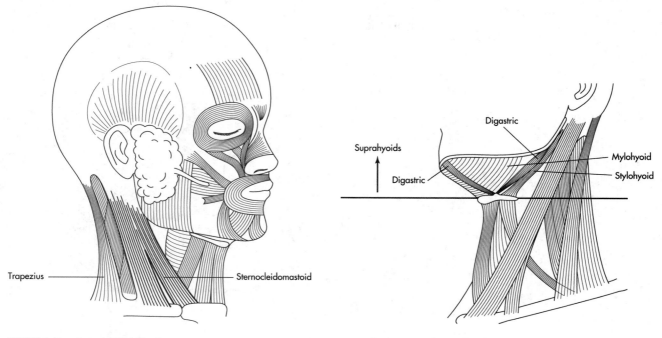

FIGURE 1-43. Posterior Neck Muscles

FIGURE 1-44. Anterior Neck Muscles

MYLOHYOID	• *Origin*—both mylohyoid lines • *Insertion*—hyoid bone • *Innervation*—CN V • *Action*—major muscle of the floor of the mouth; provides firm base for tongue and helps depress mandible
SYLOHYOID	• *Origin*—styloid process • *Insertion*—hyoid bone • *Action*—tighten or stabilize the hyoid bone during actions of other muscles

GENIOHYOID MUSCLE

• *Origin*—genial tubercles
• *Insertion*—hyoid bone
• *Action*—stabilizing hyoid

Figure 1-45

INFRAHYOID MUSCLES Figure 1-46
Action—stabilize the hyoid for depression of mandible and act as a base for the tongue

STERNOHYOID	• *Origin*—sternum • *Insertion*—hyoid
STERNOTHYROID	• *Origin*—thyroid cartilage • *Insertion*—sternum
THYROHYOID	• *Origin*—thyroid cartilage • *Insertion*—hyoid bone

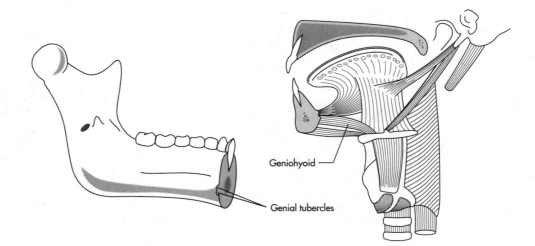

Geniohyoid

Genial tubercles

FIGURE 1-45 Geniohyoid Muscle

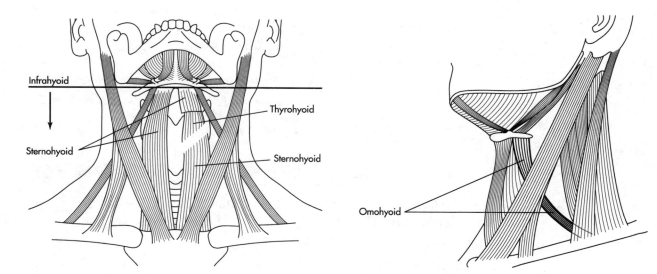

Infrahyoid

Thyrohyoid

Sternohyoid

Sternohyoid

Omohyoid

FIGURE 1-46. Infrahyoid Muscles

OMOHYOID	• *Origin*—clavicle • *Insertion*—hyoid bone

MUSCLES OF THE TONGUE

Action—movement of tongue during speech and swallowing
Innervation—CN XII (hypoglossal)

HYPOGLOSSUS	• *Origin*—hyoid • *Insertion*—tongue
GENIOGLOSSUS	• *Origin*—genial tubercles • *Insertion*—tongue
STYLOGLOSSUS	• *Origin*—styloid process • *Insertion*—tongue
PALATOGLOSSUS	• *Origin*—soft palate • *Insertion*—tongue

MUSCLES OF THE PHARYNX

STYLOPHARYNGEUS	• *Origin*—styloid process of the temporal bone • *Insertion*—lateral and posterior pharyngeal walls • *Action*—elevates the pharynx • *Innervation*—ninth cranial nerve (glossopharyngeal nerve)

CONSTRICTORS	• Superior constrictor • Middle constrictor • Inferior constrictor • ⚷ Pass bolus food from the oral cavity to the esophagus; innervated by CN X vagus nerve

PALATINE MUSCLES

Action—stretching and raising of the soft palate to seal the nasopharynx off from the oropharynx during a swallow, so that food does not pass into the nasal cavity

LEVATOR VELI PALATINI (LVP)	• *Origin*—base of cranium • *Insertion*—soft palate • *Action*—raise soft palate during swallows and function during speech • *Innervation*—CN VII
TENSOR VELI PALATINI (TVP)	• *Origin*—base of cranium • *Insertion*—soft palate • *Action*—raise soft palate during swallows, speech, and opens Eustachian tube • *Innervation*—CN V • ⚷ Two belly muscle

Salivary Glands

MAJOR SALIVARY GLANDS Figure 1-47	
PAROTID	• Directly under skin of each cheek • Mostly serous • Empties into oral cavity via stenten's duct through a papilla of buccal mucosa directly opposite the maxillary second molars • ⚷ Largest gland
SUBMANDIBULAR	• Pair of encapsulated glands below the angle of mandible directly below the surface skin and on top of the suprahyoid muscle • Mainly mucous-secreting units • Empties into Wharton's duct that travels in floor of mouth toward the anterior

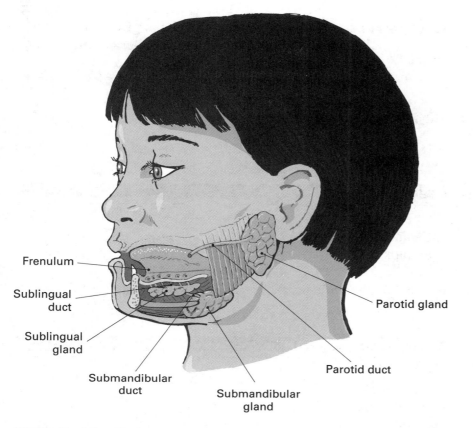

Frenulum

Sublingual duct

Sublingual gland

Submandibular duct

Submandibular gland

Parotid gland

Parotid duct

FIGURE 1-47. Salivary Glands

	midline where it empties through a mucosal papilla, a sublingual caruncle located on either side of lingual frenum
SUBLINGUAL	• Paired • Located beneath the tongue lie beneath the fold of the floor mucosa called sublingual plicae • Mainly mucous—produce thick saliva • Branch into smaller ducts called ducts of Rivinus

MINOR SALIVARY GLANDS

• Mainly mucous except Ebner's glands (serous); innervated by seventh cranial or facial nerve
• Exocrine glands scattered in the tissues of the buccal, labial, and lingual mucosa, the soft palate, the lateral portions of the hard palate, and the floor of the mouth

| EBNER'S GLANDS | Associated with the large circumvallate lingual papillae, on posterior portion of the tongue's dorsal service |

➤ DENTAL ANATOMY

Classification of Teeth

PERMANENT DENTITION

- Incisors (2)
- Canine (1)
- Premolars (2)
- Molars (3)
- ☛ Total of 8 teeth in permanent dentition quadrant

PRIMARY DENTITION

- Incisors (2)
- Canine (1)
- Molars (2)
- ☛ Total of 5 teeth in primary dentition quadrant

THREE PERIODS OF DENTITION

PRIMARY	6 months to 6 years of age ☛ Usually ends with the eruption of the permanent mandibular first molar
MIXED	6 to 12 years of age ☛ Usually ends with the exfoliation of the primary maxillary canine
PERMANENT	12 years through rest of life

NUMBERING SYSTEMS

| UNIVERSAL | Uses numbers 1–32 for the permanent dentition starting with 1 for maxillary right third molar clockwise around lower arch to 32; for the primary dentition the alphabet is used, starting with A–T |

	☛ Most widespread usage ☛ # sign alone indicates Universal numbering (i.e., #14)
PALMER	Brackets represent the four quadrants of dentition facing the patient and permanent teeth are numbered 1–8 on each side of midline; primary teeth use same bracket, but alphabet letters A–E ☛ Bracket and number or letter indicates Palmer system
INTERNATIONAL	Uses two digits for each permanent and deciduous tooth; the first digit denotes the dentition, arch, and side while the second digit denotes the tooth ☛ Federation Dentaire Internationale (FDI) System: numbers 11 through 48 represent permanent teeth and numbers 51 through 85 represent primary teeth

Maxillary Permanent Teeth

MAXILLARY PERMANENT TEETH CHARACTERISTICS

☛ On convex surfaces the clinician must roll and pivot the working end of the instrument to ensure continuity of the stroke from the convex surface into the concave area

MAXILLARY CENTRAL INCISOR	• Widest crown MD • Greatest CEJ curve and height of contour • Distal offset cingulum with shallow lingual fossa • Single cone-shape root
MAXILLARY LATERAL INCISOR	• Greatest crown variation • Prominent lingual surface • Cingulum centered • Root curves distally with sharp apex • Distal root surface concavity

MAXILLARY CANINE	• Single cusp • Facially the mesial cusp slope is shorter than distal cusp slope • Longest tooth in arch • Apex may deviate distally • Abrupt tapering of the lingual root surface • Distal coronal concavity and root surface concavity
MAXILLARY FIRST PREMOLAR	• Deeper developed groove on the mesial • Larger than second premolar with buccal cusp longer of two • Long central groove • Frequently bifurcated root trunk with larger root being the facial root • Mesial root/crown surface concavity • Distal root surface concavity
MAXILLARY SECOND PREMOLAR	• Smaller than first premolar with two cusps the same length • Increased supplemental grooves • Single-rooted that is larger in all directions than the first premolar • Mesial and distal grooved root surface concavity
MAXILLARY FIRST MOLAR	• Largest tooth in the arch • Largest crown in dentition • Four major cusps • Fifth minor cusp (•➡ Cusp of Carabelli) • Trifurcated roots • Facial concavity leading to furcation • Lingual and facial palate root concavities • Mesial concavity leading to furcation • Distal concavity with coronal extension
MAXILLARY SECOND MOLAR	• Heart-shaped crown • Oblique ridges less prominent • No fifth cusp • Distolingual cusp smaller than on first or absent • More slender trifurcated roots • Facial concavity and groove leading to furcation

MAXILLARY THIRD MOLAR	• Smaller crown than second molar • Heart-shaped crown • Three or four cusps • Usually fused roots that curve distally

Mandibular Permanent Teeth

MANDIBULAR PERMANENT TEETH CHARACTERISTICS	
MANDIBULAR CENTRAL INCISOR	• Smallest and simplest tooth • Bilaterally symmetrical • Centered cingulum • Root is longer than crown • Mesial and distal root concavity with groove
MANDIBULAR LATERAL INCISOR	• Larger than mandibular central • Appears twisted distally • Distally placed cingulum • Proximal root concavities give double-rooted appearance
MANDIBULAR CANINE	• Smooth lingual anatomy • Less sharp cusp tip • Longest root in mandibular arch • Deviation of root apex generally toward the mesial • Root generally has mesial and distal grooves • Mesial and distal root surface concavities
MANDIBULAR FIRST PREMOLAR	• Smaller than mandibular second premolar • Smaller lingual cusp • May have mesial and distal flutings • Mesial fluting more developed than distal fluting • Single-rooted • Mesial and distal horizontal root convexities • Mesial and distal apical convexities with grooves

MANDIBULAR SECOND PREMOLAR	• Larger than first premolar • Usually 3 cusps • "Y" groove pattern or two cusps (☞ Most common) • "H" or "U" groove pattern • Increased supplemental grooves • Single-rooted, which is wider facial-lingual than mesial-distal • Slight mesial and distal root surface concavities
MANDIBULAR FIRST MOLAR	• First permanent tooth to erupt • Widest crown mesiodistally • Five cusps with "Y" groove pattern • Bifurcated roots having two depressions facial and lingual • Apices of roots curved toward distal • Facial and lingual root concavities leading into furcation • Slight mesial and distal concavities • Mesial root may have two canals
MANDIBULAR SECOND MOLAR	• Smaller crown than first molar • Four cusps with cross-shape groove pattern • Bifurcated roots • Facial and lingual concavity leading to furcation with groove at the base of concavity • Mesial and distal root surface concavity with groove
MANDIBULAR THIRD MOLAR	• Single or fused roots • Apices deviate distally

Clinical Consideration and Developmental Disturbances of Permanent Maxillary Teeth

MAXILLARY CENTRAL INCISOR	
DWARFED ROOT	Tooth with very short roots in comparison to crown
HUTCHINSON'S INCISOR	Notched central incisor that develops as a result of congenital syphilis ☞ "Screwdriver shaped"

SUPERNUMERARY TEETH	Extra teeth in the jaw ☞ Most commonly located in the midline and molar regions of the maxilla, followed by the premolar region in the mandible
DIASTEMA	Any spacing between teeth in the same arch
MESIODENS	Supernumerary teeth in the midline of the maxilla ☞ Most common supernumerary teeth

MAXILLARY LATERAL INCISOR

DENS IN DENTE	An invagination of the enamel organ within the crown of the tooth ☞ "Tooth within a tooth"
MICRODONTIA	Very small, normally shaped teeth
PEG LATERAL	Conical in shape and tapers toward the incisal to a blunt point
CONGENITALLY MISSING	The condition of the teeth never having been developed ☞ Second most commonly missing tooth
GERMINATION	Splitting of a single forming tooth germ; Crown appears doubled in width

MAXILLARY CANINE

TUBERCLES	Overcalcification of enamel resulting in small cusp-like elevations on the crown
DILACERATION	A severe bend or distortion of a tooth root and crown ☞ 45-degree to more than 90-degree distortion
DENTIGEROUS CYST	Odontogenic cyst that forms from the reduced enamel epithelium ☞ Forms around the crown of an impacted or unerupted tooth

IMPACTED	Describing teeth not completely erupted that are fully or partially covered by bone and/or soft tissue
GERMINATION	Splitting of a single forming tooth germ; crown appears doubled in width

MAXILLARY FIRST PREMOLAR

Roots can occasionally penetrate the maxillary sinus

MAXILLARY FIRST MOLAR

CONCRESCENCE	A fusion or growing together of two adjacent teeth at the root through the cementum
MULBERRY MOLARS	Molars with multiple cusps that develop as a result of congenital syphilis
TUBERCLES	Overcalcification of enamel resulting in small cusp-like elevations on the crown

MAXILLARY THIRD MOLAR

IMPACTED	Describing teeth not completely erupted that are fully or partially covered by bone and/or soft tissue
CONGENITALLY MISSING	The condition of never having been developed ☛ Most commonly missing teeth
MICRODONTIA	Very small, normally shaped teeth
PEG THIRD MOLARS	Conical in shape and tapers toward the incisal to a blunt point
DENTIGEROUS CYST	Odontogenic cyst that forms from the reduced enamel epithelium ☛ Forms around the crown of an impacted or unerupted tooth
ACCESSORY ROOTS	Extra root or roots on a tooth ☛ Probably caused by trauma, metabolic dysfunction, or pressure

ANATOMIC SCIENCE ■ 55

SUPERNUMERARY TEETH	Extra teeth in the jaw ☞ More common in maxillay arch but does occur in the mandible ☞ Commonly called distomolars, paramolars, or fourth molars

Clinical Consideration and Developmental Disturbances of Permanent Mandibular Teeth

MANDIBULAR CENTRAL INCISOR

ACCESSORY ROOTS	• Extra root or roots on a tooth • Probably caused by trauma, metabolic dysfunction, or pressure

MANDIBULAR LATERAL INCISOR

ACCESSORY ROOTS	Extra root or roots on a tooth

MANDIBULAR CANINE

ACCESSORY ROOTS	Bifurcated root
DILACERATION	A severe bend or distortion of a tooth root and crown

MANDIBULAR SECOND PREMOLAR

• Premature loss of primary mandibular second molar can result in impacted second premolar
• On occasion congenitally missing

MANDIBULAR THIRD MOLAR

IMPACTED	Teeth not completely erupted that are fully or partially covered by bone and/or soft tissue
ANODONTIA	No teeth are present in the jaw
ACCESSORY ROOTS	Extra root or roots on a tooth
DENTIGEROUS CYST	Cyst around the crown of an unerupted or developing tooth

COMPARISONS BETWEEN PERMANENT AND PRIMARY TEETH

Primary teeth:
- Are wider mesiodistally relative to their incisogingival height
- Are lighter in color due to increased opacity of the enamel
- Have crowns that are constricted at CEJ, making them appear bulbous
- Have cervical ridge that is present on both the labial and lingual surfaces
- Have roots that are relatively longer and slender with more flare
- Have pulp horns that are relatively larger in proportion to those in permanent teeth
- Have greater frequency of germination occurs more frequently in primary teeth than in permanent teeth

➤ HISTOLOGY AND EMBRYOLOGY

Cells

COMPONENTS OF CELLS   Figure 1-48

NUCLEUS	Command center; contains information for its growth and reproduction within the DNA of its chromosomes

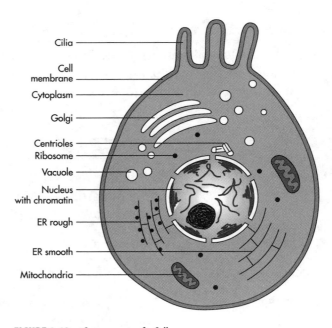

Cilia
Cell membrane
Cytoplasm
Golgi
Centrioles
Ribosome
Vacuole
Nucleus with chromatin
ER rough
ER smooth
Mitochondria

FIGURE 1-48. Components of a Cell

CELL MEMBRANE	Cytoplasm; contains all the cell's parts or organelles
ENDOPLASMIC RETICULUM (ER)	Connecting tubule system
RIBOSOMES	Line the ER or are free floating
MITOCHONDRIA	Create energy for the cells
GOLGI APPARATUS	Produces cell products
MATRIX	Environment within which cell products reside

Epithelium

TYPES OF EPITHELIUM Function to cover or line body parts; avascular	
SQUAMOUS	Flat cells
CUBOIDAL	Cube-shaped cells
COLUMNAR	Tall cells
SIMPLE	One layer of cells
STRATIFIED	Multiple layers of cells

EXAMPLES OF EPITHELIUM TYPES	
SIMPLE SQUAMOUS	Found in the peritoneum
SIMPLE CUBOIDAL	Found in the ducts of glands
SIMPLE COLUMNAR	Found in the digestive tract lining
STRATIFIED SQUAMOUS	Found in the epidermis, mucosa
STRATIFIED CUBOIDAL	Found in the liver
STRATIFIED COLUMNAR	Found in the glands
PSEUDOSTRATIFIED	Found in the respiratory epithelium

GLANDS

Classification of epithelium; developed from epithelial surfaces of the embryo

FORMED SACS	Secretory units—cells lining the unit dump their cell product to be stored
DUCTS	Lead cell products out of the gland to the surface of the epithelium
EXOCRINE	Glands with ducts
ENDOCRINE	Glands without ducts—expel secretion into surroundings

Muscle

• Only tissue that can contract

SKELETAL MUSCLE

Bulk of the muscles of the body that voluntarily move all the limbs of the body, head, and trunk
• Striated
• Needs many nuclei to operate

CARDIAC MUSCLE

- Operates involuntarily
- Intercalated discs—quick communication between cells
• Striated

SMOOTH MUSCLE

- Spindle-shaped
- Only one nucleus per cell
- Involuntary
- Found within the walls of many organs and glands
• Not striated

Nervous Tissue

Generates electrochemical signal that passes from one cell to the next

NEURONS

Basic functioning units of the nervous system that transmit messages throughout the body

Figure 1-49

SUPPORTING CELLS OR NEUROGLIA

Nourish and maintain the neurons

Connective Tissue

- Has few cells and a lot of matrix
- Begins with fibrous matrix
- Made by cells called fibroblasts

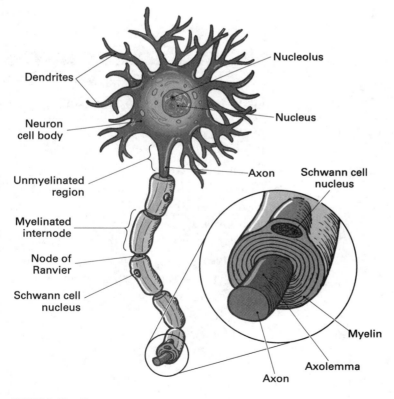

FIGURE 1-49. Neuron

GENERALIZED CONNECTIVE TISSUE Main "glue" of the body; found between and surrounding all organs of the body	
DENSE	Tightly packed connective tissue
LOOSE	Loosely packed connective tissue
REGULAR	Fibers arranged in parallel rows
IRREGULAR	Randomly arranged fibers

EXAMPLES OF GENERALIZED CONNECTIVE TISSUE	
DENSE REGULAR	Found in tendons and ligaments
DENSE IRREGULAR	Found in capsules
LOOSE REGULAR	Found in facia
LOOSE IRREGULAR	Found in facia

Specialized Connective Tissue

Cells and matrix are very unique and perform a very specialized function

BLOOD	
ERYTHROCYTES (RED BLOOD CELLS)	• Biconcave—have no nuclei • Function—transport O_2 and CO_2
LEUKOCYTES (WHITE BLOOD CELLS)	*Granulocytes* ☞ Defense cells ☞ Eosinophils (red) ☞ Basophils (blue) ☞ Neutrophils (both) *Agranulocytes* *Monocytes*—larger cells; found outside the circulatory system *Lymphocytes*—smaller cells; mainly in lymphatic and blood supply • B lymphocytes • T lymphocytes

CARTILAGE
Avascular; formed by calcification (hydroxyapatite)

CHONDROCYTES	Cells of cartilage
CHONDROBLASTS	When condrocytes are actively producing cartilage matrix ☞ "Blasts" = build
CHONDROCLASTS	Tear down cartilage or resorbs it ☞ "Clasts" = breaks down

BONE
Contains osteocytes—spider shaped

OSTEOBLASTS	Actively lay down new bone ☞ "Blasts" = build
OSTEOCLASTS	Resorption of bone (gets rid of old bone) ☞ "Clasts" = breaks down
CALCIFICATION	Fibrous matrix→calcium salts→hydroxyapatite crystals

Skin

LAYERS OF SKIN Figure 1-50

Epidermis and dermis make up skin organ (covers and protects the body)

EPIDERMIS	Outermost layer of skin; classified as epithelium (stratified squamous)
DERMIS	Below epidermis; classified as connective tissue

MUCOSA
"Internal skin"; lines the oral cavity, pharynx, and digestive tract Figure 1-51

MUCOSA PROPER	Stratified squamous epithelium
LAMINA PROPRIA	Connective tissue

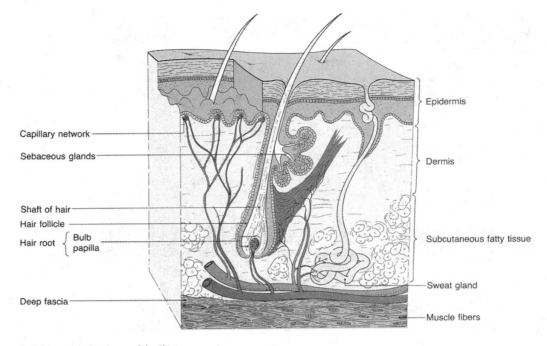

FIGURE 1-50. Structures of the Skin

Embryology

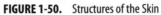

LAYERS OF EMBRYO	
ECTODERM	Forms outer covering of body and lining of oral cavity
MESODERM	Forms skeletal and muscular systems; cemetum, dentin, and pulp
ENDODERM	Forms lining of internal organs

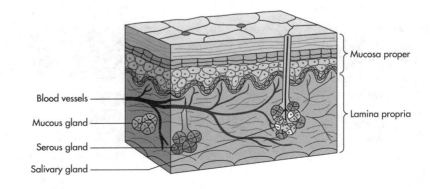

FIGURE 1-51. Mucosa

STOMODEUM

- Future mouth of embryo
- Surrounded by coalescing pharyngeal arches

TONGUE
Will develop from six processes

CIRCUMVALLATE PAPILLAE	Form the border between the ectoderm and endoderm coverings of the tongue 🗝 Mark the division between the anterior two-thirds or body of the tongue and the posterior one-third or root

Facial Development

Figure 1-52
Figure 1-53
Figure 1-54

FRONTAL PROCESS
Contains future brain; gives rise to five other processes
🗝 Begins fourth week of gestation

GLOBULAR PROCESS	• Primary palate • Philtrum and lip
LATERAL AND MEDIAN PROCESSES	• Lateral—forms sides of nose • Median—forms middle of nose 🗝 On both right and left sides
MAXILLARY PROCESS	Forms maxilla, cheeks, part of lip

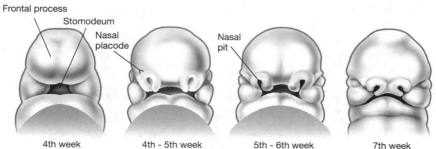

4th week   4th - 5th week   5th - 6th week   7th week

FIGURE 1-52. The Developing Face

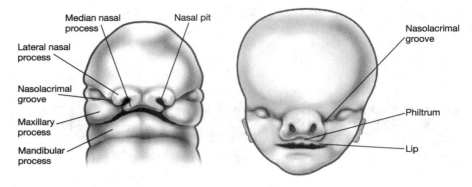

FIGURE 1-53. Face Formation

MANDIBULAR PROCESS	Forms mandible ☛ Meckel's cartilage—acts as a temporary "jawbone" until the bone of the mandible envelops it and most of it disappears
LATERAL PALATINE PROCESSES	Maxillary processes forming the sides of the palate
PALATE	Formed by three processes coalescing: two maxillary processes, lateral palatine processes, and one globular process (primary palatine) ☛ Cleft lip or cleft palate results if processes do not come together properly

Tooth Development

Teeth develop from crown to root

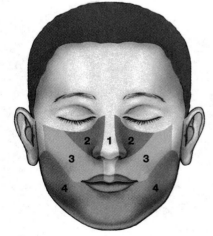

FIGURE 1-54. Development of Face: 1) Medial Nasal Process; 2) Lateral Nasal Process; 3) Maxillary Process; 4) Mandibular Process

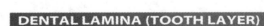

DENTAL LAMINA (TOOTH LAYER)	
INITIATION—BUD STAGE	20 thickenings of ectoderm; grows downward from oral ectoderm into surrounding lower layer of mesoderm ☛ Teeth will develop in 20 places
PROLIFERATION—CAP STAGE	Enamel organ: • Forms from the dental lamina • Inner enamel epithelium—innermost layer→cells become ameloblasts (enamel-producing cells)→responsible

	for laying down the dental tissue called enamel by a process called calcification • Layers of enamel organ **Figure 1-55** ☛ Outer three layers of the enamel organ will be pushed together to form the reduced enamel epithelium
HISTODIFFERENTIATION—BELL STAGE	Cells increase in number and take the shape of a bell
SECONDARY DENTAL LAMINA	Enamel organ makes another second enamel organ that will develop later into a second tooth→permanent teeth ☛ Succedaneous teeth
DENTAL PAPILLA	Mesoderm trapped under the enamel organ; produces dentin and pulp ☛ Odontoblasts make dentin
DENTAL SAC	• Mesoderm that surrounds the dental papilla • Forms periodontal ligament (PDL), cementum, alveolar bone ☛ Periodontal means "around the tooth" ☛ Cementoblasts make cementum
DENTINOENAMEL JUNCTION (DEJ)	Inner enamel epithelium and dental papilla are separated by basement membrane, which becomes the DEJ

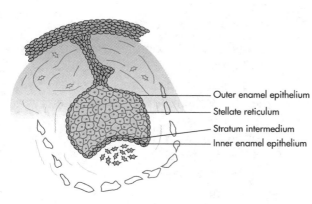

Outer enamel epithelium

Stellate reticulum

Stratum intermedium

Inner enamel epithelium

FIGURE 1-55 Layers of Enamel Organ

ROOT FORMATION

HETWIG'S EPITHELIAL ROOT SHEATH	Forms root by leaving a trail apically that will serve as a guide for other cells to follow • On one side of the sheath, odontoblasts will be attracted to form dentin • On the other side cementoblasts from PDL will cover outside of root
RESTS OF MALASSEZ	Epithelial remnants of the enamel organ left in PDL • Potential to form cysts

CALCIFICATION

ENAMEL FORMATION	Ameloblast→produces fibrous matrix→ calcium salts are attracted to the fibers from the bloodstream→larger crystals of hydroxyapatite are formed from the calcium salts→larger crystals (enamel crystals) are formed from the smaller hydroxyapatite crystals • Enamel crystals are called enamel rods • Lines of Retzius—dark lines in the enamel between layers (enamel is most likely to break along lines or between rods) • Hunter-Schreger bands—series of dark and light bands that are an optical phenomenon due to the crystalline structure of enamel • Enamel has no live cells after eruption and is not able to grow or repair itself if damaged • Enamel grows outward
DENTIN FORMATION	• Odontoblast→odontoblastic process extending off its cell body→forms a fibrous matrix→calcium salts attract from the bloodstream→hydroxyapatite crystals→form larger crystals of dentin • Ondontoblastic process remains in the calcified dentin within spaces called dentinal tubules • Predentin—earliest stage of calcification

ANATOMIC SCIENCE ■ **67**

	☛ Dentin grows inward toward pulp; odontoblastic cell bodies are located on the outer layer of the pulp
CEMENTUM FORMATION	• Cementoblasts form PDL line up outside the developing dentin of the root and Hertwig's epithelial root sheath→form a fibrous matrix around itself→attract fibers from bloodstream→hydroxyapatite crystals form from salts→larger crystals of cementum will be formed all around the cell • Formation similar to bone ☛ Spidery shape with many cell processes ☛ Each process lies in a space called a canaliculus ☛ Live tissue capable of growth and repair at the apex

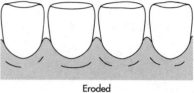

FIGURE 1-56. Erosion

Dental Histology

ENAMEL

☛ 96% inorganic; 4% water and organic materials
☛ Hardest biological tissue in body
☛ Formed from ameloblasts
☛ Hunter-Schreger bands
☛ Lines of Retzius
☛ Perikymata—horizontal lines
☛ Dentinoenamel junction (DEJ)—border between enamel and dentin

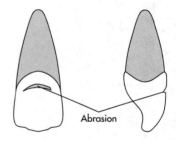

FIGURE 1-57. Abrasion

EROSION	Chemical damage to enamel **Figure 1-56**
ABRASION	Abnormal wear on enamel **Figure 1-57**
ATTRITION	Normal wear and tear **Figure 1-58**

DENTIN

• 70% inorganic; 20% organic collagen fibrous; 10% water
• Odontoblasts
• Forms bulk of tooth
• Three types:

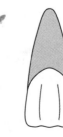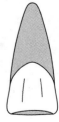

8 years · 80 years

FIGURE 1-58. Attrition

PRIMARY	Formed until tooth reaches occlusion and is functioning
SECONDARY	Formed after crown and root complete
TERTIARY	Reparative ☛ Sclerotic dentin—protective mechanism that occurs with age; made in response to trauma to seal off dentinal tubules ☛ Lines of Von Ebner—incremental lines of dentin

CEMENTUM

- Third hardest tissue in the body
- Covers roots of teeth
- Cementoblasts

CEMENTOENAMEL JUNCTION (CEJ)	Where the cementum meets the enamel around cervix of the tooth
CELLULAR CEMENTUM	Thicker cementum on the apex of the root with cells capable of growth and repair
ACELLULAR CEMENTUM	Cervical and middle portions of the root, and has no cells, therefore is not capable of growth and repair
HYPERCEMENTOSIS	Excessive amount of cementum growth, forming ball-shaped growths on the apices **Figure 1-59**

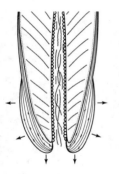

FIGURE 1-59.
Hypercementosis

PULP

- Innermost soft tissue occupying the hollowed-out inner portion of the dentin; space is called the pulp chamber and root canals
- Soft connective tissue with lots of matrix and few cells

Figure 1-60

PULP CHAMBER	Main space found under the crown of the tooth
PULP HORN	Where roof of pulp chamber comes to peaks underneath the incisal edge and under each cusp

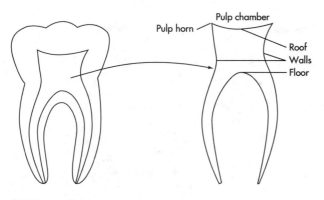

FIGURE 1-60. Pulp

ROOT CANAL	Pulp chamber space directly down into tubular spaces within each root of the tooth
APICAL FORAMEN	Opening out of the root where length of root ends
BLOOD VESSELS AND BLOOD CELLS	Provide nutrients and respiratory gases for all the cells of the pulp and the odontoblasts to keep them alive
LYMPH VESSEL AND LYMPH CELLS	Defense against foreign invaders like bacteria
PULP STONES OR DENTICLES	Odontoblasts break away from the walls of the pulp chamber and produce small stone inside the pulp **Figure 1-61**

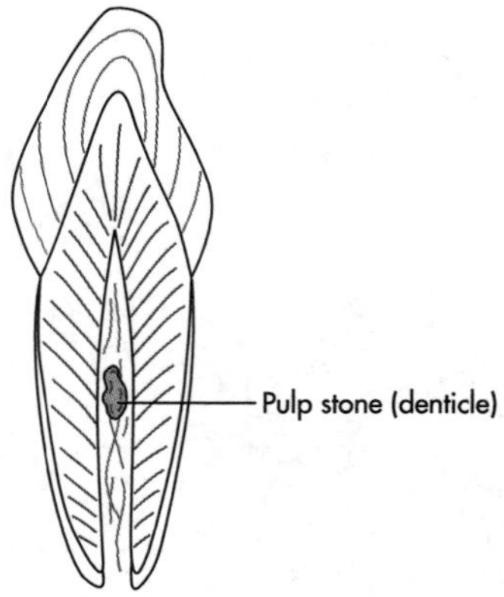

— Pulp stone (denticle)

FIGURE 1-61. Pulp Stone

Periodontal Tissues

"Peri" means around the tooth

PERIODONTAL LIGAMENT

- Derived from mesoderm
- Soft connective tissue between the tooth and the socket
- Attaches the tooth to the alveolus and provides a cushion against trauma

Figure 1-62

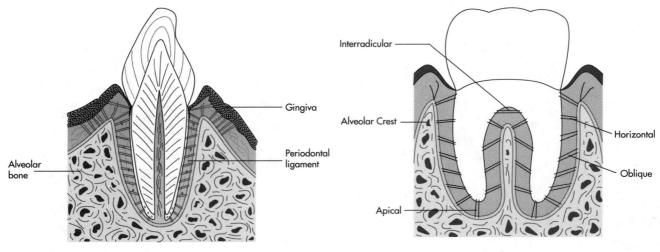

FIGURE 1-62. Periodontal Ligament

FIGURE 1-63. Periodontal Ligament Bundles

FIBROBLAST	Attach the tooth to the alveolus Two major types of fibers: • Collagen fibers • Elastic fibers ☛ Predominant cell of PDL
COLLAGEN FIBERS	Tough fibers used to support and attach the tooth in its bony socket ☛ *Principal fibers*—large collagen fiber bundles that attach the tooth to the alveolus ☛ *Sharpey's fibers*—attach PDL to cementum Do not stretch
ELASTIC FIBERS	Form network around the root; act as a cushion to traumatic forces on the teeth ☛ Like rubber bands, stretch and return to original shape
BLOOD CELLS AND VESSELS	Important to nutrition of the ligament and waste removal
LYMPH CELLS AND VESSELS	Important to the defense of the health of the ligament
NERVE FIBERS	Sense pain and regulate blood flow Proprioception—sense position of the jaw

PERIODONTAL LIGAMENT BUNDLES   Figure 1-63

ALVEOLAR CREST	Alveolar crest to cervical cementum ☛ Resists tilting, intrusive, extrusive, and rotational forces
HORIZONTAL	• Apical to alveolar crest horizontally to cementum • Resist tilting forces
OBLIQUE	Alveolar bone in an oblique manner into cementum ☛ Resists retrusive and rotational forces ☛ Most numerous of fibers
APICAL	Apical region of cementum to alveolar bone ☛ Resists extrusive forces
INTERRADICULAR	Multirooted teeth—exists between roots in the PDL ☛ Resists intrusive, extrusive, and tilting and rotational forces

ALVEOLAR BONE
Derived from mesoderm
Both compact and trabecular bone

CRESTAL BONE	Peaks at the top of the alveolus
LAMINA DURA	Hard layer that lines the socket

GINGIVA
Type of mucosa
Has epithelial layer (mucosal proper) and connective tissue layer below it (lamina propria)

SULCUS	Space or crevice created by the gingiva as it wraps around the tooth ☛ Also called periodontal pocket
ATTACHMENT EPITHELIUM	Gingiva that attaches to the tooth at the bottom of the sulcus
	Thin nonkeratinized epithelium ☛ Part of the whole epithelium of the sulcus called sulcular epithelium
FREE GINGIVA	Not attached to the alveolar bone

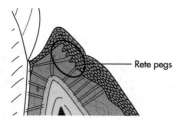

FIGURE 1-64. Rete Pegs

RETE RIDGES (PEGS)	Fingerlike extensions of epithelium into the lamina propria found in the free gingiva; help to strengthen gingiva **Figure 1-64**
ATTACHED GINGIVA	Below the free gingiva and attached to the underlying alveolar bone
FREE GINGIVAL GROOVE	Dividing line between the free gingiva and the attached gingiva
PAPILLAE	Peaks of free gingiva
MARGINAL GINGIVA	Encircling free gingiva

GINGIVAL GROUPS

DENTOGINGIVAL FIBERS	Run from the cervical tooth to surrounding gingiva located in the free gingiva above the alveolus **Figure 1-65**
ALVEOLOGINGIVAL FIBERS	Crestal bone to bottom of the alveolar bone, attaches to the gingival that covers the alveolar bone ☛ Provide very strong attachment for the gingiva below the free gingival groove or attachment gingiva **Figure 1-66**

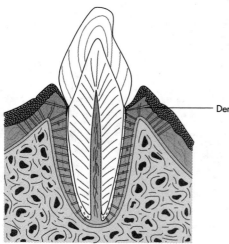

FIGURE 1-65. Dentogingival Fibers

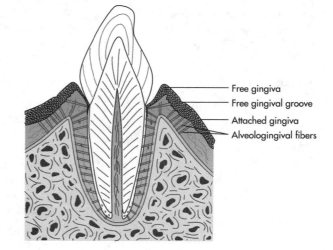

FIGURE 1-66. Alveologingival Fibers

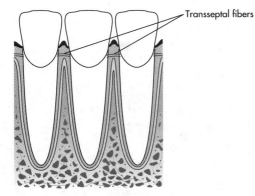

FIGURE 1-67. Transseptal Fibers

TRANSSEPTAL FIBERS	Run from cervix to cervix of the teeth across the crestal bone **Figure 1-67**
CIRCUMFERENTIAL FIBERS	Encircles each tooth to give support to the gingival collar **Figure 1-68**

MUCOSA
Soft lining of the oral cavity and the entire digestive system

☞ Resembles the skin but is very vascular

TOP (EPITHELIAL) LAYER	Mucosal proper; three layers
SECOND (CONNECTIVE TISSUE) LAYER	Lamina propria
THIRD (MUSCULAR) LAYER	Not present in the mouth

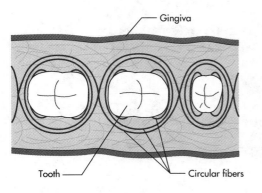

FIGURE 1-68. Circumferential Fibers

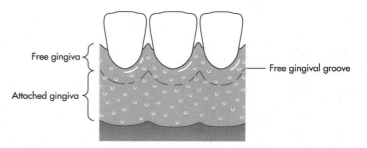

FIGURE 1-69. Gingiva

MASTICATORY MUCOSA	
GINGIVA	**Figure 1-69**
PALATAL MUCOSA	Mucosa of the palate; covers the hard palate • Soft palate—flap of soft tissue that moves during swallowing to seal off the nasal cavity from the oral cavity • Rugae—folds of palatal mucosa serve to break down food masses • Incisive papilla—covers foramen with blood vessels and nerves that extend to the lingual anterior teeth • Uvula—contains glandular tissue and is covered in palatal mucosa • Midpalatine suture—bony joint in the midline covered with palatal mucosa • Minor salivary glands—series of dots **Figure 1-70** ⚷ Keratinized

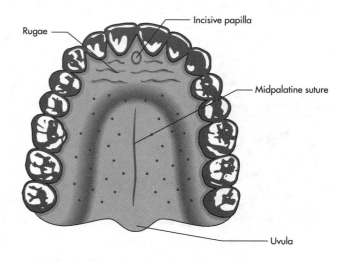

FIGURE 1-70. Minor Salivary Glands—Series of Dots

LINING MUCOSA Covers the rest of the oral cavity and pharynx (throat) Nonkeratinized mucosa	
ALVEOLAR MUCOSA	Covers the rest of the alveolar ridges • Frena—mucosal folds • Labial frena (two)—maxillary and mandibular • Buccal frena—leading into the cheek areas • Lingual frenum—under tongue **Figure 1-71** ☞ Begins where gingiva ends at the mucogingival junction
VESTIBULAR MUCOSA	Lining mucosa that continues off the mandible and maxilla turning up to line the cheeks, lips, and tongue creates a horseshoe-shaped trough Floor of the mouth—thin lining mucosal with several blood vessels • Sublingual caruncles—where Wharton's ducts from the two submandibular salivary glands empty • Sublingual plicae—folds that contain the ducts of Rivinus, tiny ducts from the sublingual salivary gland

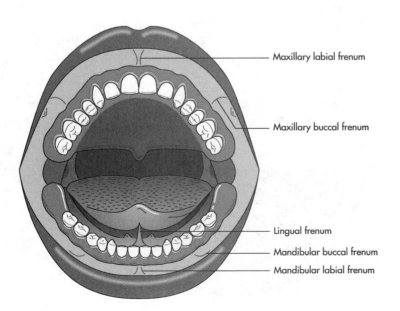

Maxillary labial frenum
Maxillary buccal frenum
Lingual frenum
Mandibular buccal frenum
Mandibular labial frenum

FIGURE 1-71. Lingual Frenum

	Figure 1-72 ☛ Several medications are administered for rapid absorption
BUCCAL MUCOSA	Lining of the cheek • Buccal frena—fold over the vestibular area and into the alveolar mucosa • Stensen's duct—comes from the parotid gland and pierces the buccinator to empty into a papilla directly opposite the maxillary second molar, the parotid papilla • Parotid glands—paired on the outermost aspect of each cheek, directly below the skin and above the muscle • Linea alba—rough horizontal fold of tissue in a line along the occlusal plane; caused by the buccal mucosa being occluded by the teeth • Pterygomandibular raphe—end of the oral cavity and buccal mucosal and is a vertical line created when a person opens his mouth widely. It is created by the buccinator and superior constrictor muscles when they come together ☛ Covers chief muscle of the cheek the buccinator muscle ☛ Landmark for the inferior alveolar injection
LABIAL MUCOSA	• Lines the lips • Vermillion border—zone of transition from skin to mucosa

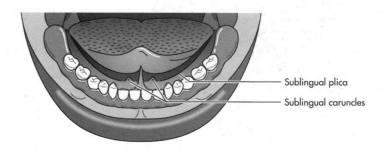

Sublingual plica

Sublingual caruncles

FIGURE 1-72. Sublingual Plicae

VENTRAL TONGUE (FLOOR OF MOUTH)	Lining mucosa underside or ventrum of the tongue and floor of the mouth • Sublingual plicae—two folds in the mucosal that have multiple ducts called the ducts of Rivinus; mucosa of the floor of the mouth that contains the opening of one of the major salivary glands, the sublingual salivary gland • Lingual mucosa—midline fold of mucosa dividing the mucosa of the floor of the mouth into right and left halves • Submandibular salivary glands—under each angle of the mandible, ducts travel under the floor of the mouth, parallel to the blood vessels and empty in the anterior area through the sublingual caruncles
PHARYNGEAL MUCOSA	• Lining mucosa of the oropharynx (food tube) • Nasopharynx—continues up into the nose • Pharynx proper—down past the tongue and leads into the esophagus • Pharyngeal pillars—two pairs of columns of mucosa-covered tissue at junction of the oropharynx and oral cavity • Glossopharyngeus and palatopharyngeus—both pairs of muscles covered with pharyngeal mucosa and form posterior border of the oral cavity • Palatine tonsils—lie in the fauces of the oropharynx • Pharyngeal tonsils (adenoids)—pair of tonsils in the nasopharynx • Lingual tonsils—found on the very back or root of the tongue; back of the throat ☛ Waldeyer's ring—all three types of tonsils that form a protective ring around the pharynx

SPECIALIZED MUCOSA Found on the top or dorsum of the tongue Help in the sensory function of the tongue, which is taste	
TONGUE	• Sac of muscles covered by mucosa • Intrinsic muscle—striated mucosa muscles inside the tongue (run in three major directions) **Figure 1-73**
DORSUM OF TONGUE	• Dorsum of tongue—top of the tongue receives the most wear and tear • Very thick, keratinized mucosa

PAPILLA OF THE DORSAL TONGUE Figure 1-74	
FILIFORM PAPILLAE	Flame-shaped papillae, scattered on the entire surface of the body of the tongue
FUNGIFORM PAPILLAE	Mushroom-shaped papillae that are not as abundant as filiform are scattered across the dorsal surface on the body of the tongue
FOLIATE PAPILLAE	Huge filiform papillae, found only on the lateral borders (sides) of the tongue
CIRCUMVALLATE PAPILLAE	Round mushroom-shaped central portion surrounded by a trough, form a "V"-shaped boarder on the tongue between the anterior two-thirds (ectoderm) and posterior one-third (endoderm) of the tongue ⚷ Von Ebner's—serous gland empties directly into the trough

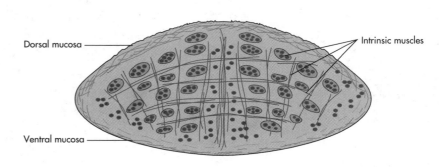

FIGURE 1-73. Tongue

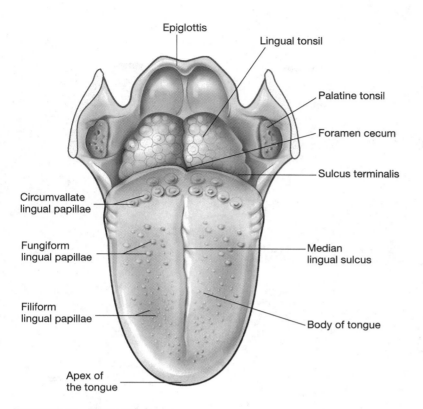

FIGURE 1-74. Papilla of the Tongue

TASTE CELLS	Sensory neurons capable of distinguishing between four major tastes scattered throughout the dorsal tongue mucosa, most are located on the walls of the circumvallate papillae **Figure 1-75**
FORAMEN CECUM	Bump or hollowed out area of tissue at the point of the "V" of the circumvallate papillae ☛ It is a reminder that the thyroid gland began its development there

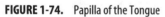

FIGURE 1-75. Taste Cells

2 Physiology

Demetra Daskalos Logothetis,
  RDH, MS

Tammy Teague, RDH, BS

➤ PHYSIOLOGY

LEVELS OF ORGANIZATION
All of the organ systems of the body

CHEMICAL LEVEL	Atoms form molecules
CELLULAR LEVEL	Molecules form organelles that perform a specific function ☛ Example: cell
TISSUE LEVEL	Similar cells work together to perform a specific function ☛ Example: cardiac muscle tissue
ORGAN LEVEL	Consists of two or more different tissues that work together ☛ Example: heart
ORGAN SYSTEM LEVEL	Organ and elements that work as a system ☛ Example: circulatory system

DIRECTIONAL TERMS

ANTERIOR	Front; before ☛ Eye is anterior to ear
VENTRAL	Belly side; on the front ☛ Lingual frenum is on the ventral side of the tongue

POSTERIOR	Back; behind ☛ Ear is posterior to the nose
DORSAL	On the back ☛ Papillae are on the dorsal surface of the tongue
MEDIAL	Toward the middle or midline of the body ☛ Scaling from molars to the anteriors move medially toward the midline
LATERAL	Toward the outside of the body ☛ Eyes are lateral to the nose
CRANIAL OR CEPHALIC	Toward the head
CAUDAL	Toward the tail
INFERIOR	Below; at a lower level ☛ Lips are inferior to the nose
SUPERIOR	Above or higher ☛ Eyes are superior to the mouth
PROXIMAL	Toward an attached base ☛ Thigh is proximal to the foot
DISTAL	Away from an attached base ☛ Fingers are distal to the wrist
SUPERFICIAL	At or near the body surface ☛ Alveolar mucosa is superficial to underlying alveolar bone
DEEP	Farther from body surface ☛ Bone is deep to surrounding muscle tissue

BODY CAVITIES Areas in the body where vital organs are suspended in chambers	
DORSAL	Fluid-filled space that includes the cranial cavity and the spinal cavity
VENTRAL	Contains three main parts: thoracic cavity, abdominal cavity, and pelvic cavity ☛ Contains organs that maintain basic life processes

COMPONENTS OF CELLS

CELL MEMBRANE	Lipid bilayer that provides isolation, protection, and support ☞ Controls the entrance/exit
CYTOSOL	Fluid component of cytoplasm ☞ Distributes materials

CHEMICAL BONDS

IONIC	Result from gain or loss of electrons between atoms ☞ Ionic bonds are broken when the substance dissolves in water
COVALENT	Produced when electrons are shared between atoms
POLAR COVALENT	• Result when sharing of electrons between atoms is unequal • Have charged portions that attract opposite charges and other polar molecules ☞ Examples: water, functional groups of most organic molecules ☞ Tend to be hydrophilic (attract water)
NONPOLAR COVALENT	Result when the sharing of electrons between atoms is equal or the molecule is symmetrical, thus canceling the polarity ☞ Examples: carbon dioxide, long chain hydrocarbons ☞ Tend to be hydrophobic (repel water)
HYDROGEN	• Electrical attractions between NH+ and C=O groups found at distances on the same molecule or on different molecules • Cause coiling of proteins and hold the strands of the DNA molecule together

NONMEMBRANOUS ORGANELLES
Cytoskeleton (microtubules or microfilaments) proteins that provide strength and materials

MICROVILLI	Microfilaments that facilitate the absorption of extracellular materials

CILIA	Membrane extensions that assist in movement of materials over the surface
CENTRIOLES	Cylindrical structure composed of microtubules that enables the movement of chromosomes during cell division
RIBOSOMES	Protein + RNA ☛ Performs protein synthesis

MEMBRANOUS ORGANELLES

ENDOPLASMIC RETICULUM (ER)	Membranous channels in cytoplasm ☛ Synthesizes secretory products and intercellular transport and storage
ROUGH ER	Has ribosomes attached
SMOOTH ER	Lacks ribosomes
GOLGI APPARATUS	Flattened chamber that stores and packages secretory products ☛ Forms lysosomes
LYSOSOMES	Vesicles containing powerful digestive enzymes ☛ Removes damaged organelles or pathogens in cells
MITOCHONDRIA	Organelles containing enzymes that regulate the reactions that provide energy for the cell ☛ Contain the enzymes and cytochromes for the Krebs cycle; produces ATP
NUCLEUS	Nucleoplasm surrounded by double membrane and connects to the endoplasmic reticulum ☛ Control center of the cell; stores and processes DNA
NUCLEOLUS	Contains the DNA and RNA, located in the nucleoplasm ☛ Synthesizes rRNA (ribosomal ribonucleic acid)

Membrane Transport

KEY TERMS	
PERMEABILITY	Determines which substances enter or leave the cytoplasm
IMPERMEABLE	No substance can cross the cell membrane
FREELY PERMEABLE	Any substance can cross the cell membrane without difficulty
SELECTIVELY PERMEABLE	Free passage of some substances and restricting passage of others ☛ Based on size, electrical charge, molecular shape, lipid solubility
PASSIVE PROCESSES	Ions or molecules move across cell membrane without needing energy ☛ Includes diffusion, osmosis, facilitated diffusion
ACTIVE PROCESSES	Require energy from the cell to move ions or molecules across the cell membrane ☛ Usually in the form of ATP

DIFFUSION Movement of molecules from area of high concentration to area of low concentration	
CONCENTRATION GRADIENT	Difference between high and low concentrations
DIFFUSION ACROSS CELL MEMBRANE	Molecules can independently diffuse across a cell membrane by lipid solubility and size of molecule ☛ Alcohol, fatty acids, steroids, dissolved gases such as oxygen and carbon dioxide enter and leave the cell by diffusion through lipid bilayers ☛ Water-soluble compounds diffuse through channels in the membrane because they are small

OSMOSIS	<ul><li>Diffusion of water molecules across a membrane</li><li>Occurs across a selectively permeable membrane that is freely permeable to water but not to solutes (dissolved materials)</li><li>Will flow toward the solution with the highest concentration of solutes</li></ul>

FILTRATION

Water and small solute molecules are forced across a membrane due to hydrostatic pressure gradient
☞ Example: heart pushes blood through the circulatory system generating blood pressure
☞ Kidney filtration is an essential step in the production of urine

CARRIER MEDIATED TRANSPORT
Process by which membrane proteins bend specific ions or organic material and move them across the cell membrane
☞ Can be passive (no ATP required) or active (ATP required)

FACILITATED DIFFUSION	Molecules that are too large to fit through membrane channels, and insoluble lipids are transported by binding to receptor sites on the protein that moves it into the cell
ACTIVE TRANSPORT	<ul><li>Utilizing ATP, the molecules or ions move across the membrane regardless of their intracellular or extracellular concentrations</li><li>Carrier proteins called ion pumps actively transport sodium (Na+), potassium (K+), calcium (Ca+), magnesium (Mg+) across the membrane</li></ul>

VESICULAR TRANSPORT
Formation of a vesicle provides movement of material in or out of the cell

ENDOCYTOSIS	Extracellular material collected in a vesicle and imported into the cell • Pinocytosis—small vesicles fill with extracellular fluid and then pinch off ☞ "Cell drinking" • Phagocytosis—pseudopodia (cytoplasmic extensions surround object)→membrane fuses to form vesicle→vesicle fuses to a lysome and breaks down contents ☞ "Cell eating"
EXCYTOSIS	• Reverse of endocytosis • Vesicle is created within cell and fuses to cell membrane discharging contents to extracellular fluid ☞ Examples: hormones, mucus, waste products

CELL DIVISION

MEIOSIS	Division of reproductive cells ☞ Produces sperm or ova
MITOSIS	Division of somatic cells ☞ Vast majority of cell division; includes four stages: prophase, metaphase, and telophase
INTERPHASE	Interval of time between cell division when DNA replication occurs

Integumentary System

- Provides mechanical protection against environmental hazards
- Contains skin, hair, sweat glands, nails, and sensory receptors

SKELETAL SYSTEM Provides mechanical support, stores energy reserves, stores calcium and phosphate reserves; 206 bones Figure 2-1	
AXIAL SKELETON	Bones of the skull, spinal column, ribs, sternum ☞ Framework of the head and trunk of the body
APPENDICULAR SKELETON	Bones of the upper and lower extremities and supporting bones ☞ Provides internal support of arms and legs, moves the axial skeleton
BONE MARROW	Red marrow—filled with blood vessels and connective tissue, manufactures RBC, WBC, and platelets ☞ Yellow marrow—contains mainly fat
SHAPES OF BONE	Long, short, flat, irregular
TYPES OF BONE	• Compact—dense, solid ☞ Example of compact—main shaft of femur • Cancellous—spongy, bony rods covered by marrow ☞ Example of cancellous—found at the end of femur (epiphysis)
CELLS OF THE BONE	• Osteocytes—mature bone cells • Osteoclasts—dissolve bony matrix, which regulates the calcium and phosphate concentrations in body fluids ☞ Osteoblasts—produce new bone
PERIOSTEUM	Fibrous covering that isolates the bone, provides a route for blood and nerves
DISEASES OR CONDITIONS	• Osteomyelitis—infection of bone-forming tissue • Osteoporosis—loss of bone mass, brittle soft bones result

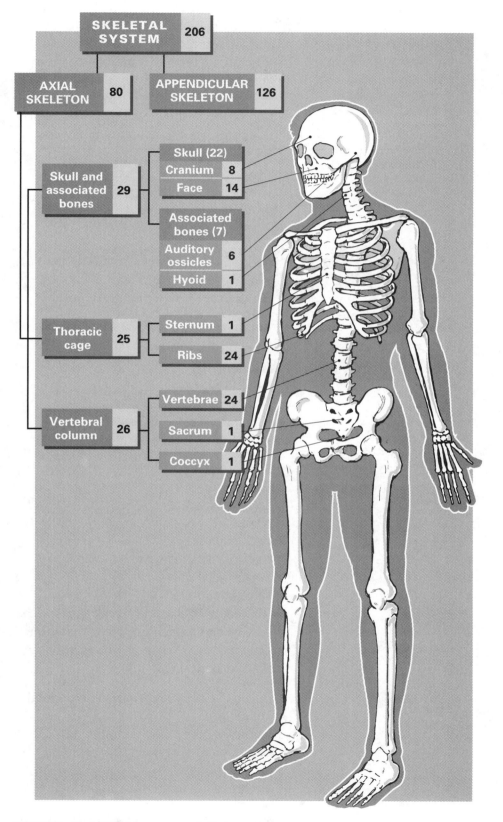

FIGURE 2-1 The Axial Skeleton

	• Cleft palate—failure of palate to form and join correctly • Fractures—breaks of the bone or cartilage • Temporomandibular joint—degeneration of the joint where the mandible articulates with the temporal bone
CARTILAGE	Nonvascular connective tissue Found where two bones join and areas such as nose and ear

BONES OF THE SKULL 22 bones that protect the brain and provide support for the sense organs	
CRANIUM (8 BONES)	• Frontal • Occipital • Sphenoid • Ethmoid • Parietal (2) • Temporal (2) ☛ Encloses the brain
FACIAL BONES (14 BONES)	• Maxillary (2) • Palatine (2) • Vomer • Zygomatic (2) • Nasal • Lacrimal (2) • Inferior nasal concha • Mandible • Hyoid ☛ Protect and support the entrances to the digestive and respiratory tract; mandible is only moveable bone; hyoid is not attached to skull
SUTURES OF THE BONE	• Coronal—between frontal and parietal bones • Sagittal—joins the parietal bones • Lambdoidal—between the occipital and parietal bones • Squamosal—temporal and parietal bones • Temporozygomatic—zygomatic and temporal bone

- Median palatine—palatine bones
- Transverse palatine—maxilla and palatine bones

BONES OF NECK AND TRUNK

- 7 cervical vertebrae—distinguished by the shape of the body
- 12 thoracic vertebrae—heart-shaped (includes ribs)
- 5 lumbar vertebrae—most massive and least mobile
- Sacrum—protects reproductive, digestive, and excretory organs; coccyx
- Ribs 1–7 are attached to sternum (true ribs)
- Ribs 8–12 are not attached (false ribs)

APPENDICULAR SKELETON Figure 2-2

PECTORAL GIRDLE	• Scapula • Clavicle
UPPER LIMB (ARM AND FOREARM)	• Humerus • Radius • Ulna • 27 bones in hand
PELVIC GIRDLE	• Coxae—hip bones, which consist of ilium, ischium, and pubis
LOWER LIMB	• Femur • Tibia • Fibula • Bones of ankle and foot

ARTICULATIONS
Joints where two or more bones meet and form a junction

FIBROUS	Immovable or fixed Example: sutures in bones of cranium
CARTILAGINOUS	Slightly movable Example: joint between bones of vertebrae
SYNOVIAL	Freely moveable, fluid in joint 6 types of synovial joints (ball and socket, hinge, pivot, gliding, saddle, and condyloid) **Figure 2-3**

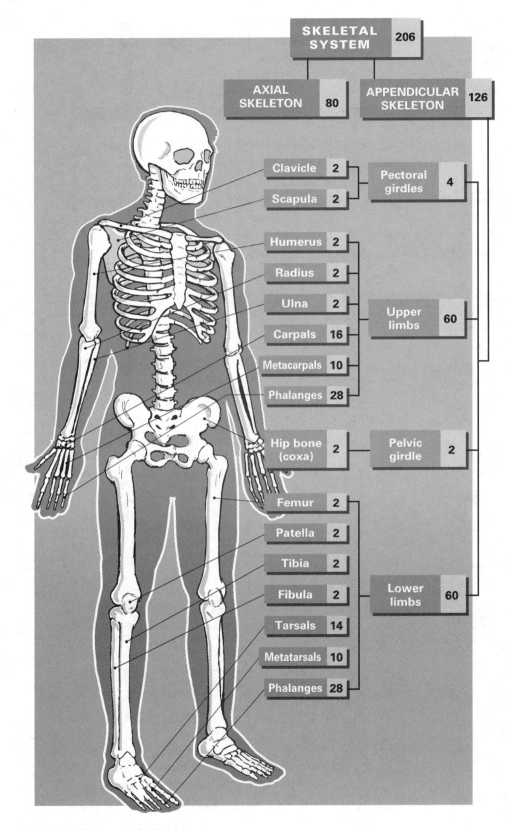

FIGURE 2-2 The Appendicular Skeleton

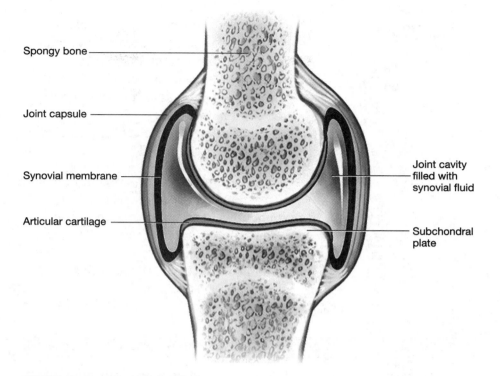

Spongy bone

Joint capsule

Synovial membrane

Articular cartilage

Joint cavity filled with synovial fluid

Subchondral plate

FIGURE 2-3 Freely Movable Synovial Joint

HORMONES IMPORTANT TO BONE GROWTH AND HOMEOSTASIS

GROWTH HORMONE (GH)	Necessary for normal growth and development of the skeleton, secreated from the anterior pituitary • Hyposecretion of GH during childhood produces a dwarf • Hypersecretion of GH produces a giant; in adulthood produces acromegaly (shape of bones, especially those in the face, become exaggerated)
THYROID HORMONES	Regulate metabolism of most cells
ESTROGEN	Important for growth in length of bone and for bone maintenance • Present in varying amounts in both sexes
TESTOSTERONE	Important for growth in mass and density of bone • Present in varying amounts in both sexes

PARATHYROID HORMONE	• Exerts the primary control in calcium homeostasis; when calcium level falls, parathyroid hormone is secreted • Raises calcium by increasing vitamin D production, increased reabsorption of calcium in the kidney • Increases osteoclastic activity to release calcium into the blood
CALCITONIN	• Normally important only in children and is secreted by special cells in the thyroid • Functions to stimulate the uptake of calcium into growing bone and the deposition of bone matrix • Can be used to aid uptake of calcium in osteoporosis patients

DISEASES RELATED TO BONES

OSTEOPOROSIS	Disorder involving demineralization of bone usually associated with older individuals and is related to several factors: • Deficiency of dietary calcium • Reduced estrogen levels common in postmenopausal women • Reduced activity and exercise • Reduced weightbearing stress on the bones (this is important in stimulating bone growth and replacement at any age)
RICKETS	• Vitamin D deficiency in children (vitamin D is necessary for absorption of calcium) • Results from improper mineralization that results in stunted growth and weakened bones
OSTEOARTHRITIS	• Noninflammatory type of arthritis resulting in degeneration of the bones and joints • Especially weight bearing
OSTEOMALACIA	• Vitamin D deficiency in adults • Causes demineralization of the bones (softening of the bones) • Periodontal disease, delayed tooth eruption

OSTEOMYELITIS	Inflammation of the bone and bone marrow due to infection
PAGET'S DISEASE	Metabolic disorder of unknown cause that involves the destruction of normal bone tissue and replaces it with tissue of irregular and unorganized structure ☛ Enlargement of bone; when in maxilla and mandible, increased spacing of teeth ☛ Radiographic manifestations: "cotton wool" appearance, hypercementosis, loss of lamina dura
RHEUMATOID ARTHRITIS	Chronic form of arthritis

DISEASE OF JOINTS

ARTHRITIS	Inflammation of a joint
GOUT	Inflammation of a joint caused by excessive uric acid

MUSCULAR SYSTEM

Locomotion, support, and heat production

TYPES OF MUSCLE Figure 2-4

SKELETAL (STRIATED)	Long thin fibers that attach to skeleton ☛ Voluntary control
SMOOTH	Forms sheets, bundles, or sheaths around other tissues found within almost every organ (not heart) ☛ Involuntary
CARDIAC	Found only in heart ☛ Involuntary

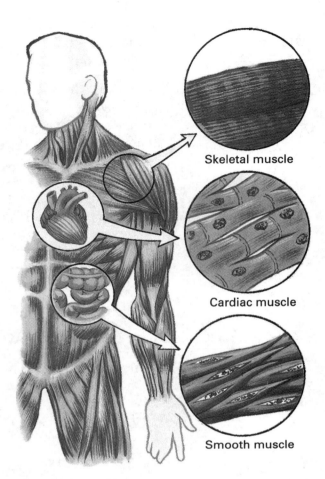

Skeletal muscle

Cardiac muscle

Smooth muscle

FIGURE 2-4 Types of Muscle

CHARACTERISTICS OF MUSCLE	
FIBER	Groups of muscle cells
FASCIA	Sheet of connective tissue that covers, supports, and separates fibers
EXCITABILITY OR IRRITABILITY	Muscle response to stimuli
EXTENSIBILITY	Ability to stretch or spread
TONE	Tension of muscular system
CONTRACTION	Become shorter and thicker • Isometric—no change in length of muscle but tension is increased • Isotonic—muscle tension remains the same but muscle shortens

RELAXATION	Release and return to normal form
TENDON	Cord that attaches muscle to bone
APONEUROSIS	Broad, flat extension that attaches muscle to bone or muscle to muscle
LIGAMENTS	Sheets of connective tissue that act to connect or support two or more bones
ANTAGONISTIC PAIRS	When one set of muscles contracts, the other relaxes ☛ Provide movement
ATP	Energy required for muscle contraction, requires oxygen or lactic acid will result ☛ Energy transfer molecule
GLYCOGEN	Stored in muscle for reserve energy, broken down by glycolysis

MUSCLE METABOLISM

ANAEROBIC GLYCOLYSIS	• Initial way of utilizing glucose in all cells to provide ATP when insufficient oxygen is available for aerobic metabolism • Does not require oxygen • Occurs in cytoplasm, not mitochondria, allowing for quick bursts of speed or strength • Slows down as pyruvic acid (product of glycolysis) builds up • Pyruvic acid is converted to lactic acid by fermentation, allowing an extension of glycolysis • Lactic buildup slows metabolism and causes muscle fatigue; lactic acid must be reconverted to pyruvic acid and metabolized aerobically in the muscle or liver

AEROBIC METABOLISM	• Performed exclusively in the mitochondria • Pyruvic acid (product of glycolysis) must be metabolized aerobically • Pyruvic acid is converted to an acetyl group and put into the Krebs cycle; energy is released in the form of ATP as high energy electrons; waste products of aerobic metabolism are CO_2 and H_2O • Aerobic metabolism is used for endurance activities

MUSCULAR CONDITIONS OR DISEASES

SPASM	Sudden involuntary muscle contraction
FIBROMYALGIA	Chronic pain in the muscle and soft tissue surrounding the joints
MUSCULAR DYSTROPHY	Congenital disorder characterized by progressive degeneration of skeletal muscle
POLYMYOSITIS	Disease causing muscle inflammation and weakness form an unknown cause
MYASTHENIA GRAVIS	Autoimmune disorder causing loss of muscle strength and paralysis

SKELETAL MUSCLES

AXIAL MUSCLES	Positions the head and spinal column and rib cage
HEAD	• Frontalis • Oribularis oris • Buccinator • Masseter • Temporalis • Pterygoids • Platysma
NECK	• Digastric • Mylohyoid • Sylohyoid • Sternocleidomastoid

TRUNK (THORACIC)	• External intercostals • Internal intercostals • Diaphragm
TRUNK (ABDOMINAL)	• External oblique • Internal oblique • Transverse abdomini • Rectus abdominis
PELVIC FLOOR (PERINEUM)	• Bulbospongiosus • Ischiocavernosus • Transverse perineus • External urethral sphincter • External anal sphincter • Levator ani

APPENDICULAR MUSCULATURE
Stabilizes and moves components

SHOULDER	• Levator scapulae • Pectoralis minor • Rhomboideus • Serratus anterior • Subclavius • Trapezius
ARM	• Coracobrachialis • Deltoid • Latissimus dorsi • Pectorails major
ELBOW	• Biceps brachii • Brachialis • Brachioradialis • Triseps brachii • Pronator teres • Supinator
WRIST	• Flexor carpi radialis • Flexor carpi ulnaris • Palmaris longus
HAND	• Extensor digitorum • Flexor digitorum

THIGH	• Gluteus maximus • Gluteus medius • Gluteus minimus • Adductor brevis • Adductor magnus • Adductor magnus • Pectineus • Gracilis • Iliacus • Psoas major
LEG	• Biceps femoris • Semimembranous • Semitendinosus • Satorius • Popliteus • Rectus femoris • Vastus intermedius • Vastus lateralis • Vastus medialis
FOOT	• Tibialis anterior • Gastrocnemius • Peroneus • Soleus • Tibialis posterior
TOES	• Flexordigitorum • Flexor hallucis

Nervous System

Transmits stimuli from outside and inside the body; it includes the brain, spinal cord, and nerve cells

FUNCTIONS OF THE NERVOUS SYSTEM

- Integration of body processes
- Control of voluntary effectors (skeletal muscles) and mediation of voluntary reflexes
- Control of involuntary effectors (smooth muscle, cardiac muscle, glands) and mediation of autonomic reflexes (heart rate, blood pressure, glandular secretion, etc.)
- Responsible for conscious thought and perception, emotions, personality, the mind

DIVISIONS OF THE NERVOUS SYSTEM   Figure 2-5

CENTRAL NERVOUS SYSTEM (CNS)	Brain and spinal cord
PERIPHERAL NERVOUS SYSTEM (PNS)	All the nerves outside the CNS
AUTONOMIC NERVOUS SYSTEM (ANS)	Specialized group of peripheral nerves that functions automatically; two divisions: sympathetic and parasympathetic

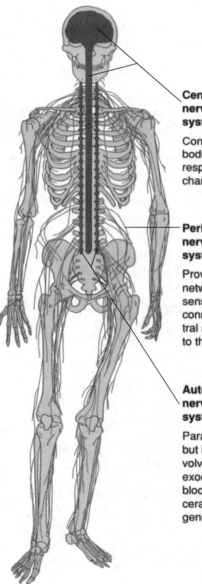

Central nervous system

Controls all basic bodily functions, and responds to external changes

Peripheral nervous system

Provides a complete network of motor and sensory nerve fibers connecting the central nervous system to the rest of the body

Autonomic nervous system

Parallels the spinal cord but is separately involved in control of exocrine glands, blood vessels, viscera, and external genitalia

FIGURE 2-5

COMPONENTS OF NERVOUS SYSTEM

NEURON	Basic structural unit of the nervous system
DENDRITES	Nerve fibers that conduct impulses toward the cell body
AXON	Nerve fibers that conduct impulses away from the cell body
SYNAPSE	Junction where chemicals are released from the ends of axons to allow the stimuli to jump to the next dendrite
MYELIN SHEATH	Layer of Schwann cells that insulate and protect the nerve
AFFERENT DIVISION OF THE PNS	Brings sensory information to the CNS
EFFERENT DIVISION	Carries motor commands to muscles and glands
SOMATIC NERVOUS SYSTEM	Part of PNS that provides voluntary control over skeletal muscles
NEUROTRANSMITTERS	Chemicals that transfer information from one neuron to another neuron or effector cell ☛ Examples: acetylcholine (Ach), norepinephrine (NE), dopamine
REFLEX	Automatic motor responses that help the body maintain homeostasis ☛ Examples: heart rate, sneezing, and swallowing
GANGLIA	Groups of neuron cell bodies
NERVES	Bundles of axons
CENTERS	Collections of neuron cell bodies that share a particular function
TRACTS	Bundles of axons inside the CNS that share common origins, destinations, and functions
PATHWAYS	Link the centers of the brain with the rest of the body

MENINGES	Specialized membranes that protect and support the brain; three layers: dura mater, arachnoid, and pia mater
BLOOD–BRAIN BARRIER	Isolates the neural tissue in the CNS from general circulation
SPINAL CORD	Serves as major highway for the passage of sensory impulses to the brain and motor impulses from the brain
EPIDURAL SPACE	Separates the spinal dural mater from the walls of the vertebral canal

BRAIN Figure 2-6
☞ 98% of neural tissue

CEREBRUM	Conscious thought, intellectual functions, memory, and complex involuntary motor patterns originate here

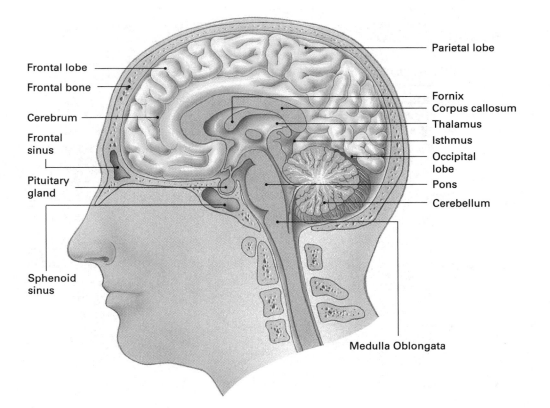

Parietal lobe
Frontal lobe
Frontal bone
Cerebrum
Frontal sinus
Pituitary gland
Sphenoid sinus
Fornix
Corpus callosum
Thalamus
Isthmus
Occipital lobe
Pons
Cerebellum
Medulla Oblongata

FIGURE 2-6

CEREBELLUM	Adjusts voluntary and involuntary motor activities on the basis of sensory and stored memories
DIENCEPHALONS	Contains relay and processing centers for sensory information, contains the thalamus and hypothalamus and epithalamus • Thalamus—receives all conscious sensations and acts as a relay center • Hypothalamus—part of the control mechanism for many of the endocrine glands
PINEAL GLAND	• Part of the epithalamus (*epi* = upon the thalamus) and receives stimuli from the hypothalamus • Secretes melatonin during the dark periods to establish our biological clock and regulates our circadian rhythm (day–night cycle) • Affects many behaviors such as sleeping, eating, sexual desire
FRONTAL LOBE	Controls motor function
PARIETAL LOBE	Receives and interprets nerve impulses from sensory receptors
OCCIPITAL LOBE	Controls sight
TEMPORAL LOBE	Controls hearing and smell
MID BRAIN	Part of brainstem that processes visual and auditory information and generates involuntary somatic motor responses
PONS	Connects the cerebellum to the brainstem; involved with somatic and visceral motor control
MEDULLA OBLONGATA	Part of brainstem that connects the brain to the spinal cord; relays sensory information and regulates autonomic functions
VENTRICLES	Four chambers of the brain

TWELVE CRANIAL NERVES
Connect to the brain

I. OLFACTORY	• Sensory nerves that conduct impulses from the nose to the brain • Only cranial nerve attached to the cerebrum
II. OPTIC	Sensory nerves that conducts impulses from the eye to the brain
III. OCULOMOTOR	Motor nerve that sends impulses to the eye
IV. TROCHLEAR	Motor impulses to external eye
V. TRIGEMINAL	Three branches: 1. Ophthalmic—sensory nerve to forehead, eyes, and nose 2. Maxillary—sensory information from the lower eye. Upper lip, cheek, nose, and maxillary region 3. Mandibular-sensory to the lower jaw and motor to the muscles of the tongue
VI. ABDUCENS	Motor nerve to the lateral rectus muscle of the eye
VII. FACIAL	Innervates the facial muscles, salivary glands, lacrimal glands, and sensation of taste to the anterior two-thirds of the tongue
VIII. ACOUSTIC	Two branches: 1. Cochlear branch—concerned with the sense of hearing 2. Vestibular branch—concerned with the sense of balance
IX. GLOSSOPHARYN-GEAL	Innervates the parotid glands, taste on the posterior third of the tongue, and part of the pharynx
X. VAGUS	Innervates part of the pharynx, larynx, and vocal cords and part of the thoracic and abdominal viscera
XI. SPINAL ACCESSORY	Innervates structures in the neck, shoulders, and back

XII. HYPOGLOSSAL	Voluntary control over muscles of the tongue

SPINAL NERVES Monitors a specific region of the body surface	
CERVICAL NERVES	C1–C8
THORACIC NERVES	T1–T12
LUMBAR NERVES	L1–L5
SACRAL NERVES	S1–S5
COCCYGEAL NERVE	Co_1

NERVE PLEXUS Networks of nerve trunks from several spinal nerves	
CERVICAL PLEXUS	Innervates the muscles of the neck and expands into the thoracic cavity to control the diaphragm
BRACHIAL PLEXUS	Innervates the shoulder and upper limbs
LUMBROSACRAL PLEXUS	Innervates the pelvis and lower limbs

DISEASES OR CONDITIONS AFFECTING THE NERVOUS SYSTEM	
NEURITIS	Inflammation of the nerves
MULTIPLE SCLEROSIS (MS)	Disease that destroys the myelin sheath of neurons in the CNS
PARKINSON'S DISEASE	Nerve disease characterized by tumors, muscle weakness, unsteady gait
BELL'S PALSY	Facial paralysis
ALZHEIMER'S	Chronic, organic mental disorder consisting of dementia ☛ More prevalent in adults between 40–60 years of age

ENCEPHALITIS	Inflammation of the brain due to disease factors such as rabies, influenza, measles, or smallpox
EPILEPSY	Recurrent disorder of the brain in which convulsive seizures and loss of consciousness occur
MENINGITIS	Inflammation of the membranes of the spinal cord and brain that is caused by a microorganism
TIC DOULOUREUX	Painful condition in which the trigeminal nerve is affected by pressure or degeneration

➤ ENDOCRINE SYSTEM

Directs long term changes in the activities of other organ systems

ENDOCRINE CELLS Glandular secretory cells that release their secretions internally	
ADENOHYPOPHYSIS	• Anterior pituitary • Secretes group of hormones called trophic hormones • Tropic hormones control other glands or act on other tissues • Controlled by hypothalamus
NEUROHYPOPHYSIS	• Posterior pituitary • Posterior pituitary stores these hormones for release on command • Controlled by hypothalamus

HORMONES

Chemical messengers that are released on one tissue and transported by the bloodstream to reach target cells in other tissues

TROPIC HORMONES Figure 2-7

GONADOTROPINS	• Follicle stimulating hormone (FSH) stimulates gametogenesis in both males and females; in females, this involves follicle development and the first stage of oogenesis, and stimulates estrogen; in males, stimulates spermatogenesis • Luteinizing hormone (LH) causes ovulation and progesterone secretion

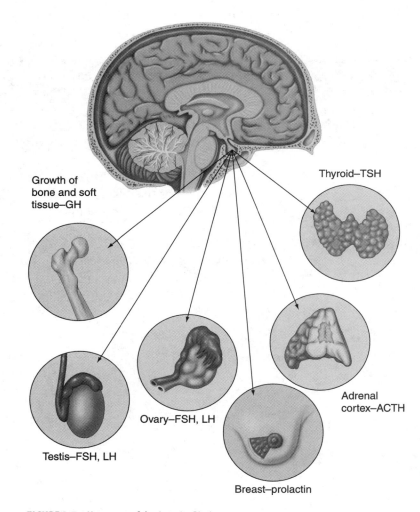

Growth of bone and soft tissue–GH

Thyroid–TSH

Testis–FSH, LH

Ovary–FSH, LH

Breast–prolactin

Adrenal cortex–ACTH

FIGURE 2-7 Hormones of the Anterior Pituitary

THYROID STIMU-LATING HORMONE (TSH)	Secreted from the hypothalamus causes the thyroid to secrete its hormones, T4 (thyroxine) and T3
ADRENAL CORTI-COTROPIC HORMONE (ACTH)	Stimulates the release of corticosteroids from the adrenal cortex
GROWTH HORMONE (GH)	• Controlled by both releasing and in hibiting hormones from the hypothalamus • Causes growth and development of the musculoskeletal system and other tissues
PROLACTIN (PRL)	Promotes breast development and milk production

NEUROHYPOPHYSIS HORMONES

Secreted by neurons from the hypothalamus

ANTIDIURETIC HORMONE (ADA)	Increases reabsorption of water from the kidney's collecting tubules in response to increasing blood osmolarity
OXYTOCIN (OT)	• Stimulates uterine smooth muscle con-tractions in labor • Triggers milk ejection by the mammary glands • Used clinically to induce labor

STRUCTURE OF HORMONES

Hormones are divided into three groups:

AMINO ACID DERIVATIVES	Epinephrine, norepinephrine, thyroid hor-mones, and melatonin
PEPTIDE HORMONES	ADH, oxytocin, growth hormone, prolactin • Largest class of hormones
LIPID DERIVATIVES	Steroid hormones and prostoglandins

GLANDS OF ENDOCRINE SYSTEM Figure 2-8

PINEAL	Controls timing of sexual maturation and sets day/night rhythms; produces mela-tonin

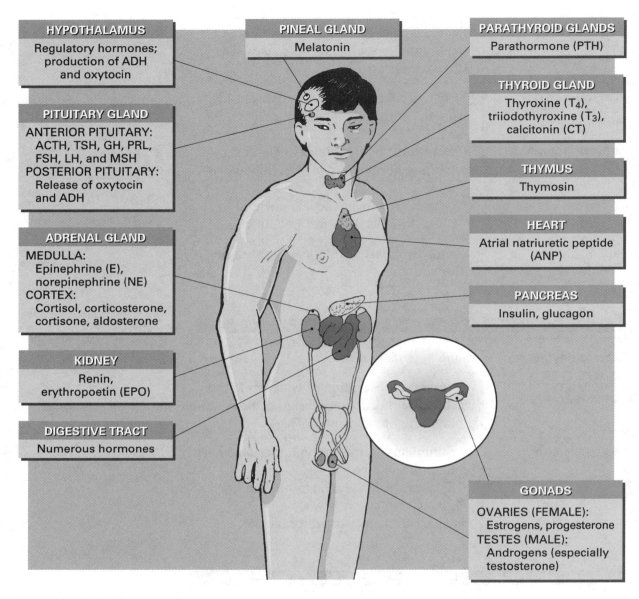

HYPOTHALAMUS
Regulatory hormones; production of ADH and oxytocin

PITUITARY GLAND
ANTERIOR PITUITARY: ACTH, TSH, GH, PRL, FSH, LH, and MSH
POSTERIOR PITUITARY: Release of oxytocin and ADH

ADRENAL GLAND
MEDULLA: Epinephrine (E), norepinephrine (NE)
CORTEX: Cortisol, corticosterone, cortisone, aldosterone

KIDNEY
Renin, erythropoetin (EPO)

DIGESTIVE TRACT
Numerous hormones

PINEAL GLAND
Melatonin

PARATHYROID GLANDS
Parathormone (PTH)

THYROID GLAND
Thyroxine (T_4), triiodothyroxine (T_3), calcitonin (CT)

THYMUS
Thymosin

HEART
Atrial natriuretic peptide (ANP)

PANCREAS
Insulin, glucagon

GONADS
OVARIES (FEMALE): Estrogens, progesterone
TESTES (MALE): Androgens (especially testosterone)

FIGURE 2-8 Glands of the Endocrine System

PITUITARY	Master gland that controls other glands, regulates growth and fluid balance; produces ACTH, TSH, GH, PRL, FSH, LH, MSH, oxytocin, and ACH
THYROID	• Controls tissue metabolic rate, regulates calcium levels; produces thyroxine, triodothyronine, and calcitonin • Hypothroidism—low thyroid function • Hyperthyroidism—Graves' disease

PARATHYROID	• Regulates calcium levels; produces parathyroid hormone (PTH) • PTH triggers increased vitamin D_3 (the active form) formation in the kidney necessary for calcium absorption • PTH increases Ca reabsorption from the kidney tubules reducing the calcium lost to the urine • PTH increases osteoclastic activity
ADRENAL	• Adjusts water balance, tissue metabolism, cardiovascular and respiratory activities; releases epinephrine, norepinephrine, cortisol, corticosterone, cortisone, aldosterone, androgens • Adrenal cortex—Outer layer of the adrenal gland and secretes corticosteroids • Cushing's syndrome—individual suffering from cortisol excess • Addison's disease—complete destruction of the adrenal cortex • Adrenal medulla—center of adrenal gland and is sympathomemetic; secretes epinephrine into the bloodstream; hypothalamus stimulates the adrenal medulla during "fight-or-flight" response, exercise, and other short-term stress situations
THYMUS	Controls WBC maturation
KIDNEYS	Controls RBC production; elevates blood pressure; secretes rennin, erythropoietin
PANCREAS	Regulated blood glucose; secretes insulin and glucagons
TESTES	Development of male sexual characteristics; secretes androgen and inhibin
OVARIES	Development of female sexual characteristics; secretes estrogens, progestins, inhibin

CONDITIONS OF ENDOCRINE SYSTEM

ACROMEGALY	Chronic disease of adults resulting in an elongation and enlargement of the bones
ADDISON'S DISEASE	Known as primary adrenal cortical insufficiency—insufficient production of adrenal steroids causes pituitary gland to increase its production of adrenocorticotropic hormones (ACTH) • Clinical manifestations—oral melonotic macules, brown pigmentation of skin
HYPOTHYROIDISM	Decreased output of thyroid hormone *Clinical manifestations:* • Children—thickened lips, enlarged tongue, delayed eruption pattern • Adults—enlarged tongue, reduced salivary flow can occur • Cretinism—during childhood • Myxedema—adults
CRETINISM	Congenital condition in which a lack of thyroid (hypothyroidism) may result in arrested physical and mental development
MYXEDEMA	Condition resulting from a hypofunction of the thyroid gland; symptoms include anemia, enlarged tongue, mental apathy
HYPERTHYROIDISM	• Excessive production of thyroid hormone; also known as Graves' disease • Children—premature exfoliation of deciduous teeth, premature eruption of permanent teeth • Adults—osteoporosis, progressive periodontal disease, burning discomfort of tongue
HYPERPITUITARISM	Excess hormone (growth hormone) production by the pituitary gland, usually caused by benign tumor known as pituitary adenoma; produces gigantism in bones during development, and acromegaly in adult life

CUSHING'S SYNDROME	Hypersecretion of the adrenal cortex; symptoms include weakness, edema, excess hair growth, skin discoloration, and osteoporosis
MYASTHENIA GRAVIS	Condition with great muscular weakness and progressive fatigue ☞ Difficulty in chewing and swallowing
DIABETES INSIPIDUS	Caused by inadequate secretion of a hormone by the posterior lobe of the pituitary gland ☞ Most common in children

Circulatory System

Internal transport of cells and dissolved materials including nutrients, wastes, and gases; maintains balance between intracellular and extracellular fluids

PULMONARY CIRCULATION

Circulates blood through the heart to the lungs and back to the heart

SYSTEMIC CIRCULATION

Carries the blood from the aorta to the smallest blood vessels and back to the heart

HEART Figure 2-9
Pump that circulates the blood throughout the body

PERICARDIUM	Outer layer, composed of a double-walled sac; exposed epithelium and connective tissue
MYOCARDIUM	Muscular wall contains cardiac muscle tissue, connective tissue, nerves, and blood vessels
ENDOCARDIUM	Epithelium that covers the inner surface
RIGHT ATRIUM	Receives blood from systemic circulation

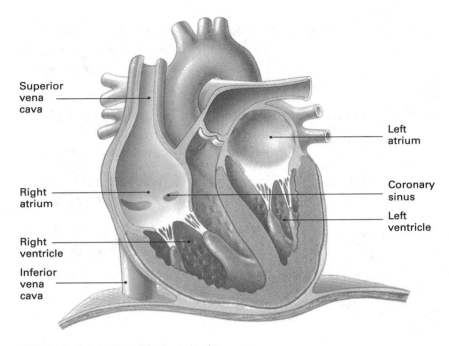

Superior vena cava

Left atrium

Right atrium

Coronary sinus

Left ventricle

Right ventricle

Inferior vena cava

FIGURE 2-9 Interior View of the Heart Chambers

RIGHT VENTRICLE	Discharges blood into the pulmonary circuit
LEFT ATRIUM	Collects blood from the pulmonary circuit
LEFT VENTRICLE	Ejects blood into the systemic circuit
INTERATRIAL SEPTUM	Separates the two atria
INTERVENTRICULAR SEPTUM	Separates the two ventricles
ATRIOVENTRICULAR VALVE	Flap of tissue that ensures a one-way flow of blood from the atria into the ventricles
SUPERIOR VENA CAVA	Large vein that delivers blood from the head, neck, upper limbs, and chest to the right atrium
INFERIOR VENA CAVA	Large vein that carries blood from the lower trunk and limbs to the right atrium
TRICUSPID VALVE	Atrioventricular valve that allows the blood to flow one-way from the right atrium to the right ventricle
BICUSPID VALVE (MITRAL VALVE)	Atrioventricular valve that allows a one-way flow of blood from the left atrium to the left ventricle

PULMONARY VALVE	Blood exits the right ventricle through the pulmonary valve into the pulmonary artery
PULMONARY ARTERY	Carries the blood to the lungs
LUNGS	Blood gets rid of waste products and picks up oxygen
PULMONARY VEIN	Carries blood from lung to the left atrium
AORTIC VALVE	Blood goes through the aortic valve from the left ventricle to the aorta and is distributed to all parts of the body
CARDIAC CYCLE	The period between the start of one heartbeat and the beginning of the next **Figure 2-10**

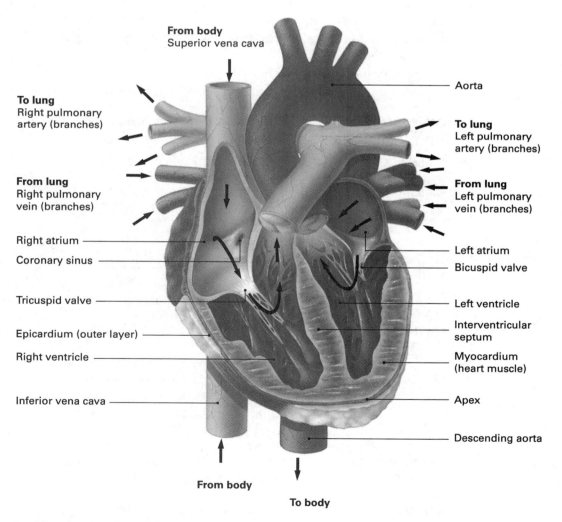

FIGURE 2-10 Cardiac Cycle—Systemic Circulation

SYSTOLE	Contraction; the chamber pushes blood into an adjacent chamber or arterial trunk
DIASTOLE	Relaxation; chamber fills with blood and prepares for the start of the next cycle
BRADYCARDIA	Slower than normal heart rate, less than 60 beats per minute
TACHYCARDIA	Faster than normal heart rate, more than 100 beats per minute
NODAL CELLS	Establish the rate of contractions; sinoatrial (SA) node and atrioventricular (AV) node

BLOOD

Three main functions:
- Transportation of nutrients, gases, waste products, and hormones
- Regulation of amount of body fluid
- Protection against pathogens and blood loss through clotting

COMPONENTS OF BLOOD	Plasma, erythrocytes, leukocytes, platelets
PLASMA	The liquid substance of blood
PLASMA PROTEINS	• Albumin—most abundant proteins responsible for blood osmolarity and viscosity • Fibrinogens (clotting proteins)—prothrombin, fibrinogen, and others • Globulin—found as antibodies, as well as storage and transport proteins
ERYTHROCYTES (RBCs)	Contain hemoglobin, which gives them the ability to carry oxygen
LEUKOCYTES (WBCs)	Defend the body against pathogens and remove toxins, wastes, and abnormal or damaged cells; neutrophils, eosinophils, basophils, monocytes, and lymphocytes
THROMBOCYTES (PLATELETS)	Fragments of cells that are necessary for blood to clot (hemostasis)
ARTERIES	Efferent vessels; carry blood away from the heart to the capillaries of the tissue

VEINS	Afferent vessels; carry blood that has drained from the capillaries back to the heart
CAPILLARIES	Connection between the arteries and veins where the exchange between blood and body cells is made

BLOOD GROUPS, TYPES

Determined by the presence or absence of specific surface antigens; A, AB, B, O, and Rh factor of − or +

Lymphatic System

Figure 2-11

FUNCTIONS OF LYMPHATIC SYSTEM

- Maintain pressure and volume of the extracellular fluid by returning excess water and dissolved substances from the interstitial fluid to the circulation
- Lymph nodes and other lymphoid tissue are the site of clonal production of immunocompetent lymphocytes and macrophages in the specific immune response

OTHER LYMPHOID TISSUE

LYMPH NODES	<ul><li>Small encapsulated organs located along the pathway of lymphatic vessels</li><li>Serve as filters through which lymph percolates on its way to the blood</li></ul>
DIFFUSE LYMPHATIC TISSUE AND LYMPHATIC NODULES	<ul><li>Nonencapsulated lymphatic tissue found in connective tissue beneath the epithelial mucosa</li><li>Intercept foreign antigens and travel to lymph nodes to undergo differentiation and proliferation</li></ul>
THYMUS	Where immature lymphocytes differentiate into T-lymphocytes

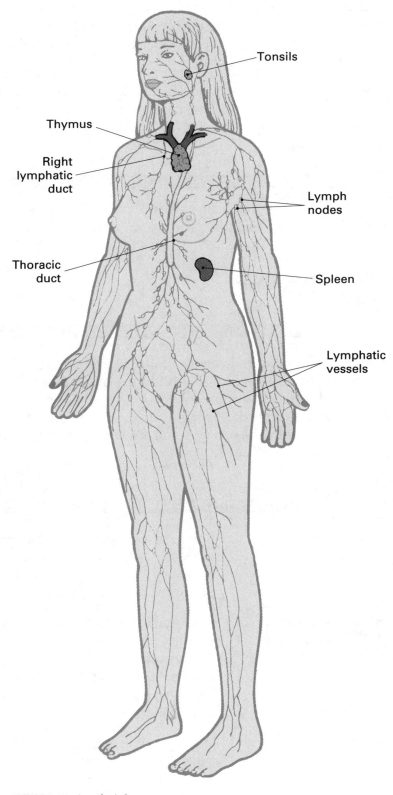

FIGURE 2-11   Lymphatic System

SPLEEN	• Filters the blood and reacts immunologically to blood-borne antigens • Function in both immune and hematopoietic systems • Immune functions include proliferation of lymphocytes, production of antibodies, and removal of antigens from the blood • Hematopoietic functions include formation of blood cells during fetal life; removal and destruction of aged, damaged, and abnormal red cells and platelets; retrieval of iron from hemoglobin degradation; storage of red blood cells

DISEASES OF LYMPHATIC SYSTEM

HODGKIN'S DISEASE	Cancer of the lymphatic cells concentrated in lymph nodes •⇥ Also called Hodgkin's lymphoma
NON-HODGKIN'S LYMPHOMA	Cancer of the lymphatic tissues other than Hodgkin's lymphoma

Digestive System

Processing of food and absorption of nutrients, minerals, vitamins, and water

Figure 2-12

COMPONENTS OF DIGESTIVE SYSTEM

INGESTION	Occurs when food enters the digestive tract through the mouth
MECHANICAL PROCESSING	Physical manipulation of solid foods • Mastication—chewing component of physical digestion • Deglutition—swallowing • Propulsion—movement of materials along the alimentary canal

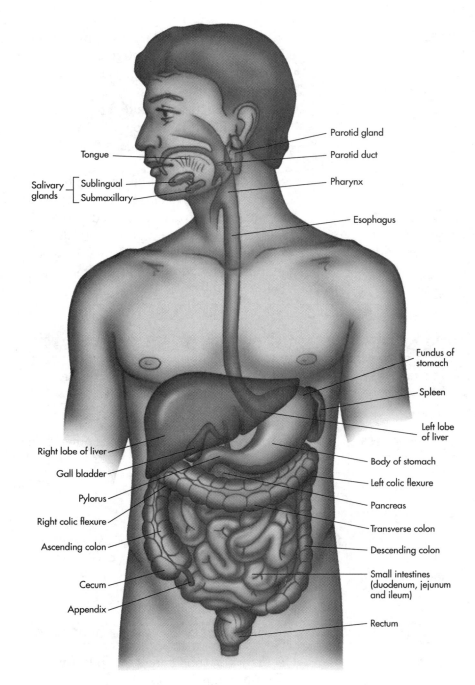

FIGURE 2-12 Digestive System

DIGESTION	Chemical breakdown of food into small fragments that can be absorbed called enzymatic hydrolysis
SECRETION	Aids digestion through the release of water, acids, enzymes, and buffers by the digestive tract and accessory organs

ABSORPTION	Movement of small molecules, electrolytes, vitamins, and water into the digestive tract
EXCRETION	Removal of waste products from the body

LAYERS OF THE DIGESTIVE TRACT

- Mucosal
- Submucosa
- Muscularis externa serosa

PERISTALSIS	Muscularis externa propels materials from one part of the digestive tract to another
SEGMENTATION	Movements that churn and fragment digestive materials in the small intestine

MAJOR COMPONENTS OF THE DIGESTIVE TRACT

Tract travels from oral cavity, pharynx, esophagus, stomach, small intestine, large intestine, rectum, and anus

ORAL CAVITY	• Analyzes material before swallowing • Mechanically processes material through the actions of the teeth, tongue, and palate • Lubricates material with mucus and salivary secretions • Salivary enzymes begin digestion **Figure 2-13**
PHARYNX	Serves as a common passageway for foods, liquids, and air ⚷ Participates in digestive and respiratory systems
ESOPHAGUS	Muscular tube that begins at pharynx and ends in the stomach
STOMACH	• Temporary storage of ingested food • Mechanical breakdown of resistant materials • Acids and enzymes break down chemical bonds • Production of intrinsic factor; necessary for vitamin B_{12} absorption ⚷ Digestion on proteins and carbohydrates

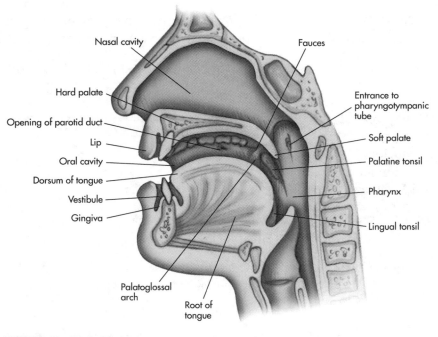

FIGURE 2-13 The Oral Cavity

SMALL INTESTINE	Three parts: the duodenum, jejunum (where the bulk of digestion and absorption occurs), and ileum
LARGE INTESTINE	Reabsorption of water and compaction of feces, absorption of vitamins, and storage of fecal material

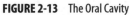

ACCESSORY ORGANS

LIVER	Performs metabolic and hematological regulation and produces bile which breaks down fats 🔑 Largest organ (excluding skin); has over 200 known functions
PANCREAS	• Secretes insulin and glucagons into the blood • Secretes water, ions, and digestive enzymes into the small intestine
GALLBLADDER	Stores and concentrates bile for release into the small intestine

Respiratory System

- Moves air to and from the gas exchange surfaces where diffusion occurs between air and circulation blood
- Provides nonspecific defenses against pathogens
  - Permits vocal communication
  - Controls pH of body fluids
- Includes the nose, nasal cavity, sinuses, pharynx, larynx, trachea, and lungs

COMPONENTS OF RESPIRATORY SYSTEM Figure 2-14

RESPIRATORY TRACT	Conduction passageway that carries air to and from the alveoli
NOSE	Air enters respiratory tract; hairs and mucus aid in defense
PHARYNX	Throat; allows for passage of air into the larynx ☞ Shared by the digestive tract
LARYNX	Surrounds and protects the glottis; as air passes through, it vibrates the true vocal cords, which produce sounds
TRACHEA	Windpipe; C-shaped cartilages protect the airway
BRONCHI	Branches enter the lung and narrow to form bronchioles
BRONCHIOLES	Supplies lobule; delivers air to the respiratory surfaces of the lungs
LUNGS	Bronchi branches into bronchioles, which open into expansive chambers called alveolar ducts that end in alveolar sacs and connects individual alveoli, the exchange surfaces of the lungs ☞ Made up of 5 lobes; the right lung has 3 lobes and the left lung has 2 lobes
RESPIRATORY MEMBRANE	Where gas exchange occurs in the alveoli
PLEURAL CAVITIES	House each lung; lined by a serous membrane

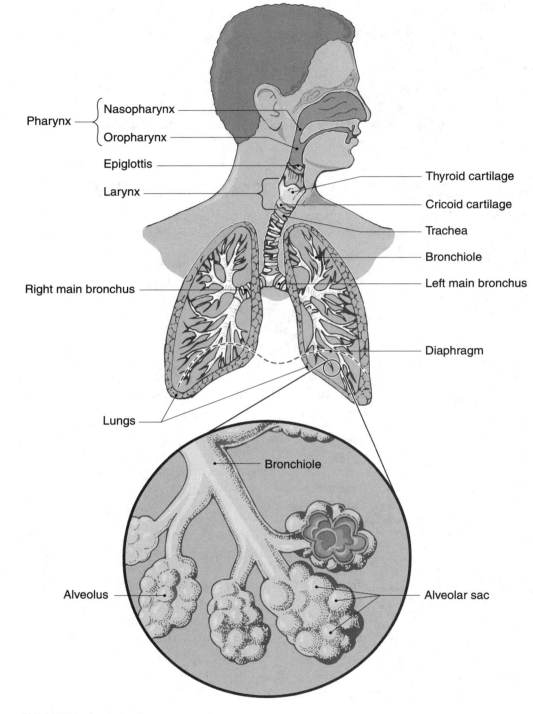

FIGURE 2-14 Respiratory Organs

PULMONARY VENTILATION	Movement of air into and out of lungs; breathing ☛ Before birth, fetal lungs are fluid filled and collapsed; after the first breath, alveoli normally remain inflated for the life of the individual
HYPOXIA	Oxygen content in tissues is decreased
ANOXIA	No oxygen supply to tissue; will result in tissue death
RESPIRATORY CYCLE	Single breath; consisting of inhalation (inspiration) and exhalation (expiration)
ALVEOLAR VENTILATION	Amount of air reaching the alveoli each minute
RESPIRATION CENTERS OF THE BRAIN	Nuclei in the pons and medulla oblongata

DISEASES OF THE RESPIRATORY SYSTEM

EMPHYSEMA	Pulmonary condition that occurs as a result of long-term heavy smoking
PLEURISY	Inflammation of the pleura
PNEUMONIA	Inflammatory condition of the lung resulting from a bacterial and viral infection
TUBERCULOSIS	Infectious disease caused by tubercle bacillus, *Mycobacterium turberculosis*

Urinary System

- Regulation of blood volume and blood pressure
- Regulation of the concentration of plasma ions
- Hemostasis of blood pH
- Conservation of valuable nutrients
- Includes the kidneys, mucosal, bladder, and urethra

COMPONENTS OF URINARY SYSTEM   Figure 2-15

NEPHRON	Basic functional unit of the kidney; responsible for production of filtrate, reabsorption of nutrients, water, and ions

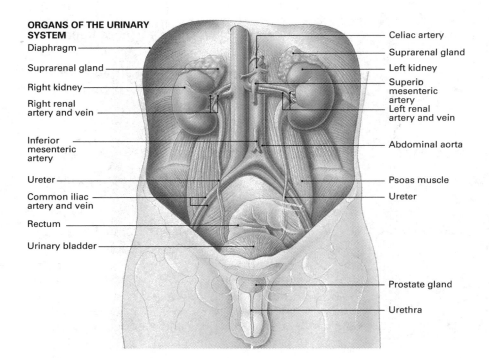

ORGANS OF THE URINARY SYSTEM

Diaphragm

Suprarenal gland

Right kidney

Right renal artery and vein

Inferior mesenteric artery

Ureter

Common iliac artery and vein

Rectum

Urinary bladder

Celiac artery

Suprarenal gland

Left kidney

Superior mesenteric artery

Left renal artery and vein

Abdominal aorta

Psoas muscle

Ureter

Prostate gland

Urethra

FIGURE 2-15 The Urinary System

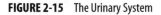

AFFERENT ARTERIOLE	Delivers blood to the renal tubule
EFFERENT ARTERIOLE	Blood departs from the renal tubule
PROXIMAL CONVOLUTED TUBULE	Actively resorbs nutrients, plasma proteins, and electrolytes from the filtrate
LOOP OF HENLE	Ascending and descending limbs
URINATION	Excretion and elimination of dissolved solutes 🔑 Examples of waste products are urea, creatinine, and uric acid
URINE FORMATION	Involves filtration, reabsorption, and secretion
GLOMERULAR FILTRATION RATE (GFR)	Amount of filtrate produced in the kidneys each minute
HORMONES THAT REGULATE KIDNEY FUNCTION	Angiotenison II, aldosterone, ADH, and ANP
URETERS	Move urine from the renal pelvis to the bladder

URINARY BLADDER	Distensible sac for urine storage; the detrusor muscle compresses the bladder to expel urine into the urethra
FLUID BALANCE	Maintained through intracellular and extracellular fluid balance
FLUID SHIFT	Water movement between the intracellular and extracellular fluids
ELECTROLYTE BALANCE	Total electrolyte concentrations can affect a variety of cell functions ☞ Imbalance usually results from sodium gains and losses; potassium balance problems are less common but more dangerous
ACID-BASE BALANCE	Normal pH is between 7.35 and 7.45
ACIDOSIS	pH falls below 7.35
ALKALOSIS	pH exceeds 7.45
PROTEIN BUFFER SYSTEM	Blood plasma proteins and hemoglobin in red blood cells help prevent drastic changes in pH
CARBONIC ACID-BICARBONATE BUFFER SYSTEM	Prevents pH changes due to organic acids in the extracellular fluids
PHOSPHATE BUFFER SYSTEM	Prevents changes in the intracellular fluids
RENAL COMPENSATION	Kidneys vary their rates of hydrogen ion secretion and bicarbonate ion resorption depending on the pH of extracellular fluids

DISORDERS OF THE URINARY TRACT

PYELONEPHRITIS	Inflammation of the renal pelvis and the kidney
GLOMERULONEPHRITIS	Inflammation of the kidney
URINARY RETENTION	An inability to fully empty the bladder ☞ Blockage in the urethra

Reproductive System

Produces, stores, nourishes, and transports gametes

REPRODUCTIVE SYSTEM	
FERTILIZATION	Fusion of sperm from the father and an ovum from the mother to create a zygote
ZYGOTE	Fetus
GAMETES	Reproductive cells

MALE REPRODUCTIVE SYSTEM Testes produce sperm cells; spermatozoa travel along epididymis, ductus deferens, the ejaculatory duct, and urethra before leaving the body	
SEMINAL VESICLE	Secretory gland
PROSTRATE GLAND	Secretory gland
SEMEN	Ejaculate that contains sperm
EJACULATION	Release of semen
ERECTION	Dilation of erectile tissue in the penis
HORMONES	Follicle stimulation hormone, luteinizing hormone, and gonadotropin-releasing hormone

FEMALE REPRODUCTIVE SYSTEM Ovaries produce ovum monthly as part of the ovarian cycle; an oocyte is released during ovulation	
FERTILIZATION	Occurs 12–24 hours after its passage into the uterine cavity if it encounters a spermatozoa
UTERUS	Provides mechanical protection and nutritional support to a developing embryo
UTERINE CYCLE	Typical 28-day cycle; menstruation cycle
MENSTRUATION	1–7 days; menses and the destruction of the functional zone of endometrium

PROLIFERATIVE PHASE	Functional zone undergoes repair and thickens
SECRETORY PHASE	Endometrial glands are active and the uterus is prepared for the arrival of an embryo
MENARCHE	Menstrual activity begins
MENOPAUSE	Menstrual activity ends
MAMMARY GLANDS	Produce milk for infant consumption
HORMONES	Estradiol, estrogen, LH, GnRH, FSH, progesterone

CHAPTER

3 Biochemistry and Nutrition

Catherine Bosiljevac Sovereign, MS, RDH, RD

➤ NUTRITION

Nutrients

DEFINITIONS	
NUTRIENT	Biochemical substance used by the body for growth, maintenance, and repair
ESSENTIAL NUTRIENT	Substance that the body cannot make or cannot make in sufficient quantities and must be obtained from an outside source
CLASSES OF NUTRIENTS	Carbohydrates, lipids, proteins, vitamins, water, and minerals

CALORIE	
KILOCALORIE (KCAL)	• The measure of energy in food used by the body to work and generate heat ☛ Kilocalorie is the actual unit of measure • Common practice is to use the lowercase term "calorie" to mean the same thing ☛ There is no empty-calorie food since the term "calorie" means a measure of food

NUTRIENT DENSITY

Nutrients a food provides relative to the calories it provides
•━ Many snack foods and desserts are low in nutrient density

CLASSIFICATION OF NUTRIENTS

ORGANIC	Have carbon–carbon or carbon–hydrogen bonds; carbohydrate, lipid, protein, vitamins
INORGANIC	Do not have carbon bonds: minerals, water
ENERGY-YIELDING	Contain calories: carbohydrate, lipid, protein

CURRENT NUTRIENT AND ENERGY STANDARDS

DRI	• Dietary reference intakes, as of 2000 • Revised and expanded RDA information includes Estimated Average Requirements (EAR), tolerable upper intake levels (UL), and adequate intakes (AI) guidelines
RDA	• Recommended Dietary Allowances, revised 1989 • Designed to cover the needs of virtually all healthy people • Used to evaluate the diets of populations • Not intended as requirements for individuals • Averaged over several days of food intake •━ Set high, not an average except for energy (calories) •━ Grouped according to age ranges **Figure 3-1**
EAR	• Estimated Average Requirement • Used to set the RDA • Nutrient intake level estimated to meet 50% of people

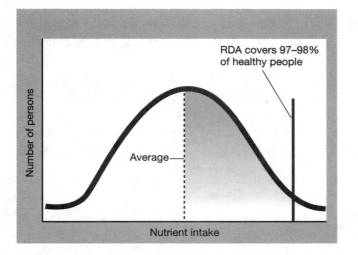

FIGURE 3-1 Recommended Dietary Allowance

AI	• Used if not enough data is available to set EAR • Used for infants and for other age groups for calcium, vitamin D, fluoride, panthothenic acid, biotin, and choline
DV	Daily values Reference values developed specifically for use on food labels ⚬ Compared to a 2,000-calorie diet

Dietary Guidelines for Americans

DIETARY GUIDELINES	
AIM FOR FITNESS	• Aim for a healthy weight • Be physically active every day ⚬ For healthy children over 2 years of age and adults of any age
BUILD A HEALTHY BASE	• Choose according to the Food Guide Pyramid • Choose a variety of grains, especially whole grains • Choose a variety of fruits and vegetables • Keep foods safe to eat

CHOOSE SENSIBLY	• Choose a diet low in saturated fat and cholesterol with total fat in moderate amounts • Choose foods and beverages with moderate amounts of natural and added sugars • Choose and prepare foods with less salt • If you drink alcoholic beverages, do so in moderation

Diet-Planning Guides

FOOD GUIDE PYRAMID Figure 3-2 Foods that provide similar kinds of nutrients are grouped together	
BREAD, CEREAL, RICE, & PASTA GROUP	6–11 servings
VEGETABLE GROUP	3–5 servings
FRUIT GROUP	2–4 servings
MILK, YOGURT & CHEESE GROUP	2–3 servings
MEAT, POULTRY, FISH, BEANS, EGGS & NUTS GROUP	2–3 servings
FATS, OILS & SWEETS GROUP	Sparingly (this is the tip of the pyramid)

EXCHANGE LISTS Originally designed for use by people with diabetes Foods are grouped by their proportion of carbohydrate, fat, and protein	
CARBOHYDRATE GROUP	• Starch—includes starchy vegetables • Fruit • Milk—nonfat, lowfat, and whole • Other carbohydrates—desserts and snacks with added sugars and fats • Vegetables ⚬╾ Portion sizes vary to equal 15 grams of carbohydrate per serving; grams of fat varies ⚬╾ Milk also contains protein

Food Guide Pyramid
A Guide to Daily Food Choices

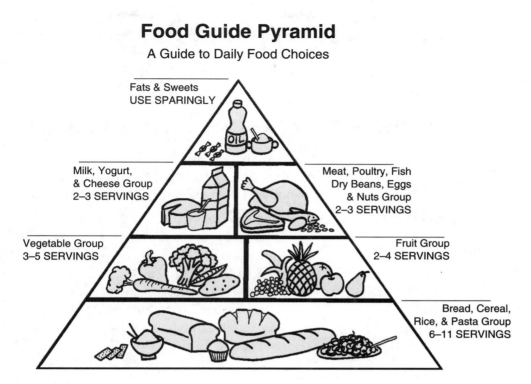

Fats & Sweets
USE SPARINGLY

Milk, Yogurt,
& Cheese Group
2–3 SERVINGS

Meat, Poultry, Fish
Dry Beans, Eggs
& Nuts Group
2–3 SERVINGS

Vegetable Group
3–5 SERVINGS

Fruit Group
2–4 SERVINGS

Bread, Cereal,
Rice, & Pasta Group
6–11 SERVINGS

FIGURE 3-2

MEAT AND MEAT SUBSTITUTE GROUP	Meat, poultry, fish, legumes, peanut butter, eggs, cheeses; very lean, lean, medium-fat, high-fat ☛ Portion sizes vary to equal 7 grams of protein per serving
FAT GROUP	☛ Provides 5 grams of fat per serving

Carbohydrates (CHO)

BIOCHEMISTRY	• Compounds composed of carbon, hydrogen, and oxygen (CHO) • Usually found in a ratio of 1:2:1, respectively • Atoms are arranged to form monosaccharides, which are the basic units of sugars and starch
AVAILABLE CHO	Sugars and starches that can be digested by the enzymes in the human digestive system ☛ Provide 4 calories per gram

UNAVAILABLE CHO	Fiber in foods that the human body cannot digest ☞ Does not provide calories

FUNCTIONS OF CHO

PRIMARY	Available carbohydrates serve as the primary energy for all of the cells in the body by being converted to glucose
SECONDARY	• Spare protein from being used for energy and glucose production • Fiber benefits the body by providing bulk in the intestines • Helps the elimination and prevention of some dietary lipids from being absorbed • In excess, can be made into triglycerides and stored as fat

SIMPLE CHO (SUGARS)
Monosaccharides and disaccharides

HEALTH EFFECTS	• Do not cause diabetes or hyperactivity but may need to be restricted in the control of these conditions; if eaten in excess, sugar may contribute to obesity and heart disease because of its conversion to lipids in the body and the fact that foods with added sugar are often high in fat • Nutrient deficiencies may occur if the diet is high in sugars because more nutritious foods are not consumed • Dental caries is the only disease that is confirmed to be associated with sugar consumption; starchy foods can also contribute to decay because they are often more retentive than sugars ☞ Humans are born with the preference for sweets and human breast milk tastes sweet to infants

> ☞ Sugar, primarily sucrose, is only one of the factors involved in the formation of caries

MONOSACCHARIDES

CHEMICAL STRUCTURE	Consists as a single ring that is one sugar in size; three are important in human nutrition; all contain six carbon atoms (hexoses); structure varies ☞ Saccharide = sugar ☞ Mono = one ☞ -ose = sugar
GLUCOSE	• Type of sugar used in the body; blood sugar or dextrose; not usually consumed in the diet directly; half of each disaccharide and the product of starch digestion • The liver converts all other sugars to glucose ☞ Does not taste very sweet ☞ Normal fasting blood glucose levels are 80–120 mg/dL **Figure 3-3**
GALACTOSE	Part of the lactose molecule; not usually found free in food ☞ Does not taste sweet

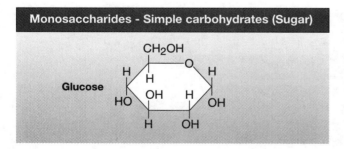

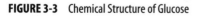

FIGURE 3-3 Chemical Structure of Glucose

FRUCTOSE	• Called fruit sugar or levulose • ⚷ Tastes very sweet • Sweetest of the sugars; found naturally in fruits and honey • ⚷ May be of some benefit for persons with hypoglycemia and diabetes • Used to make high-fructose corn syrup (HFCS) • ⚷ Because fructose, like other sugars, is converted to glucose in the liver, there is a delay in the rise of blood glucose when this sugar is eaten by people with true hypoglycemia and diabetes

DISACCHARIDES

CHEMICAL STRUCTURE	• Two monosaccharides joined together by a bond • Three are important in human nutrition: sucrose, lactose, and maltose • ⚷ Di = two **Figure 3-4**

CONDENSATION

• Chemical reaction that joins two molecules together; a molecule of water is formed as a result of this reaction
• This reaction is also used to make lipids and proteins
• ⚷ Also called dehydration synthesis

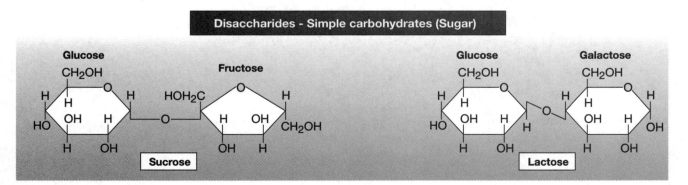

FIGURE 3-4 Chemical Structure of Sucrose and Lactose

SUCROSE	• Consists of one glucose molecule and one fructose molecule; table sugar or granulated sugar; made from sugarcane or sugar beets • The main type of sugar in honey, maple sugar, turbinado sugar, light and dark brown sugar, confectioners' sugar, and raw sugar ☛ These other sugars are not more nutritious than white sugar and could contain microorganisms ☛ Fructose is responsible for the very sweet taste
LACTOSE	Consists of one glucose molecule and one galactose molecule; milk sugar; primary carbohydrate for infants consuming breast milk and milk-based formula • Food sources are milk and milk products such as yogurt, cheese, and ice cream
	• Lactose intolerance is the inability to digest all of the lactose because of a decline in the enzyme lactase that often occurs in adulthood; symptoms include bloating, gas, abdominal discomfort, and diarrhea ☛ Lact = milk; ase = enzyme ☛ Intestinal bacteria feed off the undigested lactose, which causes these symptoms ☛ Intolerance is not the same as an allergy ☛ An allergy to milk is a reaction to one or more of the proteins in milk; can be life threatening; foods with casein and/or whey need to be avoided ☛ Because milk and milk products are the primary dietary source of calcium, eliminating these foods from the diet due to lactose intolerance can result in a calcium deficiency; eating foods with a lower lactose content than milk, such as yogurt and cheese, may reduce symptoms

MALTOSE	• Consists of two glucose molecules; malt sugar • Not usually consumed in foods directly • Produced when starch is broken down during digestion and during the fermentation process that yields alcohol

COMPLEX CHO (STARCH)

AVAILABLE CHO	Long chains of glucose molecules; polysaccharides that can be digested by human digestive enzymes ☞ poly = many
CHEMICAL STRUCTURE	• Hundreds or thousands of glucose molecules linked together, with or without branching • The number of glucose and the degree of branching determines the type of starch ☞ Two main groups of starch: plant starch and glycogen

PLANT STARCH

FOOD SOURCES	Grains (wheat, rice, barley, etc.), legumes (cooked dried beans and peas), and tubers (potatoes, yams, etc.) **Figure 3-5**

GLYCOGEN

• The storage form of glucose for humans and animals
☞ Only small amounts in meat
• Made in the liver from glucose after the ingestion of starch and/or sugar that is not immediately needed by the body
• Stored in the liver and muscle cells for use when glucose is needed by the brain or other cells in the body
☞ For physical activity or to raise blood glucose levels
• Highly branched for the quick release of glucose
Figure 3-6

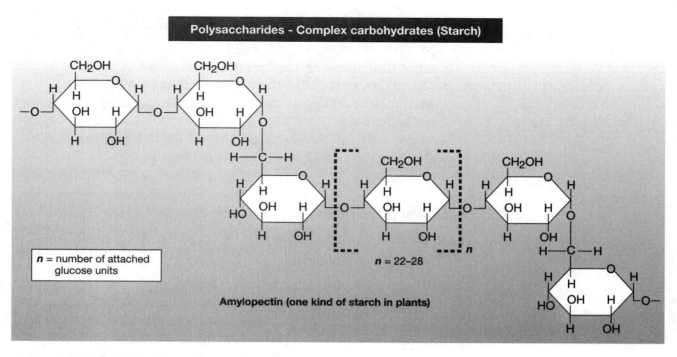

FIGURE 3-5 Chemical Structure of Plant Starch

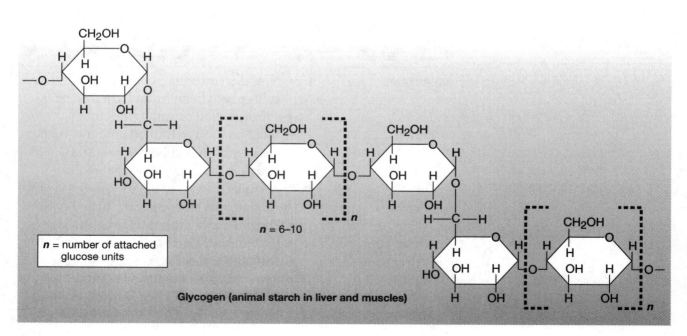

FIGURE 3-6 Chemical Structure of Glycogen

RECOMMENDED INTAKE OF CARBOHYDRATES

- 55–60% of total calories per day
- Only 10% recommended from sugars
- 45–50% recommended from complex CHO/starch
- Minimum of 100 grams of CHO to provide adequate glucose for the body
- ☞ Food Guide Pyramid groups that provide CHO are the grain/cereal group, the vegetable group, and the fruit group

Sugar Alternatives

Natural and artificial substances that taste sweet but are chemically different from mono- and disaccharides

NATURAL

SUGAR ALCOHOLS	• Sorbitol, mannitol, and xylitol • Occur naturally in foods; provide 4 calories per gram • Noncariogenic: not fermented by oral bacteria • Have a laxative effect on the intestines even if eaten in small amounts causing gas, bloating, and diarrhea • ☞ Limit their use • Used in sugar-free gums and candies

ARTIFICIAL; FDA-APPROVED

ASPARTAME	• NutraSweet/Equal; contains the amino acids phenylalanine and aspartic acid • ☞ A dipeptide or small protein • Must be used in limited amounts by persons with PKU (phenylketonuria), which is the inability to metabolize phenylalanine • ☞ Usually diagnosed at birth • Digested as a protein • Provides 4 calories per gram • 180–200 times sweeter than sucrose • ☞ Only small amounts needed • Does not promote decay or raise blood glucose levels

	• Not stable at high temperatures; use limited to foods not heated such as gum, candies, sodas, puddings, yogurt, and frozen desserts; can be added to foods and beverages once they have been heated • Considered safe and not associated with serious adverse health effects 🔑 Not recommended for pregnant women, infants, or children
ACESUFAME K	• Sunette/Sweet One; a derivative of ace-toacetic acid; also contains potassium (K) • Not digested; no calories • 200 times sweeter than sucrose 🔑 Only small amounts needed • Does not promote decay or raise blood glucose levels • Heat stable; uses include gum, nondairy creamers, sodas, puddings, gelatin desserts, dry mixes, and baked goods • Some aftertaste when used alone; improved taste when blended with other artificial sweeteners
SACCHARIN	• Sweet'N Low • Not digested; no calories • 300–400 times sweeter than sucrose • Does not promote decay or raise blood glucose levels • Only small amounts needed • Research now demonstrates it is unlikely to cause cancer in human

Fiber

UNAVAILABLE CHO

• Polysaccharides that cannot be digested by human digestive enzymes
• Includes cellulose, hemicelluloses, pectins, gums, mucilages, and nonpolysaccharides such as lignins
• Intestinal bacteria can digest some fibers and ferment them to form short-chain fatty acids that are absorbed by intestinal cells
🔑 Nonstarch polysaccharides
🔑 Noncariogenic; not used by oral bacteria

RECOMMENDED INTAKE	
ADULTS	20–35 grams of fiber per day ⚷ Includes both types of fiber
CHILDREN	Age of the child plus 5 grams per day is recommended by the American Health Foundation for children over the age of 2 years ⚷ Example: A 7-year-old child needs 7 + 5 or 12 grams per day

EXCESSIVE INTAKE OF FIBER More than 40 grams per day for adults	
EFFECTS OF EXCESS	• Fiber binds up minerals; intake above the recommended amount can negatively affect mineral status • A sudden intake of a lot of fiber, even to the recommended levels, can cause diarrhea or constipation and may even cause an obstruction of the GI tract • May displace energy-dense and nutrient-dense foods ⚷ Requires an increase in fluid intake

WATER-SOLUBLE FIBER Forms a gel in water; used to make jams and jellies	
FUNCTIONS	• Slows down the transit time of the GI tract; provides satiety ⚷ Delays hunger • Delays the absorption of glucose which can help keep blood glucose levels from rising rapidly ⚷ Helpful in glucose control for people with diabetes • Lowers blood cholesterol by binding up some dietary lipids so that they are not absorbed in the small intestine and prevents bile from being reabsorbed in the large intestine; the liver takes cholesterol from the blood to make more bile ⚷ May reduce the risk of heart disease

FOOD SOURCES	Fruits (apple, citrus), oats, oat bran, barley, and legumes

WATER-INSOLUBLE FIBER
Does not dissolve in water but attracts and holds water

FUNCTIONS	• Provides bulk and promotes regularity; helps prevent and treat constipation, hemorrhoids, and diverticulosis • Speeds up the transit time of the GI tract • Increases the muscle tone of the intestines • May protect against colon cancer
FOOD SOURCES	Vegetables, wheat and rice bran, fruits, nuts, whole grains

Lipids

BIOCHEMISTRY

- Lipids contain the same three elements as carbohydrates: carbon (C), hydrogen (H), and oxygen (O), but they contain less oxygen in proportion to hydrogen and carbon
- Includes fats, oils, phospholipids, and sterol

FUNCTIONS IN FOOD

- Provide 9 calories per gram
- Carry many of the compounds that give foods their aroma and flavor
- Provide satiety by slowing the rate of gastric emptying
- Carry the fat-soluble vitamins A, D, E, K

FUNCTIONS IN THE BODY

- The body's chief form of stored energy; energy reserves
- The major component of cell membranes
- Insulate the body from extremes of temperature
- Cushion and protect internal organs
- Fuel cellular activities
- Spare protein from being used for energy
- Where some of the fat-soluble vitamins are stored

FATS

- Lipids that are usually solid at room temperature
- Composed mostly of triglycerides
- Includes butter, margarine, shortening, animal fat, eggs

OILS

- Lipids that are liquid at room temperature and composed of triglycerides
- Includes vegetable and nut oils

TRIGLYCERIDES
The chemical form of fats and oils in the diet and the fat stored in the body

CHEMICAL STRUCTURE	
	• Three fatty acid molecules attached to one molecule of glycerol as a result of the condensation reaction
	☛ Tri = three
	• Glycerol is a three-carbon molecule and one fatty acid is attached to each of the three C atoms
	• Fatty acids are chains of C atoms with attached H atoms
	• The number of C atoms are even numbers, 4–24 in length; fatty acids in commonly eaten foods have 18–22 C atoms
	• The fatty acids may be saturated or unsaturated

RECOMMENDED INTAKE OF TOTAL FATS

Total fat intake should be 30% or less of total calories per day

SATURATED FATTY ACIDS

Fatty acids that contain the maximum number of H atoms and have no double bonds.
- ☛ "Saturated" with H atoms
- ☛ An example of a saturated fatty acid is stearic acid

SATURATED FATS
Triglycerides composed mostly of fatty acids that are saturated; usually solid at room temperature

RECOMMENDED INTAKE OF SATURATED FATS	• 10% or less of total calories per day
FOOD SOURCES	• Includes animal fats, butter, egg yolks, cocoa butter, whole milk, cheese, chocolate, stick margarine, hydrogenated and tropical oils • Tropical oils are very saturated but are liquid at room temperature because of their short carbon chains ☛ Tropical oils include coconut, palm, and palm kernel oils
HEALTH EFFECTS	Saturated fats raise total cholesterol levels and raise low-density lipoprotein (LDL) or "bad cholesterol" levels

POINTS OF UNSATURATION

• At the double bond where H atoms can easily be added
• Important in converting liquid oils to solid fats
☛ See Hydrogenation

UNSATURATED FATS

• Triglycerides composed mostly of unsaturated fatty acids
• Include monounsaturated and polyunsaturated fats/oils
• Fatty acids that do not contain the maximum number of H atoms
☛ Not "saturated" with H atoms
• Where H are missing, the C atoms form double bonds with one another
• Have one or more double bonds, monounsaturated and polyunsaturated fatty acids, respectively
☛ MUFA = monounsaturated fatty acids; an example is oleic acid
☛ PUFA = polyunsaturated fatty acids; an example is linoleic acid

MONOUNSATURATED FATS
Triglycerides composed mostly of fatty acids that have one double bond

MUFA	10% or less of total calories per day

FOOD SOURCES	Includes olives, olive oil, canola oil, peanuts, peanut oil, peanut butter, cashews, and avocados
HEALTH EFFECTS	Monounsaturated fats may lower total cholesterol levels and raise HDL or "good cholesterol" levels

POLYUNSATURATED FATS

PUFA	• 10% or less of total calories per day • Triglycerides composed of mostly fatty acids with two or more double bonds
FOOD SOURCES	Includes corn, soybean, cottonseed, safflower, sesame, and sunflower oils, almonds, filberts, pecans, walnuts, liquid margarine, and fish
HEALTH EFFECTS	Polyunsaturated fats lower total cholesterol levels and they may also lower both LDL and HDL cholesterol levels

OMEGA-3 FATTY ACIDS

• Omega-3 fatty acids are another class of polyunsaturated fatty acids that have been shown to be beneficial to health
• They have many double bonds but the location of the first double bond is located three carbon atoms from the omega end of the fatty acid, called the omega-3 carbon
⊶ Also called n-3 fatty acids
⊶ Include eicosapentaenoic acid (EPA) and docosahexaenoic acid (DHA)

FOOD SOURCES	Ocean fish, shellfish, canola oil, soybeans/tofu, walnuts, wheat germ, and some vegetables
HEALTH EFFECTS	• Omega-3 fatty acids may lower total cholesterol and LDL cholesterol levels and raise HDL cholesterol levels • Other potential health benefits from omega-3 fatty acids include the prevention of blood clots, lowered blood pressure, and reduced inflammation

- Negative effects include bruising, increased bleeding time, and increased risk of stroke if consumed in high amounts
- 🔑 There is no recommended level of intake, however, one to two meals including fish per week may be beneficial

ESSENTIAL FATTY ACIDS (EFA)
The body can make all of the necessary fatty acids except two: linoleic acid and linolenic acid; these two fatty acids must be supplied by the diet and are therefore considered essential

FOOD SOURCES	• Both of the essential fatty acids are polyunsaturated and are found in a wide variety of foods, especially plant and fish oils; they can be stored in the body • Deficiency symptoms include a skin rash, reproductive failure, growth retardation, kidney and liver disorders, and subtle visual and neurological disturbances
RECOMMENDED INTAKE EFA	Together, linoleic acid and linolenic acid are recommended to make up at least 3% of total calories per day, equal to approximately 1 tablespoon of oil high in PUFA for adults

OXIDATION OF FATTY ACIDS

- MUFA and PUFA have double bonds where H atoms are not attached called points of unsaturation; oxygen atoms can attach at the points of unsaturation resulting in the oxidation of the fatty acid
- Oxidation causes the oils to smell and taste rancid, which shortens the shelf life of oils and foods made with oils
- Saturated fatty acids are more resistant to oxidation and therefore less likely to become rancid

HYDROGENATION

- A chemical process using metal catalysts to add H atoms to PUFA to reduce the number of double bonds
- This process makes PUFA more resistant to oxidation; hydrogenation also makes the oil more saturated and solid at room temperature, which makes the fat more spreadable
- Hydrogenated oils also have the negative health effects associated with saturated fats

FOOD SOURCES	Include shortening, stick and soft margarine, baked goods, and commercial frying fats

CIS AND TRANS FORMATION OF FATTY ACIDS

- The way in which the H atoms are attached at the points of unsaturation (double bonds) determines whether a fatty acid is a cis-fatty acid or a trans-fatty acid
- If the H atoms are attached on the same side of the points of unsaturation, the arrangement is called cis
- If the H atoms are attached on opposite sides of the points of unsaturation, the arrangement is called trans

TRANS-FATTY ACIDS

- Small amounts of trans-fatty acids occur naturally in food
- Trans-fatty acids occur whenever oils are hydrogenated, especially when oils are only partially hydrogenated
- Partially hydrogenated oils are the predominant type of fats used in processed and fried foods

FOOD SOURCES	Hard and soft margarine, cakes, cookies, doughnuts, crackers, meat and dairy products, snack chips, peanut butter, shortening and other fats used for frying

PHOSPHOLIPIDS

CHEMICAL STRUCTURE	Compounds similar to triglycerides but contain only two fatty acids attached to one glycerol molecule; the third fatty acid is replaced by a phosphate group and some other molecule

LECITHIN
Lecithin is the most common type of phospholipid; it contains a molecule of choline in place of the third fatty acid

FUNCTIONS OF PHOSPHOLIPIDS	• Soluble in both fat and water, serving as important constituents of cell membranes, moving back and forth across the lipid-containing membranes of cells into the watery fluids on both sides • Allow fat-soluble substances such as vitamins and hormones to pass in and out of cells • Act as emulsifiers in the body and in foods, keeping fats dispersed in watery fluids
FOOD SOURCES	Egg yolk and soybeans ☛ There is no recommended level of intake

STEROLS

CHEMICAL STRUCTURE	• C, H, and O molecules arranged in a multiring structure • Sterols include bile acids, sex hormones, adrenal hormones, vitamin D, and cholesterol
CHOLESTEROL	• A fat-like waxy substance that is made in the body by the liver and obtained from foods of animal origin • The majority of cholesterol is made by the body from fragments of carbohydrate, lipid, and protein; only a small percent is obtained from the diet
FUNCTIONS OF CHOLESTEROL IN THE BODY	The major function is to form bile acid which is needed to digest lipids; cholesterol is also a structural component of cell membranes, myelin, steroid hormones, and vitamin D
RECOMMENDED INTAKE OF CHOLESTEROL	300 mg or less per day ☛ This is not the same as blood cholesterol levels

FOOD SOURCES	• Animal tissues: meats, fish, poultry and organ meats • Animal byproducts: egg yolk and dairy products

FAT ALTERNATIVES

CARBOHYDRATE-BASED	• Oatrim and TrimChoice: made from oat flour; provides 1–4 calories per gram • Z-Trim: made from the seed hulls of oats, soybeans, peas, and rice and the bran of corn or wheat; no calories provided
PROTEIN-BASED	Simplesse and K-Blazer: made from egg white or milk proteins; processed by microparticulation to give them the "mouth feel" of fat; provides 1–2 calories per gram
FAT-BASED	• Salatrim (Benefat): made from triglycerides with short- and long-chain fatty acids; provides 5 calories per gram • Caprenin: made from triglycerides that contain fatty acids that are not well absorbed; provides 5 calories per gram
ARTIFICIAL	Olestra (Olean): made from sucrose and fatty acids in the chemical form known as a sucrose polyester (having many ester bonds) ☛ Cannot be digested: no calories provided

Proteins

BIOCHEMISTRY

Compounds that contain carbon, hydrogen, oxygen, and nitrogen (N) atoms

AMINO ACIDS

• Molecules made up of a central carbon with an amino group, an acid group, a hydrogen atom, and a distinctive side group (or side chain; also called the R group) attached
• The building blocks of proteins

- The amino group (NH_2) contains the N
- There are 20 different amino acids important in human nutrition; the side group is different on each of the 20 different amino acids, the rest of the molecule is the same
- ☞ amino = contains nitrogen
- ☞ Think of the different 20 amino acids like the letters of the alphabet; each amino acid can be used many times

CHEMICAL STRUCTURE	Proteins are made by joining many amino acids together and in different sequences
PEPTIDE BOND	The bond formed between each adjoining amino acid as an acid result of the condensation reaction ☞ peptide = amino
DIPEPTIDE	When two amino acids are joined together by a peptide bond, the resulting structure is called a dipeptide
TRIPEPTIDE	Three amino acids bonded together
OLIGOPEPTIDE	Four to nine amino acids bonded together
POLYPEPTIDE	• Ten or more amino acids bonded together • Proteins are polypeptides containing up to several hundred amino acids
ESSENTIAL AMINO ACIDS	• Amino acids that cannot be made by the body or that cannot be made in sufficient quantities and therefore must be obtained from foods • There are 9 essential amino acids: histidine, isoleucine, leucine, lysine, methionine, phenylalanine, threonine, tryptophan, and valine
NONESSENTIAL AMINO ACIDS	• Amino acids that the body can make if nitrogen in acids is available to make the amino group; fragments from carbohydrate and triglycerides are used to make the rest of the amino acid molecule • There are 11 nonessential amino acids: alanine, arginine, asparagine, aspartic acid, cysteine, glutamic acid, glutamine, glycine, proline, serine, and tyrosine

PROTEIN SHAPE

- Determined by the types of amino acids used, the number of amino acids, and the sequence of the amino acids
- Polypeptide chains twist into complex shapes to make them stable in the body's watery fluids
- The shape of a protein determines its function

FUNCTIONS OF PROTEIN	<ul><li>Building new tissues during growth, maintenance, and repair from wounds and illness (collagen)</li><li>Fluid and electrolyte balance</li><li>Constituents of antibodies, enzymes, and hormones</li><li>Transportation of compounds through the body and in and out of cells</li><li>DNA and RNA (genetic material)</li><li>Neurotransmitters</li><li>Regulation of pH (acid-base balance)</li><li>Blood clotting (fibrin)</li><li>Vision (opsin)</li><li>Pigments (melanin)</li><li>Providing energy (if necessary): 4 calories per gram</li></ul>

DENATURING OF PROTEINS

- Proteins are denatured or change shape when subjected to heat, acid, base, alcohol, heavy metals, or other agents
- When they are denatured they lose their function
- Denaturing occurs when foods containing protein are cooked and digested; the proteins can no longer perform the functions that they did in the animal or plant that was eaten, but once the individual amino acids are absorbed by the body, new functional proteins are made
- Denature = change shape
- Think of the shape, color, and texture of raw verses cooked egg whites

TRANSAMINATION

Transferring the amino group from one amino group to another amino group so that a new protein can be made

DEAMINATION

- Removal and excretion of the amino group
- Occurs when proteins are used for making compounds other than new proteins; occurs when protein is used to make glucose, triglycerides, and ATP
- Deamination produces ammonia, which is converted to urea by the liver and excreted by the kidneys as urine

GLUCONEOGENESIS

Making glucose from a noncarbohydrate sources; occurs when glucose is made from protein

NITROGEN BALANCE
The amount of nitrogen consumed (N in) compared to the amount of nitrogen excreted (N out)

ZERO N BALANCE OR NITROGEN EQUILIBRIUM	When N in = N out; occurs when adequate protein is consumed by healthy adults
POSITIVE N BALANCE	When N in > N out: protein is used to promote growth; seen in pregnant women, infants, children and adolescents and in persons recovering from illnesses, surgery, burns, trauma, or protein deficiency ⊶ > = greater than
NEGATIVE N BALANCE	When N in < N out: protein is broken down to provide energy (calories) and glucose; seen in persons who are starving or suffering from burns, infections, injuries, or fever ⊶ < = less than

PROTEIN QUALITY
A high-quality protein contains all 9 essential amino acids in sufficient amounts and is easily digested

REFERENCE PROTEIN	• Egg protein is one of the most complete and easily digested proteins for humans, therefore it is used as the standard against which other proteins are compared • Includes the egg yolk and the egg white

COMPLETE PROTEIN	• Protein from foods that contains all of the essential amino acids in the amounts that the body requires; they may also contain some or all of the nonessential amino acids • Includes animal tissues and animal by-products: meat, fish, poultry, eggs, milk, cheese • Gelatin is one animal product that is not a complete protein • A small number of plant proteins are complete, such as soy
INCOMPLETE PROTEIN	• Protein from foods that does not contain all of the essential acid or does not contain them in sufficient quantity • There is one or more limiting amino acid; many grains are low in lysine and isoleucine; legumes are low in methionine and tryptophan
COMPLEMENTARY PROTEINS	• Combining plant foods so that the amino acids low in one will be supplied by the other and visa versa; the protein quality of the combined foods is higher than if either food were eaten alone • The mainstay of a strict vegetarian diet • ☛ Eating grains (rice, corn, wheat) with legumes (beans, peas, peanuts)

RECOMMENDED INTAKE

PROTEIN	• Protein has an RDA, unlike carbohydrates and lipids, which do not have an RDA • The RDA for adults is 0.8 grams of protein per kilogram of appropriate or ideal body weight; a person with excess body fat does not require additional protein • The RDA for pregnant or lactating women, infants, and children is higher • The RDA assumes that people are healthy—eating some complete protein foods and eating sufficient carbohydrates and lipids to provide adequate calories so that protein will not be needed to provide energy
PERCENT OF CALORIES	10–15% of total calories per day

PROTEIN-ENERGY MALNUTRITION (PEM)

- A deficiency of both calories and protein
- Two classic forms are kwashiorkor and marasmus

KWASHIORKOR	• A condition that results from an infection superimposed on malnutrition; now thought to be a form of food poisoning caused by aflatoxin from moldy grain • Develops rapidly; acute PEM • Characterized by onset between ages 1–3 years when the child is weaned from nutrient- and protein-rich breast milk to a protein-poor, starchy cereal • Adequate energy with inadequate high-quality protein • Some weight loss and muscle wasting but some body fat is retained; growth is slowed • Fluid and electrolyte balance are affected resulting in edema of the abdomen and limbs • The liver enlarges with fat • Hair is dry and brittle with a loss of color • Iron is unbound in the body and unavailable for use, which promotes bacterial growth and free-radical damage • The child is apathetic, sad, and irritable with a loss of appetite
MARASMUS	• A condition resulting from severe food deprivation or impaired absorption over a long time period; chronic PEM • Inadequate energy, protein, vitamins, and minerals • Occurs in infancy up to the age of 2 years; severe weight loss and muscle wasting with no fat stores • Severe growth retardation and impaired brain development • No edema or enlarged, fatty liver present • Hair is sparse, dry, and thin; skin is dry and thin • The child is anxious and apathetic but has a good appetite

MARASMUS-KWASIORKOR MIX	• The child with marasmus may later develop kwashiorkor, suggesting that the adaptation to starvation seen in marasmus may fail, resulting in kwashiorkor

EXCESS PROTEIN INTAKE
Often described as protein intake greater than 2 times the RDA; often from protein intake of animal origin
⊶ Includes meat, eggs, and dairy products

HEALTH EFFECTS	• Heart disease can result because foods high in protein are also often high in fat, saturated fat, and cholesterol • High protein diets may result in low intakes of other nutrients from fruits, vegetables, and grains; weight gain may also occur when high-fat, protein-rich foods are eaten often • A diet high in animal proteins has been correlated to an increase risk of some types of cancer • Calcium excretion increases with high protein diet, possibly increasing the risk of developing osteoporosis • A sudden, high intake of protein can result in dehydration because water is needed by the kidneys to dilute urea

Vegetarian Diets

VEGAN

- A dietary pattern that excludes animal tissues (meat, fish, poultry) and animal by-products (eggs, dairy products)
- Includes vegetables, fruits, grains, nuts, and seeds only
- Complementary protein combining is necessary to get adequate amounts of the essential amino acids
- May be low in high-quality protein, vitamin B_{12}, vitamin D, calcium, iron, and zinc
- ⊶ Also called strict vegetarian or pure vegetarian

LACTOVEGETARIAN

- A dietary pattern that excludes animal tissues (meat, fish, poultry) and eggs
- Includes dairy products, vegetables, fruits, grains, nuts, and seeds
- If sufficient amounts of dairy products are consumed, along with complementary protein combinations, calcium, vitamin B_{12}, and high-quality protein intake are usually adequate
- ⚷ Lacto = milk

OVOVEGETARIAN

- A dietary pattern that excludes animal tissues (meat, fish, poultry) and dairy products
- Includes eggs, vegetables, fruits, grains, nuts, and seeds
- If egg yolks are consumed often along with complimentary protein combinations, iron, zinc, high-quality protein, and vitamin B_{12} intake are usually adequate
- ⚷ Ovo = egg
- ⚷ The egg yolk contains iron, zinc, and other nutrients; the egg white contains mainly protein

LACTO-OVO VEGETARIAN

- A dietary pattern that only excludes animal tissues (meat, fish, poultry)
- Includes dairy products and eggs in addition to vegetables, fruits, grains, nuts, and seeds
- Calcium, iron, zinc, and high-quality protein are usually adequate if sufficient amounts of dairy products and egg yolks are consumed

➤ DIGESTION

GASTROINTESTINAL (GI) TRACT

- The GI tract is about 30 feet in length
- Includes the mouth (oral cavity), esophagus, stomach, small intestine, and large intestine (colon)
- Accessory organs involved in digestion are the liver, gallbladder, and pancreas

Figure 3-7

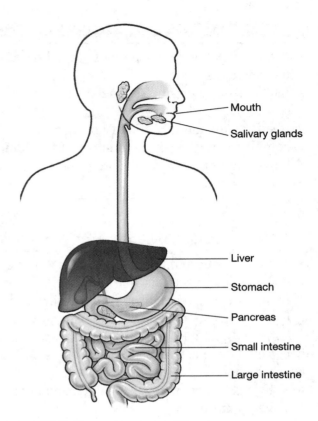

FIGURE 3-7   Human Gastrointestinal Tract

HYDROLYSIS
Chemical reaction that splits molecules apart with the addition of water; occurs during the digestion of carbohydrates, lipids, proteins   ☞ Hydro = water   ☞ Lysis = breaking

MOUTH **Mastication occurs**	
STARCH DIGESTION BEGINS	Salivary amylase breaks starch, which is composed of chains of glucose molecules, into dextrin and maltose

ESOPHAGUS

- Food pipe
- Allows food to pass from the mouth to the stomach
- Goes through the diaphram

STOMACH

- Holding tank
- Muscular, elastic, saclike organ
- Holds each bolus of food swallowed; secretes hydrochloric acid (HCl), some enzymes, and fluids
- Churns, mixes, and grinds food to form chyme
- Stretches to give the message of fullness after eating
- The carbohydrate, lipid, and protein content of the chyme determines the emptying time of the stomach

PROTEIN DIGESTION BEGINS	HCl causes protein strands to uncoil and pepsin breaks the strands into smaller fragments of protein
INTRINSIC FACTOR	The glycoprotein "intrinsic factor" is secreted by the stomach and attaches to vitamin B_{12}, which facilitates the absorption of B_{12} in the small intestine

SMALL INTESTINE

SIZE AND FUNCTION	- The small intestine is about 10 feet in length with an absorptive surface area equal to a quarter of a football field - Where digestion of carbohydrate and protein is completed; where lipids are digested; the principal site of nutrient absorption ☞ "Small" because its diameter is small compared to the large intestine ☞ Villi and microvilli line the small intestine

THREE SEGMENTS	• *Duodenum*—the top portion, about 10 inches long, where sodium bicarbonate and bile are secreted into the small intestine via the common bile duct • *Jejunum*—the first two-fifths of the small intestine beyond the duodenum • *Ileum*—the remaining segment of the small intestine ☞ deuodenum = twelve fingers width ☞ Bile is secreted only if chyme contains lipid

LARGE INTESTINE (COLON)

SIZE AND FUNCTION	• The remaining portion of the GI tract; about 5 feet in length • Water, some minerals, and undigested residues such as fiber pass into the large intestine where most of the water, electrolytes, and bile salts are absorbed ☞ "Large" because of its diameter ☞ Most bile is recirculated in the body
THREE SEGMENTS	• *Ascending colon*—goes up the right side of the abdomen • *Transverse colon*—passes across the front to the left side • *Descending colon*—down the left side of the abdomen and includes the sigmoid colon and rectum where waste products, fiber, bacteria, and any unabsorbed nutrients are stored until they are excreted ☞ Sigmoid = S-shaped

MECHANICAL DIGESTION

MASTICATION	The actions of the teeth, tongue, and muscles of mastication that tear and grind food into small pieces and blend it with saliva ☞ Xerostomia affects taste and the ability to swallow foods easily

SALIVA	Lubricates food to facilitate taste and swallowing
EPIGLOTTIS	Cartilage in the throat that closes off the airway when food or liquids are swallowed
BOLUS	Each portion of food that is swallowed and enters the esophagus
PERISTALSIS	• Involuntary wavelike muscular contractions of the esophagus, stomach, small intestine, colon, and rectum • It involves circular and longitudinal muscles that rhythmically contract and relax, mixing and churning food as it digests
CARDIAC SPHINCTER	The circular muscle at the junction between the esophagus and the stomach that closes after a bolus is swallowed to prevent the reflux of stomach contents ☛ Also called the gastroesophageal sphincter
CHYME	The semiliquid mass of partly digested food, mixed with HCl and expelled from the stomach to the small intestine
PYLORIC SPHINCTER	The circular muscle at the junction between the stomach and small intestine that regulates the flow of chyme into the small intestine ☛ Also called the pylorus
SEGMENTATION	Periodic squeezing by the circular muscles of the intestines that momentarily forces the chyme back a few inches to maximize contact with digestive juices and the absorptive surface of the intestinal walls
IIEOCECAL VALVE	The circular muscle at the junction of the small intestine and the colon ☛ A sphincter muscle
ANUS	The last circular muscle of the GI tract that controls the release of waste products (feces) ☛ A sphincter muscle

CHEMICAL DIGESTION	
SALIVA	Salivary amylase initiates the chemical digestion of starch
HYDROCHLORIC ACID (HCl)	• Gastric glands secrete HCl into the stomach, which causes the pH of the stomach to be very acidic; HCl is needed to prepare minerals to be absorbed in the small intestine • Most enzymes, including salivary amylase, are denatured in the stomach but pepsinogen is activated to pepsin, which initiates the chemical digestion of protein ☞ Gastro = stomach ☞ Mucin protects the stomach mucosa from HCl **Figure 3-8** ☞ No significant chemical digestion of carbohydrate or lipid occurs in the stomach
SODIUM BICARBONATE	Secreted by the pancreas to neutralize the acidic chyme as it enters the small intestine

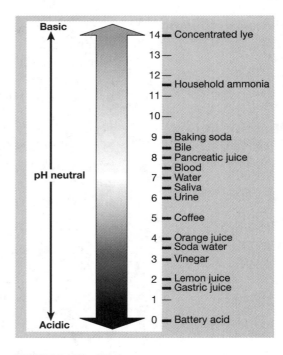

FIGURE 3-8 The pH Scale

BILE	• Made in the liver, stored in the gallbladder and secreted into the small intestine (duodenum) when dietary lipids are mixed in the chyme • Made from the cholesterol that the liver produces • An emulsifier that has both water-soluble and fat-soluble portions; allows lipids to mix with a watery solution where lipases can break them down into smaller particles
PANCREATIC ENZYMES	Secreted into the small intestine to digest carbohydrate (carbohydrases), lipid (lipases), and protein (proteases)

Vitamins

VITAMINS

- Substances that the body cannot make at all or that it cannot make in sufficient quantities to sustain life
- The first vitamins discovered contained nitrogen, however not all vitamins contain nitrogen
- The amounts needed are measured in milligrams (mg) or micrograms (mcg)
- Vitamins do not contain energy/calories but are needed for the body to metabolize carbohydrates, lipids, and proteins, which do contain calories
- ☛ vita = life
- ☛ amine = contains nitrogen
- ☛ 28 grams (g) = about 1 ounce
- ☛ 1 g = 1000 mg; 1 mg = 1000 mcg

WATER-SOLUBLE VITAMINS

- Eight B vitamins and vitamin C
- Absorbed directly into the blood from the small intestines
- Travel freely in the watery fluids of the body
- Not usually stored in large amounts; short-term storage in the body fluid "pool"
- Required in frequent doses every 1 to 3 days
- Excreted by the kidneys in the urine
- Toxicity is uncommon from food intake; may occur from supplement use

B VITAMINS	• Many B vitamins are coenzymes; without them certain enzymes are inactive • Some are needed to release the energy in foods for use by the body; others are needed in cellular metabolism • The B vitamins were originally numbered as they were discovered; later some were not found to be essential so the numbers vary • Some B vitamins have a name and a number and others do not have a number • Deficiencies of single B vitamins rarely occur; if a person shows signs of a deficiency they are often deficient in more than one B vitamin; one exception is vitamin B_{12} • In this text, we will use the most common term followed by any other terms in parentheses ☛ Enzymes = various types of proteins needed to cause chemical reactions to occur or to occur at a faster rate

THIAMIN (B_1)

FUNCTIONS	• Part of the coenzyme thiamin pyrophosphate (TPP) • Used for energy metabolism, appetite regulation, nerve and heart function
DEFICIENCY	Beriberi; symptoms include edema, enlarged heart, abnormal heart rhythms, heart failure, muscle weakness and wasting, loss of appetite, mental confusion, paralysis ☛ loss of appetite = anorexia
TOXICITY	Rare
DRI	1.1–1.2 mg per day; based on caloric intake
FOOD SOURCES	Pork products, liver, whole or enriched grains, legumes, and nuts ☛ Easily destroyed by heat

RIBOFLAVIN (B₂)

FUNCTIONS	• Part of the coenzyme flavin mononucleotide (FMN) and flavin adenine dinucleotide (FAD) • Used for energy metabolism normal vision, skin health the mouth
DEFICIENCY	Ariboflavinosis: cheilosis, glossitis, inflamed eyelids, photophobia, and skin lesions with greasy scales ☛ Cheilosis = cracks at the corners of the mouth ☛ Glossitis = painful, smooth, burning, inflamed tongue
TOXICITY	Rare
DRI	1.1–1.3 mg per day; based on caloric intake
FOOD SOURCES	Milk, cheese, yogurt, cottage cheese, leafy green vegetables, whole or enriched grains ☛ Easily destroyed by ultraviolet light and irradiation; dairy products are packaged in opaque plastic or cardboard containers to prevent light exposure; heat stable

NIACIN (B₃, NICOTINIC ACID, NIACINAMIDE)

FUNCTIONS	• Part of the coenzyme nicotinamide adenine dinucleotide (NAD and NADP) • Used for energy metabolism and the health of the skin, nervous system, and the GI tract
DEFICIENCY	Pellagra: the 3 Ds—diarrhea, dermatitis, dementia; also glossitis, depression, fatigue, and memory loss
TOXICITY	From the use of supplements: "niacin flush" characterized by burning, tingling, and itching especially on the neck and face; caused by taking high doses of nicotinic acid, which is used to treat high blood cholesterol

DRI	14–16 mg per day; based on caloric intake
FOOD SOURCES	Protein-containing foods such as meat, fish, poultry, milk, eggs, and nuts because these foods contain the amino acid tryptophan, which can be made into niacin; whole and enriched grains, mushrooms, and leafy green vegetables ☛ 60 mg tryptophan = 1 mg niacin

PANTOTHENIC ACID

FUNCTIONS	Part of coenzyme A (CoA) used in energy metabolism, synthesis of lipids, steroids, neurotransmitters, hemoglobin
DEFICIENCY	Rare
TOXICITY	Rare
DRI, AI	5 mg per day
FOOD SOURCES	Widespread in foods ☛ Easily destroyed by heat

VITAMIN B₆ (PYRIDOXINE, PYRIDOXAL, PYRIDOXAMINE)

FUNCTIONS	All three forms can be used by the body to make the coenzyme pyridoxal phosphate (PLP) used in amino acid and fatty acid metabolism, and the synthesis of red blood cells, nucleic acids, lecithin, and neurotransmitters
DEFICIENCY	Microcytic anemia (small red blood cells), glossitis, weakness, insomnia, growth failure, convulsions, dermatitis, and kidney stones ☛ Micro = small; cytic = cell
TOXICITY	• High doses may be taken by people experiencing carpal tunnel syndrome and women for PMS symptoms • Excess B₆ can cause bloating, depression, fatigue, headaches, and nerve damage that may be irreversible

DRI	1.3 mg per day; based on grams of protein eaten
FOOD SOURCES	Vegetables, meat, fish, poultry, shellfish, legumes, whole and enriched grains, bananas, and some other fruits ☛ Destroyed by heat

FOLATE (FOLIC ACID, FOLACIN, PTEROYLGLUTAMIC ACID)

FUNCTIONS	• The term "folate" is used to describe food sources of this vitamin while the term "folic acid" refers to the form added to fortified grain products and supplements • Part of the coenzymes dihydrofolate (DHF) and tetrahydrofolate (THF) • Used in DNA synthesis and new cell formation; includes cells of the fetus, especially for closure of the neural tube, which develops into the brain and spinal cord; also for cells with a high turnover rate such as those of the oral tissues, GI tract, and RBC maturation • Important in the prevention of heart disease by breaking down homocysteine, a compound that promotes fatty plaques to form on the walls of blood vessels ☛ May also prevent cleft lip/palate ☛ RBC = red blood cell
DEFICIENCY	• Neural tube defects of the fetus, glossitis, deterioration of the tract causing heartburn, diarrhea, and malabsorption • Heart disease, macrocytic anemia, weakness, insomnia, and depression • Deficiencies can be caused from burns, blood loss, skin diseases, damage to the GI tract, multiple pregnancies • Medications used to treat cancer, oral contraceptives, aspirin, antacids, and smoking increase the need for folate ☛ Macro = large
TOXICITY	Taking over 1,000 mcg daily can mask the signs of a B_{12} deficiency

RDA	• 400 mcg per day for women of child-bearing age (15–45 yr) to prevent neural tube defects and to support fetal growth • 400 mcg per day for all adults to help prevent heart disease
FOOD SOURCES	• Primarily plant foods such at leafy green vegetables and legumes; also found in seeds, oranges, and grapefruit • Grain products such as cereals, pasta, and breads must be fortified with additional folic acid • Liver is the only animal tissue that provides high amounts of folate • Heat and exposure to oxygen destroy folate • ⚷ The name suggests the word "foliage"

VITAMIN B_{12} (COBALAMIN)

FUNCTIONS	• Part of the coenzymes deoxyadenoslycobalamin and methylcobalamin • Needed to activate one of the folate coenzymes, DNA and RNA synthesis, maintenance of the myelin sheath, bone cell activity, fatty acid and amino acid metabolism • ⚷ Works closely with folate • ⚷ Contains cobalt
INTRINSIC FACTOR	Vitamin B_{12} is released from food proteins by pepsin and hydrochloric acid in the stomach; then the intrinsic factor, a glycoprotein secreted by parietal cells in the stomach, attaches to B_{12}, allowing it to be absorbed in the intestine
DEFICIENCY	• Macrocytic anemia is the term used if caused by a low intake of B_{12}; deficiency may occur in people who eat a vegan diet for a long period of time • Pernicious anemia, the same as macrocytic anemia; it is an older term that is still used to describe severe anemia related to low levels of intrinsic factor and/or low HCl

- Many adults have low levels of HCl, atrophic gastritis, from the aging process, iron deficiency, the overuse of antacids or from infection with *H. pylori* (the bacteria that causes most ulcers)
- Degeneration of nerves causing a "creeping" paralysis of the extremities and moves inward and up the spine
- If not detected early and treated with adequate B_{12}, the nerve damage becomes permanent
- Treatment usually requires an injection of B_{12} monthly
- ☞ Excess folate will prevent the macrocytic anemia but not nerve damage caused by low B_{12} status
- ☞ The same type of anemia caused by a folate deficiency

TOXICITY	Rare
RDA	2.4 mcg per day
FOOD SOURCES	Animal tissue and animal byproducts (meat, fish, poultry, eggs, milk, yogurt, cheese)

BIOTIN

FUNCTIONS	Part of a coenzyme used in energy metabolism, fat and glycogen synthesis, and amino acid metabolism
DEFICIENCY	Rare; can occur when greater than two dozen egg whites are consumed daily for several months (often seen in people who do body building) because avidin, a protein in raw egg whites, binds biotin; cooking denatures avidin
TOXICITY	Rare
DRI, AI	30 mcg per day
FOOD SOURCES	Widespread in foods; also some is synthesized by bacteria in the intestines

NON-B VITAMINS

Choline, inositol, carnitine, PABA, lipoic acid, laetril, and other substances are not essential nutrients

VITAMIN C (ASCORBIC ACID)

FUNCTIONS	Collagen synthesis necessary for wound healing, scar tissue formation, ligaments, tendons, and the foundation for bones and teeth; an antioxidant to prevent cell damage; synthesis of the thyroid hormone thyroxin; amino acid metabolism; and enhances the absorption of iron
DEFICIENCY	• Scurvy, which is characterized by pinpoint hemorrhages, bleeding gums, failure of wounds to heal, rough skin, muscle degeneration and pain, depression, atherosclerotic plaques in blood vessels, joint pain, suppression of the immune system, and microcytic anemia • Severe scurvy can lead to tooth loss, hysteria, heart attack, and massive internal bleeding
TOXICITY	• From supplement use • Includes nausea, abdominal cramps, diarrhea, headache, fatigue, insomnia, hot flashes, skin rashes, kidney stones, and the aggravation of gout • May interfere with some medical tests and the action of anticoagulants
DRI, AI	75–90 mg per day; more for people who smoke
FOOD SOURCES	Citrus fruits, strawberries, kiwi fruit, mangoes, watermelon, red and green bell peppers, spinach, sweet potatoes, tomatoes, lettuce, potatoes, fortified cereals, vegetables of the cabbage family (brussel sprouts, cabbage, broccoli) ⚷ Easily destroyed by heat and exposure to air

FAT-SOLUBLE VITAMINS

- Vitamins A, D, E, and K
- Digested and absorbed like lipids; require bile and are first absorbed into the lymph and then enter the blood
- Many require protein carriers to transport them in the body
- Stored in fatty tissues of the body and in the liver
- Needed in periodic doses; average intake over several days
- Toxicity can easily occur from supplement use
- Not readily excreted

VITAMIN A (RETINOL, RETINAL, RETINOIC ACID)

FUNCTIONS	• The three different forms are all active in the body • They are commonly known as retinoids • Beta-carotene is a precursor to vitamin A • Cell differentiation; maintenance of epithelial cells, mucous membranes, the cornea, and skin; bone and tooth growth; vision; reproduction; immunity • ☛ Precursor = inactive form
DEFICIENCY	• Hypovitaminosis A • Impaired enamel and dentin formation, poor bone growth, anemia, night blindness, xerophthalmia, hyperkeratosis of the skin, diarrhea, infections, kidney stones
TOXICITY	• Hypervitaminosis A (from preformed vitamin A) • Birth defects; skin rashes; hair loss; bone abnormalities; dry, cracked lips; nosebleeds; brittle nails; nausea; vomiting; diarrhea; muscle weakness; liver damage; death • Excess intake of beta-carotene causes it to be stored in the fatty tissues of the body; palms of hands turn orange • ☛ Beta-carotene does not cause severe toxicity symptoms

RDA	800–1,000 mcg per day
FOOD SOURCES	• Foods contain either pre-formed vitamin A or the precursor beta-carotene • Preformed: fortified milk and other dairy products, fortified margarine, egg yolk, liver, and fortified cereals • Beta-carotene: dark green leafy vegetables (spinach, turnip greens, broccoli), deep orange vegetables and fruits (pumpkin, winter squash, sweet potatoes, carrots, apricots, cantaloupe) • ☞ Heat stable

VITAMIN D (CALCIFEROL)

FUNCTIONS	• Vitamin D is a hormone as well as vitamin • Enhances the absorption of calcium and phosphorus; if intake is low, it draws these minerals out of the bones and stimulates their retention by the kidneys • ☞ Hormone = compound made by one organ of the body that affects another part of the body
DEFICIENCY	• Rickets (children), osteomalacia (adults) • Both cause soft bones • Loss of muscle tone, increased excretion of calcium in the feces, malformed teeth; associated with osteoporosis
TOXICITY	• Hypervitaminosis D • Nausea, vomiting, increased blood levels of calcium and phosphorus, calcification of soft tissues (blood vessels, kidneys, heart, lungs), kidney stones and kidney damage, headache, joint pain, fatigue, excessive thirst, muscle weakness
DRI, AI	5–10 mcg per day
FOOD SOURCES	Beef, liver, egg yolks, fatty fish and fish oils, fortified milk, margarine, butter, and fortified cereals

SELF-SYNTHESIS	• It can be manufactured by the body from skin exposure to ultraviolet light; light on the face, neck, and hands daily for 10–15 minutes is usually adequate; where sun exposure is limited due to weather, sunscreen, or being home-bound, dietary sources must supply total need or a supplement may be recommended • Dark skin pigments block vitamin D synthesis and requires longer exposure times to ultraviolet light

VITAMIN E (ALPHA-TOCOPHEROL)

FUNCTIONS	An antioxidant; stabilizes cell membranes and protects PUFA and vitamin A in foods and in the body
DEFICIENCY	Erythrocyte hemolysis (breaking of RBC), hemolytic anemia, impaired vision, speech, and muscular functioning
TOXICITY	Rare; can interfere with blood clotting; can enhance the effects of anticoagulant medications
RDA	15 mg per day
FOOD SOURCES	Polyunsaturated plant oils, leafy green vegetables, wheat germ, whole grain breads and cereals, liver, egg yolks, nuts, and seeds ☞ Easily destroyed by heat and exposure to air

VITAMIN K

FUNCTIONS	Synthesis of blood-clotting proteins and a bone protein that is involved in the regulation of blood calcium ☞ Vitamin K is named for *koagulation,* a Danish word
DEFICIENCY	Hemorrhaging

TOXICITY	Interferes with anticoagulant medications; jaundice, red blood cell hemolysis, and brain damage
DRI, AI	90–120 mcg per day
FOOD SOURCES	Liver, milk, leafy green vegetables, and vegetables of the cabbage family; bacterial synthesis in the intestines supplies some of the body's need; may be affected by the use of antibiotic drugs

WATER

- Water is part of the fluid of every cell; it constitutes about 60 percent of the adult body (higher for infants, children)
- Water is associated with lean tissue, which is the weight of the body minus the weight of body fat
- Intercellular fluid—inside of the cells; about two-thirds of the water in the body
- Extracellular fluid—fluid that is outside of the cells and includes interstitial fluid that is between the cells

FUNCTIONS	• The major component of the blood and lymph that carries nutrients throughout the body and helps the body get rid of waste products via the urine and feces • A solvent for amino acids, glucose, minerals, and vitamins • Involved in chemical reactions including hydrolysis and condensation • Maintains the structure of large molecules including proteins and glycogen • Helps in the regulation of body temperature • Involved in maintaining blood volume and blood pressure • Acts as a lubricant between cells and around joints • Helps to cushion the joints and the eye; during pregnancy, amniotic fluid protects the fetus
WATER BALANCE	Controlled mainly by the hypothalamus in the brain and the kidneys by the hormones ADH, angiotensin, and aldosterone ☛ ADH = antidiuretic hormone

DEHYDRATION	When water output exceeds intake; causes thirst, dry skin and dry mouth, low blood pressure, rapid heart rate, fatigue, headache, impaired physical performance, low urine output, dizziness, and exhaustion
WATER IOTOXICATION	Rare; can be caused by kidney disease or severe food restriction, as seen in the eating disorder anorexia nervosa when large amounts of water are consumed in the place of food ⚷ Causes a dilution of electrolytes affecting nerve conduction
MINIMUM INTAKE	In adults, the body must excrete about 2 cups (480 mL) of urine each day to get rid of waste products, therefore, the minimum intake is 2 cups (16 ounces) ⚷ mL = milliliters
OPTIMAL INTAKE	Depends on activity level, environmental temperatures, composition of the diet, etc.; approximately one half cup per 100 calories expended or roughly 2 1/2 quarts
SOURCES OF WATER	Water itself, other beverages, fruits, vegetables, meats, cheeses, and the water produced during metabolism in the chemical reaction condensation ⚷ Caffeine and alcohol act as diuretics

➤ MAJOR MINERALS

Minerals needed in the body in amounts greater than 500 mg per day; includes the electrolytes

ELECTROLYTES

- Mineral salts that dissolve in water and dissociate into charged particles called ions
- Includes sodium, chloride, potassium, and calcium

GENERAL FUNCTIONS	Maintain fluid balance, acid-base balance, blood pressure, nerve transmission, and muscle contraction

SODIUM (Na)

FUNCTIONS	• Fluid balance, nerve transmission, muscle contraction • The main cation in extracellular fluid • Na = natrium, a term for sodium • cation = positively charged ion
DEFICIENCY	Muscle cramps, loss of appetite, apathy
TOXICITY	Edema, acute hypertension
FOOD SOURCES	Table salt (NaCl), soy sauce, processed foods, some vegetables and meats, dairy products, baking powder and baking soda, condiments • NaCl = sodium chloride; 40% is sodium, 60% chloride
REQUIREMENT	500 mg per day minimum • 1 tsp salt = 2,000 mg sodium

CHLORIDE (Cl)

FUNCTIONS	• Occurs in association with sodium in the extracellular fluid where it is the major anion; the ionic form of chlorine • Fluid balance, part of hydrochloric acid • anion = negatively charged ion
DEFICIENCY	Can be caused by vomiting; disrupts acid-base balance
TOXICITY	In dehydration, blood levels of chloride are concentrated
FOOD SOURCES	Table salt, and foods containing NaCl
REQUIREMENT	750 mg per day minimum

POTASSIUM (K)

FUNCTIONS	Fluid balance, nerve transmission, muscle contraction • K = kalium, a term for potassium
DEFICIENCY	• Muscle weakness, leg cramps, loss of appetite, paralysis, confusion; occur with dehydration

	• Can occur with the use of some types of diuretics used in the treatment of high blood pressure; potassium-sparing diuretics are available
TOXICITY	• Muscle weakness, tingling and numbness in extremities, diarrhea, bradycardia, abdominal cramps • Can occur with the use of potassium salt (KCl) in place of table salt in the treatment of high blood pressure
FOOD SOURCES	Whole, fresh foods (not processed), especially milk, fruits, vegetables, and legumes
REQUIREMENT	2,000 mg per day minimum

CALCIUM (Ca)

FUNCTIONS	• The most abundant mineral in the body; found primarily in the bones and teeth along with phosphorus-forming hydroxyapatite crystals; provide strength and rigidity • A small amount (1%) of calcium is in the blood and other fluids where it participates as an electrolyte in nerve transmission and muscle contraction; also involved in blood clotting, hormone secretion, and calmodulin, which is needed for normal blood pressure
DEFICIENCY	• Stunted growth in children, osteoporosis in adults • Osteoporosis is also influenced by other factors such as hormone levels, smoking, dieting, lack of exercise, steroid intake, genetics, alcohol and caffeine intake, excessive amounts of fiber, protein, or sodium, or a vitamin D defiency • Blood calcium levels are tightly controlled by hormones; if levels rise, rigor occurs; if levels decrease, tetany occurs • rigor = stiffness of the muscles • tetany = inability to maintain muscle contractions, spasms

TOXICITY	Constipation, urinary stones, kidney dysfunction, and interference with the absorption of other minerals
FOOD SOURCES	Milk, cheese, yogurt, cottage cheese, fish with bones (sardines, salmon), oysters, green vegetables (broccoli, bok choy, turnip and mustard greens, kale), almonds, legumes, seeds, tofu and corn tortillas if processed with calcium, and calcium-fortified orange juice and other fortified foods
FACTORS THAT ENHANCE ABSORPTION	Vitamin D, lactose, hydrochloric acid, phosphorus in optimal amounts
FACTORS THAT INHIBIT ABSORPTION	High phosphorus intake (meats, carbonated sodas), very high fiber intake (binds minerals), phytates (in nuts, seeds, and grains), oxalates (in spinach and beets), low levels of lactose, vitamin D, and hydrochloric acid
DRI, AI	• 19–50 years of age—1,000 mg per day • 51 yr and older—1,200 mg per day • Postmenopausal women not on HRT—1,500 mg per day • HRT = hormone replacement therapy

PHOSPHORUS (P)

FUNCTIONS	Mineralization of teeth and bones; part of phospholipids in cell membranes; used in making ATP; acid-base balance; DNA and RNA • ATP = adenosine triphosphate
DEFICIENCY	Bone pain, weakness
TOXICITY	• Low blood levels of calcium; affects bone health • Often seen with a high intake of sodas and low intake of dairy products including milk

FOOD SOURCES	Meat, fish, poultry, milk, cheese, yogurt, legumes, liver, carbonated sodas, and food additives
RDA	700 mg per day

MAGNESIUM (Mg)

FUNCTIONS	Bone mineralization, as a component of many enzymes, energy metabolism, blood clotting, nerve transmission, muscle relaxation, maintenance of enamel, and immunity
DEFICIENCY	Weakness, tetany, bizarre eye and facial movements, difficulty swallowing, hallucinations, confusion, convulsions
TOXICITY	Rare in the past, now seen more often with the use of magnesium-containing laxatives
FOOD SOURCES	Legumes, nuts, seeds, whole grains, green vegetables, seafood, cocoa, chocolate, watermelon, milk, yogurt
RDA	310–420 mg per day
UPPER LEVEL	350 mg from nonfood sources (see Toxicity)

SULFUR (S)

FUNCTIONS	Found in two essential amino acids: cysteine and methionine
DEFICIENCY	Rare; occurs along with a protein deficiency
TOXICITY	Rare
FOOD SOURCES	All protein-containing foods
RDA	None; only needed as part of 2 essential amino acids

Trace Minerals

IRON (Fe) Minerals needed in the body in amounts less than 500 mg per day	
FUNCTIONS	The part of hemoglobin that carries oxygen; part of myoglobin, a protein in muscles that holds oxygen; a cofactor in many enzymes; involved in ATP formation; protects against heavy metal poisoning ☞ Fe = ferrous/ferris ☞ myo = muscle ☞ metalloenzyme = an enzyme that contains one or more minerals
STORAGE PROTEINS	Ferritin and hemosiderin
DEFICIENCY	• Microcytic hypochromic anemia (small, pale RBCs) • Reduced ability to work, weakness, fatigue, reduced learning ability, lowered immunity, frequent infections; pale nailbeds, gingiva, and eye membranes; blue sclera; impaired wound healing; reduced resistance to cold; pica • Can be caused by a low intake or absorption of iron; blood losses (menstruation, ulcers, parasitic infections, aspirin), pregnancy, high-milk diets, rapid growth ☞ hypo = too little; chromic = color ☞ Pica = a craving for nonfood substances
TOXICITY	• Iron overload (hemochromatosis) causing organ damage and aggravating heart disease, diabetes, arthritis, and liver cancer; infections; death • Occurs from supplement use or poisoning; multiple blood transfusions, high alcohol intake, and metabolic disorders
FOOD SOURCES	Red meat, fish, dark meat of poultry, shellfish, egg yolks, liver, legumes, tofu, dried fruits, and fortified grains
HEME IRON	Most absorbable form of iron in foods, found in animal tissues; enhances the absorption of nonheme iron

NON-HEME IRON	Least absorbable form of iron in foods, found in plant foods and animal tissue
FACTORS THAT ENHANCE ABSORPTION	The MFP (meat, fish, protein) factor in animal tissues enhances the absorption of non-heme iron; sugars, vitamin C, HCl and citric and lactic acids
FACTORS THAT INHIBIT ABSORPTION	Phytates and fiber; calcium and phosphorus; EDTA; tannic acid in tea; polyphenols (found in coffee, tea, and many plants) ☛ EDTA is in many food additives
NONFOOD SOURCE	Iron cookware releases iron into acidic foods ☛ Called contamination iron
DRI	• Men: 8 mg per day • Women: 19–50 years—18 mg per day 51 years + —8 mg per day

ZINC (Zn)

FUNCTIONS	Immune function, growth, part of many enzymes, blood clotting; associated with insulin and thyroid function; needed for normal taste perception, sperm production, and fetal development; helps protect the body from heavy metal poisoning; wound healing
DEFICIENCY	Growth retardation, impaired cell division; taste alterations; low sperm counts; rough, dry skin; night blindness; low insulin; altered metabolic rate; impaired immune response
TOXICITY	Even a small amount above the DRI on a regular basis can lower the body's copper content, which can lead to the degeneration of the heart muscle; very high doses can cause diarrhea, vomiting, decreased absorption of calcium and copper; muscle pain, degeneration of the heart muscle, anemia; reproductive and renal failure

FOOD SOURCES	Shellfish, meat, poultry, liver, legumes, whole grain cereals and breads, milk, yogurt, and cheese
DRI	8–11 mg per day

IODINE/IODIDE (I)
The term *iodine* is used to refer to food; *iodide* refers to when it is in the body

FUNCTIONS	Required as part of two thyroid hormones
DEFICIENCY	• Simple goiter—an enlargement of the thyroid gland due to a low iodine intake by adults • Cretinism—impaired fetal development; physical and mental retardation
TOXICITY	Also an enlarged thyroid gland
FOOD SOURCES	Iodized salt, seafood, dairy products, plants grown in iodine-rich soil
DRI	150 mcg per day

SELENIUM (Se)

FUNCTIONS	An antioxidant that works with vitamin E
DEFICIENCY	Predisposition to heart disease; an enlarged, fibrous heart
TOXICITY	Disorders of the GI tract, loss of hair and nails, skin lesions, nerve disorders, and tooth damage
FOOD SOURCES	Seafood, meat, whole grains
DRI	55 mcg per day

COPPER (Cu)

FUNCTIONS	Part of many enzymes including antioxidants and iron metabolism
DEFICIENCY	Rare; anemia, bone abnormalities
TOXICITY	Nerve disorders; some genetic disorders cause toxicity

FOOD SOURCES	Seafood, nuts, seeds, whole grains, legumes, organ meats
DRI	900 mcg per day

MANGANESE (Mn)

FUNCTIONS	The body contains only a very small amount of this trace mineral; it is a cofactor in many enzymes involved in metabolism
DEFICIENCY	Rare; can be caused if intake of phytates iron or calcium is very high
TOXICITY	Disorders of the nervous system; often caused by environmental contamination
FOOD SOURCES	Widespread in foods, especially organ meats
DRI, AI	1.8–2.3 mg per day

FLUORIDE (F)
The ionized form of fluorine

FUNCTIONS	Forms fluoroapatite crystals, along with calcium and phosphorus, in the bones and teeth; fluoride replaces the hydroxyl portions of hydroxyapatite crystals, making teeth more resistant to dental caries
DEFICIENCY	High rates of dental caries
TOXICITY	Acute intake causes nausea, vomiting, diarrhea, abdominal pain, and tingling or numbness of the extremities; chronic intake can cause fluorosis, making teeth weak and permanently stained
FOOD SOURCES	Fluoridated water and water with naturally occurring fluoride; foods and beverages prepared with fluoridated water; tea, seafood
OTHER SOURCES	Swallowing of fluoridated toothpastes, rinses, or prescription fluoride pastes and gels; fluoride supplements (drops or tablets)

DRI	3–4 mg per day

CHROMIUM (Cr)

FUNCTIONS	Needed for normal insulin activity and blood glucose control
DEFICIENCY	Elevated blood glucose levels, impaired insulin response, and glucogon response
TOXICITY	Rare; can occur from occupational exposure
FOOD SOURCES	Unprocessed foods such as whole grain breads and cereals, brewer's yeast, nuts, cheese, liver
DRI, AI	25–35 mcg per day

MOLYBDENUM (MO)

FUNCTIONS	A cofactor in many enzymes involved in metabolism
DEFICIENCY	Rare
TOXICITY	Rare; can be caused by occupational exposure; gout-like symptoms
FOOD SOURCES	Legumes, whole grain breads and cereals, leafy green vegetables, milk, and liver
DRI	45 mcg per day

BORON

FUNCTIONS	Needed in very small amounts; needed for mineral metabolism
DEFICIENCY	Mineral metabolic disorders of unknown etiology
TOXICITY	Rare
FOOD SOURCES	Plant foods such as fruits, vegetables, nuts, and legumes
DRI	None

CHAPTER

4 Microbiology and Immunology

Demetra Daskalos Logothetis, RDH, MS

➤ BASIC CELL TYPES

Life forms are composed of one of two basic cell types

PROKARYOTIC CELLS Chemicals like penicillin specifically interfere with the function of prokaryotic cells, treating diseases caused by these cells	
SHAPES	• *Cocci* (singular, *coccus*)—spherical bacteria • *Bacilli* (singular, *bacillus*) or rods—cylindrical-shaped bacteria • *Spirilla* (singular, *spirillum*)—helical-shaped bacteria
COMPONENTS OF PROKARYOTIC CELLS	• Most species are divided into two different categories based on their reaction to gram stain • Gram stain—cell staining procedures that differentiates between gram-positive and gram-negative cell walls • Gram-positive = purple • Gram-negative = pink **Figure 4-1**

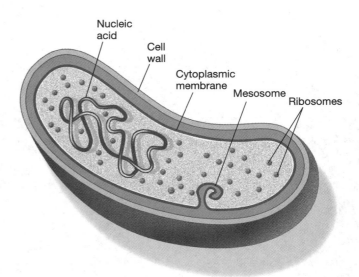

FIGURE 4-1 Components of a Prokaryotic Cell

CELL ENVELOPE STRUCTURE	Cytoplasmic membrane—innermost structure—same in all cells ☞ Functional barrier between inside and outside of the cell Energy producing system for prokaryotic cells
	Cell wall—differs from gram (+) and gram (−) cells ☞ Gram (+)—peptidoglycan; thick (multilayered) ☞ Gram (−)—more complex; lipopoly-saccharide outer membrane and very thin peptidoglycan layer between outer and inner cell membrane
	Glycocalyx—external to cell wall; varies from species to species Bacteria secrete polysaccharides to produce slimy gel-type matter ☞ Have ability to exclude ink during staining procedures
EXTERNAL APPENDAGES	• Flagella—provides movement for the cell to sites between bacteria and surface • Pili—tubes DNA to pass from cell to cell; attachment

ENDOSPORES	• Bacillus, clostridium, sporosarcina form endospores • Resistant protein layer protecting cell material from harsh environments

EUKARYOTIC CELLS
Figure 4-2

CELL WALLS	Simple polysaccharide, fungi, algae, plant cells have cell walls ☞ Animal (human) cells have no cell wall
FLAGELLA AND CILIA	More complex than on prokaryotic cells—perform same functions
CYTOPLASMIC MEMBRANE	Similar to prokaryotic cells

BACTERIAL MORPHOLOGY
Figure 4-3

COCCI	Usually appear in chains of various lengths • Pairs (diplococci) • Chains (streptococci) • Clusters (staphylococci) ☞ Predominates in oral health

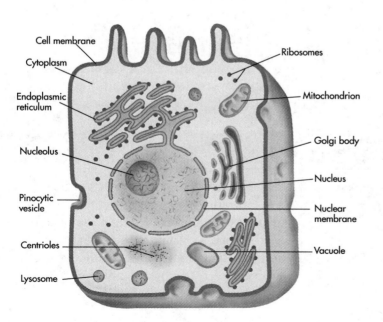

FIGURE 4-2 Main Structured Components of a Eukaryotic Cell

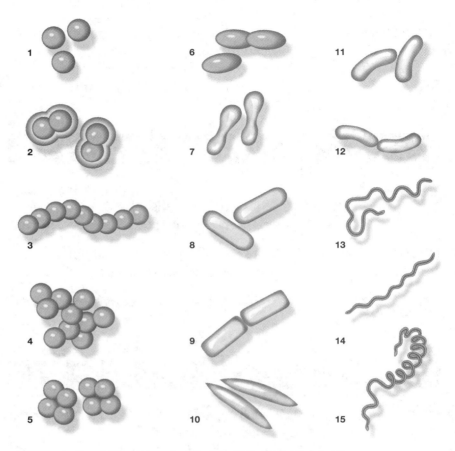

FIGURE 4-3 Bacterial Morphology: Cocci (1–5), Bacilli (6–12), Spirilla (13–15)

BACILLI	• Cylindrical-shaped bacteria or rods • Most occur as single cells
SPIRILLA	• Helical-shaped bacteria • Spiral or curved

➤ METABOLIC FUNCTIONS

ENERGY METABOLISM **Any chemical change or reaction that occurs within the cell**	
PHOTOSYNTHESIS	Process by which autotrophic organisms convert radiant energy from the sun into a form of chemical energy that they use or can be used by living organisms that require organic matter as their energy source (heterotrophic organisms)

	☞ Green plants on land and algae growing in water are responsible for most of the photosynthetic activity on earth
CATABOLISM	Carbohydrates, proteins, and lipids store energy in their chemical bonds that are available for biosynthesis through catabolic reactions ☞ Glucose or a polymer of glucose such as starch is the main source of energy for most cells
METABOLIC ENERGY	Energy obtained by metabolic processes is stored in adenosine triphosphate (ATP) molecules that contain three phosphate groups; two are connected to high-energy bonds readily available for cellular functions ☞ Energy released → ATP loses phosphate group → adenosine diphosphate (ADP) → energy and phosphate available; ATP regenerated through the cell respiration process **Figure 4-4**
GLYCOLYSIS	Splitting of glucose—series of reactions involving the catabolism of glucose, causing the production of pyruvic acid **Figure 4-5**
FERMENTATION	The conversion of pyruvic acid into alcohol and organic acids
CELL RESPIRATION	Krebs cycle and electron transport chain: regenerate ATP $(ADP = P \rightarrow ATP)$

BIOSYNTHESIS

Metabolic activities of cells engaged in producing building blocks needed for the formation of new cellular components

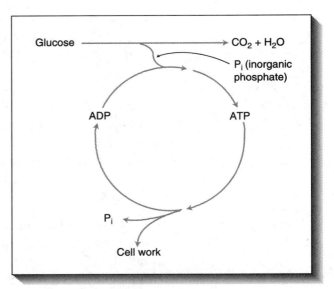

FIGURE 4-4   The ATP-ADP Cycle

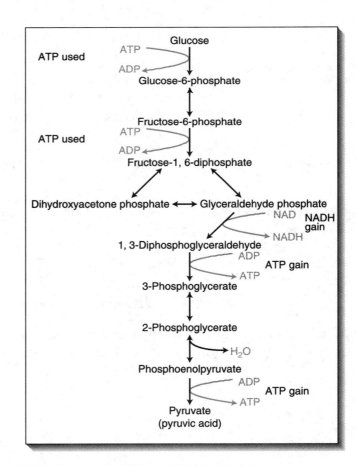

FIGURE 4-5   Simplified Schematic of the Glycolytic Pathway

➤ MICROORGANISMS

Staphylococci

BACTERIA

- Spherical-shaped bacterium occurring in grape-like clusters
- Causative agent of a wide variety of human infections
- *S. aureus* has the ability to clot plasma by secreting enzyme called coagulase
- Staphylococci that do not secrete coagulase are of no or low virulence
- Pyogenic bacteria (pus-producing)

STAPHYLOCOCCAL DISEASES	
VIRULENCE MECHANISM	• Hemolysins—breaking of blood cells • Leukocidens—bacterial toxin that destroys leukocytes • Fibrinolysin—biochemical reactions for lysis of clots in the vascular system • Enterotoxins—toxins produced by bacteria that act on the intestinal living cells • Toxic shock toxins • Exfoliatin—toxins produced by *S. aureus* causing dermatological changes (scalded skin)
DISEASES	• Skin and wound infections ☛ Example: boils, impetigo • Internal infections • Toxic shock syndrome • Scalded skin syndrome • Food poisoning ☛ Foods that are not cooked after preparation ☛ Example: potato salad, cream pies
TRANSMISSION	• Person to person—direct or indirect contact • Endogenous—originates with patient ☛ Example: burn on hand is infected with bacteria carried on patient's own skin or in nose

DIAGNOSIS	Based on isolation of organism from lesion ☛ *S. aureus* on blood agar produces a zone of clear hemolysis (breaking of blood cells) around its typically golden yellow colony
TREATMENT	Antibiotics ☛ *S. aureus* has ability to develop resistance against chemotherapeutic agents ☛ Methicillin—bacteria with the enzyme penicillinase are resistant

Streptococci

CHARACTERISTICS

- Gram positive, coccal-shaped bacteria appearing in chains of various lengths
- Part of normal bacterial flora of skin, nose, mouth, and mucosal surfaces
- *Streptococcus pyogenes, streptococcus pneumoniae, streptococcus agalactiae* are responsible for most streptococcal infections in humans

STREPTOCOCCUS PYOGENES

VIRULENCE MECHANISMS	• Hemolysins • Fibrinolysin • M-protein—a major virulence factor of streptococci; located on the cell surface, this antigen can be used to separate group A streptococci into over 80 serotypes • Erythrogenic toxin—produce the fever and rash associated with scarlet fever • Protein F—promotes adherence to pharyngeal cells • Hyaluronidase—the spreading factor, enzyme that breaks down hyaluronic acid that acts as an intracellular glue

DISEASES	• *Sore throat*—"strep throat" • Group A streptococci are the major cause • *Scarlet fever*—results from production of erythrogenic toxin called pyrogenic exotoxin • *Toxic shock-like syndrome* • Group A beta-hemolytic streptococci • *Puerperal fever*—(child bed fever) • Group A streptococci • *Infections of the skin*—lesions of the skin where prior injuries have occurred • Example: impetigo • *Poststreptococcal disease*—disease that occurs as a direct result of streptoccocal infection • Example: glomerulonephritis and rheumatic fever—onset 1 to 4 weeks after an acute streptococcal infection
TRANSMISSION	• Person to person • Airborne contact
DIAGNOSIS	Clinical and laboratory findings • Culture material on blood agar plate for 24 hours for the presence of beta-hemolytic colonies
TREATMENT	• Penicillin • Erythromycin • Cephalosporin • Beta-hemolytic streptococci are highly susceptible to most antimicrobial agents

STREPTOCOCCUS PNEUMONIAE

VIRULENCE MECHANISMS	• Capsule—retards the rate of phagocytosis • Pneumolysin—cytoplasmic protein of bacteria that binds to cholesterol of host cells, disrupting their cell membrane forming pores

DISEASES	• Pneumonia • Pleurisy—pneumococci that spread from the lungs into the pleural cavity and cause abscesses • Otitis media—middle ear infection • Meningitis
DIAGNOSIS	• Physical examination • Lung x-rays • Laboratory diagnosis—microscopic examination and culturing on artificial media •̄ Differentiation of pneumococci from streptococci is by their bile solubility pneumococci contains autolytic enzymes that are activated in the presence of bile
TRANSMISSION	• Person-to-person aerosol transmission • Opportunists
TREATMENT	Penicillin or other antibiotics

Neisseria

BACTERIA

• Gram-negative diplococci (paired cocci)
• Environmentally fragile and readily killed by exposure to drying, chilling, sunlight, acids, or alkalies

NEISSERIA MENINGITIDES
Leading cause of young adult meningitis

VIRULENCE MECHANISMS	• Capsule • Endotoxin
DISEASES	• Spinal meningitis • Disseminated infection
DIAGNOSIS	• Microscopic examination • Inoculation on nutrient agar
TRANSMISSION	• Airborne • Person to person
TREATMENT	• Penicillin • Broad-spectrum antibiotics • Sulfonamides

NEISSERIA GONORRHOEAE
Cause of most frequent reported sexually transmitted disease, gonorrhea

VIRULENCE MECHANISMS	• Attachment pili to mucosal tissues of humans • Induces inflammation • Endotoxins
DISEASE	• Gonorrhea
DIAGNOSIS	• Easier in males than in females • Purulent discharge examined with microscope for presence of intracellular gram-negative diplococci
TRANSMISSION	• Sexually • Mother to newborn
TREATMENT	• Penicillin • Ceftriaxone and doxycycline

Spirochetes

CHARACTERISTICS

Spiral-shaped, long, slender, motile microorganisms—include Borellia, Leptospira, Treponema; only Borellia can be visualized using light microscopy

TREPONEMA PALLIDUM

VIRULENCE MECHANISMS	Avoids immune responses
DISEASE	Syphilis
DIAGNOSIS	• Appearance of primary chancre or secondary lesions • Presence of spirochetes in exudates from lesion followed by serological tests
TRASMISSION	• Sexually • Congenital
TREATMENT	• Penicillin • Erythromycin

BORRELIA	
VIRULENCE MECHANISM	Antigenic variants
DISEASES	• Relapsing fever—*Borrelia recurrentis* • Lyme disease—*Borrelia burgdorferi*
TRANSMISSION	• Ticks • Animals to humans
TREATMENT	• Penicillin • Broad-spectrum antibiotics • Tetracyclines

Anaerobic Bacteria

CLOSTRIDIA All gram-positive, spore-forming, anaerobic bacilli; produce powerful exotoxins	
CLOSTRIDIUM TETANI	Produces an exotoxin causing tetanus ☛ **Tet**anus is **tet**anic paralysis (blocks glycine, an inhibitory neurotransmitter)
C. BOTULINUM	Produces a preformed, heat-labile toxin that inhibits Ach release, causing botulism
C. PERFRINGENS	Produces α toxin, a hemolytic lecithinase that causes myonecrosis or gas gangrene ☛ **Perf**ringens **perf**orates a gangrenous leg

NON-SPORE-FORMING BACTERIA	
BACTEROIDES	• Gram-negative bacilli • Infections—peritonitis, liver abscesses, pulmonary, upper respiratory, wounds, bacteremia
FUSOBACTERIUM	• Gram-negative bacilli • Infections—liver abscesses, pulmonary, upper respiratory, wounds, bacteremia

Gram-Positive Bacilli

CORYNEBACTERIUM DIPHTHERIAE

- Causes diphtheria via exotoxin
- Symptoms incluse pseudomembranous pharyngitis (grayish-white membrane) with lymphadenopathy
- Lab diagnosis based on gram-positive rods with metachromatic granules
- ☞ Grows on tellurite agar

BACILLUS ANTHRACIS

- Causes anthrax
- Inhalation of spores can cause life-threatening pneumonia
- Transmitted from animals to humans

Mycobacteria and Related Microorganisms

MYCOBACTERIA

☞ All mycobacteria are acid-fast organisms

M. TUBERCULOSIS	• Major cause of human tuberculosis • Non-spore-forming bacillus • Transmission—airborne, person to person • Symptoms—fever, night sweats, weight loss, hemoptysis • Treated with various anti-microbial agents
M. LEPRAE	• Causes leprosy (Hansen's disease) • Acid-fast bacillus that likes cool temperatures (infects skin and superficial nerves) • Cannot be grown *in vitro* • Treat with long-term oral dapsone • Two forms: lepromatous (failed cell-mediated immunity and is worse) and tuberculoid, which is self-limited ☞ LEpromatous = LEthal

ACTINOMYCETES Gram-positive bacteria; some are acid-fast and related to the mycobacteria	
ACTINOMYCES ISRAELII	Gram-positve anaerobe, causes oral/facial abscess with "sulfur granules" that may drain through sinus tract in skin; normal oral flora ☛ Head and neck infections following injury to mouth or jaw, such as tooth extractions

Enterobacteriaceae

CHARACTERISTICS Gram-negative bacilli, a large family containing more than 100 species of bacteria; inhabit primarily the large intestine; referred to as the enteric bacilli	
SALMONELLA TYPHI	Not killed by macrophages, can actually multiply within macrophages ☛ Causes typhoid fever and is transmitted in contaminated water by feces
SALMONELLA	• One of the most common infectious diseases in United States • Found as normal flora in the intestinal tract of animals and birds • When ingested by humans proliferates in the intestines causes gastroenteritis • Symptoms include fever, nausea, abdominal pain, and diarrhea • Motile • Transmitted by ingesting salmonella through contaminated foods ☛ Has animal reservoir; common sources are poultry products
SHIGELLA	Primarily pathogens of humans and is transmitted through human fecal contamination of food, water, fingers, feces

Vibrio and Helicobacter

VIBRIO **Gram-negative, motile bacilli that is highly virulent and causes a variety of human diseases**	
VIBRIO CHOLERAE	• Causative agent of human cholera • Multiplies rapidly in intestinal tract and ruptures, releasing potent enterotoxin, causing violent diarrhea • Transmitted via contaminated food or water • Treated with tetracycline and rehydration

HELICOBACTER	

Causes gastritis and up to 90% of duodenal ulcers; risk factor for peptic ulcer and gastric carcinoma

H. PYLORI	• Causes gastrointestinal infections • Gram-negative bacillus • One of few organisms adapted to live in the stomach of humans; creates alkaline environment • Urease positive—a breath test gives strong indication of infection • Treatment—triple therapy: bismuth (Pepto-Bismol), metronidaxole, and amoxicillin

Haemophilus and Bordetella

Both genera are capable of producing human respiratory disease

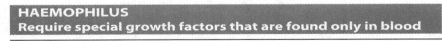

HAEMOPHILUS **Require special growth factors that are found only in blood**	

- ☞ Haemo = blood
- ☞ Philus = loving

HAEMOPHILUS INFLUENZAE	<ul><li>Requires blood products specifically hemin (X factor), and NAD (V factor) for growth on chocolate agar</li><li>Causes epiglotitus, meningitis, otitis media (ear infections), and pneumonia</li><li>Transmission via airborne and person to person</li><li>Treat with ampicillin, and prevent with vaccine</li></ul>☛ Ha**EMOP**hilus = **E**piglotitus, **M**eningitis, **O**titis media, **P**neumonia ☛ Does not cause the flu (influenza virus does)

BORDETELLA PERTUSSIS

- Causative agent of pertussis ("whooping cough")
- Transmitted airborne and person to person
- Treat with respiratory support and antimicrobials, prevent with vaccine
- ☛ Vaccination has greatly reduced the number of cases

Rickettsiae and Chlamydiae

RICKETTSIAE

- Obligate intracellular parasites of animal cells
- Transmitted to humans by vectors and produce serious generalized infections

RICKETTSIA RICKETTSII	<ul><li>Causes Rocky Mountain spotted fever</li><li>Symptoms—rash on palms and soles, headache, fever</li><li>Transmitted by tick bites</li><li>Treat with tetracyclines</li></ul>

CHLAMYDIAE

- Obligate intracellular parasites that cause mucosal infections. Cause conjunctivitis, pneumonia
- Transmitted by human to human, direct contact, sexually
- Treat with erythromycin or tetracycline

Viruses

Acellular, obligate intracellular "parasites"—need a host cell to replicate

VIRAL GENOME Genetic material	
DNA VIRAL GENOMES	All DNA viruses are dsDNA except parvoviridae ☞ Double stranded = dsDNA
RNA VIRAL GENOMES	All RNA viruses are ssRNA except reoviridae ☞ Single stranded = ssRNA

VIRAL REPLICATION

- All DNA viruses replicate in the nucleus (except poxvirus)
- All RNA viruses replicate in the cytoplasm (except influenza virus and retroviruses)

DNA Viruses

ADENOVIRUS

- DS linear, no envelope
- Causes upper respiratory diseases, sore throat, pneumonia, conjunctivitis (pink eye)

HEPADNAVIRUS

STRUCTURE	DS-partial circular, has envelope
MEDICAL CONCERNS	Causes Hepatitis B

HERPESVIRUSES

STRUCTURE	DS-linear, has envelope
MEDICAL CONCERNS	- HSV 1—oral and some genital lesions - HSV 2—genital and some oral lesions - Varicella-zoster virus—chickenpox, zoster, shingles - Epstein-Barr virus—mononucleosis, Burkitt's lymphoma

- Cytomegalovirus—infection in immuno-suppressed patients (transplant recipients)
- HHV 6—roseola
- HHV 8 (KSHV)—Kaposi's sarcoma-associated herpesvirus

POXVIRUS

STRUCTURE	DS-linear, has envelope
MEDICAL CONCERNS	Smallpox

RNA Viruses

PICORNAVIRUSES

STRUCTURE	SS + linear, no envelope
MEDICAL CONCERNS	- Rhinovirus—common cold - Coxsackievirus—herpangina (febrile pharyngitis; hand, foot, and mouth disease) - Hepatitis A—acute viral hepatitis

TOGAVIRUSES

STRUCTURE	SS + linear, has envelope
MEDICAL CONCERNS	Rubella (German measles)

RETROVIRUSES

STRUCTURE	SS + linear, has envelope
MEDICAL CONCERNS	HIV/AIDS

ORTHOMYXOVIRUSES

STRUCTURE	SS − linear, has envelope
MEDICAL CONCERNS	Influenza virus

PARAMYXOVIRUSES

STRUCTURE	SS – linear, has envelope
MEDICAL CONCERNS	• Parainfluenae—croup • Measles • Mumps

RHABDOVIRUSES

STRUCTURE	SS + linear, has envelope
MEDICAL CONCERNS	Rabies

CORONAVIRUSES

STRUCTURE	SS + linear, has envelope
MEDICAL CONCERNS	Coronavirus—common cold

BUNYAVIRUSES

STRUCTURE	SS – circular, has envelope
MEDICAL CONCERNS	• California encephalitis • Hantavirus—hemorrhagic fever, pneumonia

FLAVIVIRUSES

STRUCTURE	SS + linear, has envelope
MEDICAL CONCERNS	• Hepatitis C • Yellow fever

HEPATITIS SEROLOGIC MARKERS

IgM HAVAb	IgM antibody to HAV: best test to detect active Hepatitis A
HBsAg	Antigen found on surface of HBV: continued presence indicates carrier state
HBsAb	Antibody to HbsAg: provides immunity to hepatitis B

HBcAg	Antigen associated with core of HBV
HBcAb	Antibody to HbcAg: positive during window period; IgM HBcAb is an indicator of recent disease
HBeAg	A second, different antigenic determinant in the HBV core; important indicator of transmissibility ☞ (**BE**ware)
HBeAb	Antibody to e antigen; indicates low transmissibility

Fungi

- Eukaryotic organisms
- Fungal diseases are called mycoses

YEASTS

CANDIDA ALBICANS	• Candidiasis more prevalent in persons on broad-spectrum antibiotic therapy • Causative agent for thrush mouth

➤ IMMUNOLOGY

ACQUIRED IMMUNITY

Specific immunity that develops as a result of exposure to an antigen
☞ Improves with each exposure to an antigen

HUMORAL ANTIBODY RESPONSE	• Mediated by antibodies that circulate with body fluids • Refers to the production of B lymphocytes (B cells)
CELL-MEDIATED IMMUNE RESPONSE	• Mediated by specialized cells • Involves production of T cells and natural killer cells

IMMUNE RESPONSE COMPONENTS (LYMPHOCYTES)

B CELLS	• Respond to antigens by producing a protective protein (antibody) that combines with the antigen to form an antigen–antibody complex that marks the foreign substance for phagocytosis • Present in blood ⌐ Antigen determinants must have complimentary configuration
T CELLS	• Leave bone marrow as pre-T cells and mature in thymus into T cells • Defense cells that are cytotoxic and physically attack and destroy pathogenic cells

CYTOKINES

INTERLEUKIN 1 (IL-1)	• Secreted by macrophages • Chemotactic for monocytes and neutrophils • Induces granulocyte-monocyte colony-stimulating factor (GM-CSF) • Induces fever
INTERLEUKIN 2 (IL-2)	• Secreted by helper T cells • Stimulates growth of active T and B cells
INTERLEUKIN 3 (IL-3)	• Secreted by activated T cells, mast cells • Supports the growth and differentiation of bone marrow stem cells
INTERLEUKIN 4 (IL-4)	• Secreted by helper T cells • Promotes growth of B cell • Enhances the synthesis of IgE and IgG
INTERLEUKIN 5 (IL-5)	• Secreted by helper T cells • Induces differentiation of activated B cells into antibody-producing cells • Enhances the synthesis of IgA

TUMOR NECROSIS FACTOR - α	<ul><li>Secreted by macrophages</li><li>Increases IL-2 receptor synthesis by helper T cells</li><li>Increases B-cell proliferation</li><li>Attracts and activates neutrophils</li></ul>
TUMOR NECROSIS FACTOR - β	<ul><li>Secreted by activated T lymphocytes</li><li>Activation of phagocytic cells</li><li>Functions similar to those of TNF - α</li></ul>

CLASSES OF ANTIBODIES (IMMUNOGLOBULINS)

IgG	<ul><li>Present in circulation</li><li>Long-term antibody that protects the host against infections and toxins</li><li>Crosses placenta</li><li>Fixes complement</li></ul>
IgM	<ul><li>Produced in early response to antigen</li><li>Found predominately in blood</li><li>Does not cross placenta</li><li>Fixes complement</li></ul>
IgA	<ul><li>Found in blood, tears, saliva, mucosal secretions, breast milk</li><li>Protection against infections of superficial tissues</li><li>Does not fix complement</li></ul>
IgD	<ul><li>Antigen receptor on B cells</li><li>Found in serum</li></ul>
IgE	<ul><li>Mediates immediate type I hypersensitivity</li><li>Attaches to mast cells and basophils</li></ul>

HYPERSENSITIVITY

TYPE I IMMEDIATE HYPERSENSITIVITY	<ul><li>Ag cross-links IgE on presensitized mast cells and basophils, triggering release of vasoactive amines</li><li>Reaction occurs rapidly after Ag exposure</li><li>☛ First and Fast = anaphylaxis</li></ul>

TYPE II CYTOTOXIC HYPERSENSITIVITY	• IgM, IgG bind to Ag on "enemy" cell, leading to lysis (by complement) or phagocytosis • Example is hemolytic disease of the newborn (erythroblstosis fetalis), where maternal anti-Rh IgG crosses the placenta nad binds the Rh antigen on fetal red blood cells
TYPE III IMMUNE COMPLEX HYPERSENSITIVITY	• Caused by the deposition of immune complexes (antigen-antibody complexes) at various body locations • Common sites affected are blood vessels, kidneys, joints, lungs, and skin • Diseases in immune complexes include rheumatoid arthritis, systemic lupus erythematosus, and fibrosing alveolitis
TYPE IV DELAYED HYPERSENSITIVITY	• Immune reaction that develops begin ning 18 to 24 hours following contact with antigen • Sensitized T lymphocyte encounters antigen and then releases lymphokines (leads to macrophage activation) • Examples include TB skin test, transplant rejection, contact dermatitis ☛ Fourth and Last = delayed

CHAPTER

5 Pathology

Demetra Daskalos Logothetis,
RDH, MS

➤ GENERAL PATHOLOGY

Inflammation

Vascular response to injury

STEPS IN THE ACUTE INFLAMMATORY RESPONSE Injury is brief and source is removed from tissue Figure 5-1	
VASOCONSTRICTION	First brief inflammatory response
VASODIALATION	Relaxation of the smooth muscles caused by chemical mediators at time of injury; process known as active hyperemia and is responsible for erythema and heat
EXUDATE	Increased vascular permeability allows fluid and plasma proteins to leave the blood vessels into injured tissues to help dilute the injurious agents
SEROUS EXUDATE	Associated with mild inflammation and composed of plasma fluids, proteins, and a few white blood cells ☛ Example: fluid in a blister

Adapted from Ibsen, O. & Phelan, J. *Oral Pathology for the Dental Hygenist,* 3rd ed. Philadelphia: WB Saunders, 2000.

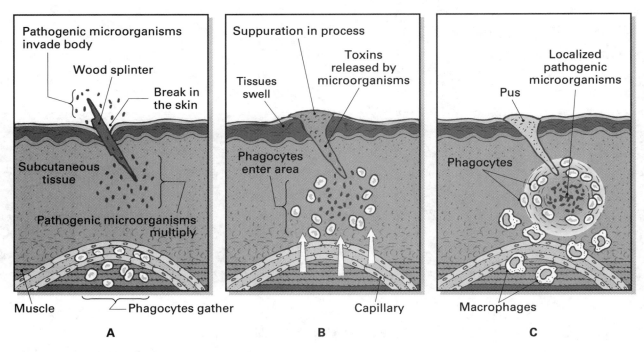

FIGURE 5-1 Steps in Acute Inflammatory Response

FIBROUS EXUDATE	Rich in protein (fibrinogen) causes the exudates to close due to the formation of fibrin ☞ Example: pleurisy—exudates on the surface of lung caused by pneumonia
PURULENT EXUDATE (SUPPURATION)	Contains many white blood cells—neutrophils (polymorphonuclear leukocytes, or PMNs) ☞ Example: pus
EDEMA	Exudate escapes from the blood vessels into the tissues
FISTULA	Exudate drains, forming a passage through the tissue
MARGINATION	Movement of white blood cells to the periphery of the venule
ADHESION (PAVEMENTING)	White blood cells become sticky and adhere to walls of blood vessels
EMIGRATION	Following adhesion the white blood cells emigrate from the blood vessels with plasma fluids and enter the injured tissue due to chemotactic factors

CHEMOTAXIS	Moving of white blood cells toward the target area for the body's defense against the injury
OPSONIZATION	Serum factors called opsonins help neutrophils recognize and attach to the pathogens ☛ Enhance phagocytosis
PHAGOCYTOSIS	Ingesting of the foreign substance

WHITE BLOOD CELLS INVOLVED IN ACUTE INFLAMMATORY RESPONSE (LEUKOCYTES)

NEUTROPHIL (POLY-MORPHONUCLEAR LEUKOCYTE, PMN) MONOCYTE (MACROPHAGE)	• First cell to emigrate to site of injury • Primary cell • Main goal is to kill infectious agent • Second cell involved in inflammation • Removes dead and dying cells to help pave the way for fibroblasts to heal wounds
EOSINOPHIL AND MAST CELL	Involved in inflammation and immunity

CHRONIC INFLAMMATION

- Results from injury that persists for weeks or months
- Cells involved are lymphocytes, plasma cells, and macrophages
- Repair is simultaneous as chronic inflammation proceeds, but cannot be complete until source of injury is removed

GRANULOMATOUS INFLAMMATION	Microscopic grouping of macrophages form granulomas

CHEMICAL MEDIATORS OF INFLAMMATION
Chemical agents called chemical mediators that start or amplify the inflammatory response control inflammation; they can be exogenous or endogenous

HISTAMINE	• Vasoactive amine • Initiates the early phases of acute inflammation, and mediates the increased vascular permeability

KININ SYSTEM	• Mediate inflammation by causing increased permeability of the venules • Limited to early phases of inflammation • Bradykinin produces pain
CLOTTING MECHANISM	• Functions to clot blood • Mediates inflammation • Important in repair process
COMPLEMENT SYSTEM	• Mediates vascular response (releases histamine) • Provides phagocytic leukocytes (chemotaxis) • Opsonizing targets of phagocytic cells
PROSTAGLANDINS	Increases vasodilatation, permeability, pain, redness

Regeneration and Repair

REPAIR **Body's attempt to restore injured tissues by replacing damaged cells with new cells; usually completed within 2 weeks**	
DAY OF INJURY	Clot forms (locally produced fibrin) as blood flows to site of injury
ONE DAY FOLLOWING INJURY	• Neutrophils emigrate to injured tissues • Phagocytosis of foreign substances
TWO DAYS FOLLOWING INJURY	• Monocytes emigrate to injured tissues • Macrophages continue phagocytosis • Neutrophils reduce in number as chronic inflammation proceeds • Fibroblasts increase in connective tissue • Granulation tissue forms in connective tissue
SEVEN DAYS FOLLOWING INJURY	Fibrin is digested by tissue enzymes and initial repair is completed
TWO WEEKS FOLLOWING INJURY	• Granulation tissue forms scar tissue • Increased number of collagen fibers and decreased vascularity

TYPES OF REPAIR

HEALING BY PRIMARY INTENTION	• Healing of tissue with little loss of tissue • Small clot with little granulation tissue • Example: surgical incision
HEALING BY SECONDARY INTENTION	• Injury with loss of tissue • Large clot forms slowly resulting in increased formation of granulation tissue • Causes extensive scarring of skin

➤ ORAL PATHOLOGY

Oral Lesions: Normal Variations

FORDYCE'S GRANULES

Description: Clusters of ectopic sebaceous glands
Location: Usually on buccal mucosal or vermilion border of the lips, commonly bilateral
Clinical manifestation: Yellow lobules
TX: No treatment needed

Figure 5-2

TORI

Description: Overgrowth of bone
• Grow gradually
• Inherited—generally in women
• Various shapes and sizes

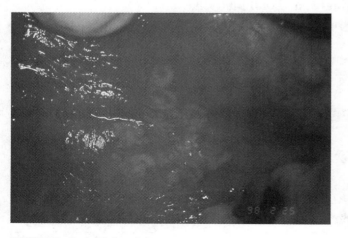

FIGURE 5-2 Fordyce's Granules

PALATAL TORI	*Location:* At midline of palate *Clinical manifestations:* Asymptomatic *TX:* No treatment needed
MANDIBULAR TORI	*Location:* on the lingual aspect of the mandible above the mylohyoid ridge, usually bilateral *TX:* No treatment needed

LINEA ALBA

Description: Predominate in patients with clenching or bruxing habit
Location: Buccal mucosa at occlusal plane, usually bilateral
Clinical manifestations: White line that extends from anterior buccal mucosal to posterior buccal mucosa
TX: No treatment needed

LEUKOEDEMA

Description: Benign anomaly common in African Americans caused by thickening of epithelium
Location: Buccal mucosal, occurs bilaterally
Clinical manifestations: Gray/white film that causes the buccal mucosal to look opaque
TX: No treatment needed

MELANIN PIGMENTATION

Description: Prominent in dark-skinned individuals
Location: On gingiva and oral mucosal
Clinical manifestations: Melanin pigment on gingiva and oral mucosa
TX: No treatment needed

LINGUAL VARICOSITIES

Description: Prominent lingual veins commonly seen in individuals over 60 years
Location: On ventral and lateral surfaces of the tongue
Clinical manifestations: Red to purple vessels
TX: No treatment needed

LINGUAL THYROID NODULE

Description: Thyroid tissue remnant during developmental stages; may be the only functioning thyroid tissue
Location: On tongue posterior to circumvallate papillae
Clinical manifestations: Nodular mass
TX: Must do thyroid testing before removal

FISSURED TONGUE

Description: Cause is unknown; may be due to vitamin deficiency
Location: Dorsal of tongue
Clinical manifestations: Deep fissures or grooves
TX: Instruct patient to keep clean to prevent irritation

MEDIAN RHOMBOID GLOSSITIS

Description: Possibly caused by fungal infection from *Candida albicans*
Location: In midline of dorsal tongue
Clinical manifestations: Raised erythematous rhomboid-shaped area of papillary atrophy
TX: No treatment needed

GEOGRAPHIC TONGUE

Description: Most likely stress related
Location: Dorsal and lateral borders of tongue
Clinical manifestations: Depapillated erythematous patches (map-like appearance) with white boarders
TX: No treatment needed
Figure 5-3

HAIRY TONGUE

Description: Elongation of filiform papillae
Location: Dorsal of tongue
Clinical manifestations: White, black, yellow or brown filiform papillae due to chromogenic bacteria, smoking, food, and some drugs
☛ Most notably caused by antacids, oxygenating rinses, corticosteroids, and systemic antibiotics
TX: Brush tongue

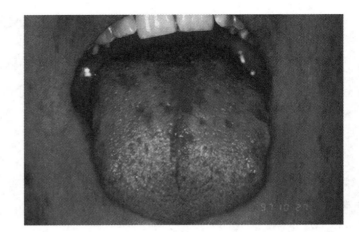

FIGURE 5-3 Geographic Tongue

Lesions Caused by Physical and Chemical Injuries

INJURIES TO THE TEETH	
ATTRITION	*Description:* Normal wearing away of tooth structure as an individual ages and is accelerated by bruxism (grinding and clenching the teeth for nonfunctional purposes) *Location:* Occlusal and incisal surfaces *Clinical manifestations:* Wear facets, hypertrophy of masseter muscle and muscle fatigue, TMJ sensitivity *TX:* Fabrication of night guard
ABRASION	*Description:* Pathologic wearing away of tooth structure from mechanical habits (repetitive habit or improper tooth brushing technique) *Location:* At site of wear, varies upon cause *Clinical manifestation:* Loss of tooth structure *TX:* Inform patient of cause and correct habit; restorative work may be needed to repair defect
EROSION	*Description:* Chemical action that causes loss of tooth structure (bulimia, sucking on lemons)

Location: Varies upon cause
Clinical manifestation: Involves several teeth and gives a smooth, polished appearance
TX: Prevention, and restorative work as needed
Figure 5-4

ABFRACTION	*Description:* Wedge-shaped lesions of teeth caused by malocclusion, biomechanical forces *Location:* At the cervical areas of teeth *Clinical manifestations:* Wedge-shaped notches *TX:* Restoration or no treatment needed **Figure 5-5**

INJURIES TO SOFT TISSUE

ASPIRIN BURNS	*Description:* chemical exposure to soft tissue causing necrosis of the oral mucosal; aspirin (acetylsalicylic acid) placement directly on painful tooth causes tissue to become necrotic and white *Location:* Site of aspirin placement *Clinical manifestations:* Necrotic white painful ulcer *TX:* Treatment of painful tooth, and medication for ulcer

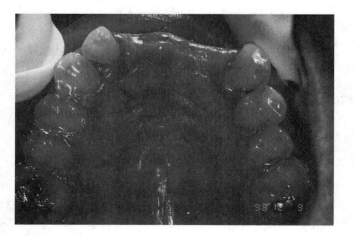

FIGURE 5-4 Erosion

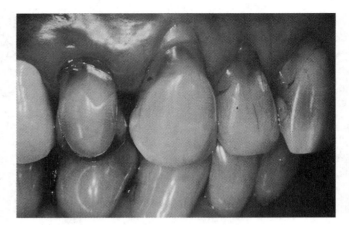

FIGURE 5-5 Abfraction

ELECTRICAL BURNS	*Description:* Often caused by young children biting on live electric cord *Location:* Area of contact *Clinical manifestations:* Destruction of tissue *TX:* Repair damaged tissue
HEMATOMA	*Description:* Results from an accumulation of blood within the tissue due to trauma *Location:* Area of trauma on buccal/labial mucosa *Clinical manifestation:* Red/purple mass, and may vary in size *TX:* No treatment required, will resolve with time ⚬─ Commonly induced following IA and PSA injections
NICOTINE STOMATITIS	*Description:* Benign lesion associated with smoking *Location:* On the hard palate *Clinical manifestations:* Characterized by raised ret dots at opening of minor salivary glands *TX:* Eliminate cause (smoking)

TOBACCO CHEWER'S LESION	*Description:* Lesion in area where chewing tobacco is placed; long-term use will increase risk of squamous cell carcinoma *Location:* Site where tobacco is placed *Clinical manifestations:* Wrinkled white tissue *TX:* Eliminate cause (chewing tobacco)
TRAUMATIC ULCER	*Description:* Occurs from trauma such as: biting of the cheek, lip, or tongue, irritation from partial or complete denture, injury from food or sharp edges *Location:* At site of trauma *Clinical manifestations:* Ulceration at site of trauma *TX:* None if lesion heals within 7 to 14 days; biopsy recommended after 14 days
AMALGAM TATTOO	*Description:* Caused by amalgam particles embedded into the tissues secondary to dental restorative treatment *Location:* Commonly found on the gingiva *Clinical manifestations:* Bluish-gray flat lesion *Radiographic manifestations:* Particles may be seen radiographically *TX:* No treatment required **Figure 5-6**
SOLAR CHEILITIS	*Description:* Degeneration of the tissue of the lips due to excessive sun exposure; may increase risk of basal cell carcinoma or squamous cell carcinoma *Location:* Lips, with lower lip usually more involved *Clinical manifestations:* Color of vermilion border appears pale pinkish and mottled *TX:* No treatment required

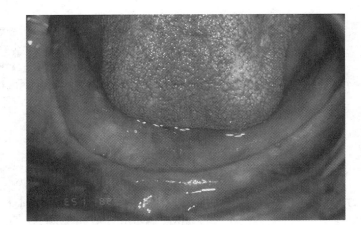

FIGURE 5-6 Amalgam Tattoo

MUCOCELE	*Description:* Forms from severed salivary gland →mucous salivary gland secretion spills into adjacent connective tissue→ granulation tissue forms cyst-like structure *Location:* Lower lip is most common site *Clinical manifestations:* May appear bluish if near the surface, and the color of mucosal if deeper in the tissue *TX:* Excision • Not a true cyst because space is not lined by epithelium **Figure 5-7**
RANULA	*Description:* Obstruction of salivary duct caused by sialolith or local trauma *Location:* Associated with sublingual and

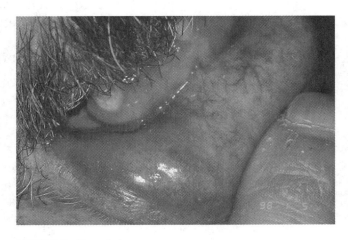

FIGURE 5-7 Mucocele

submandibular glands on the floor of the mouth
Clinical manifestations: Swelling
TX: Surgery to remove cause of obstruction
Figure 5-8

SIALOLITH	*Description:* Salivary gland stone *Location:* Occurs in both major and minor salivary glands *Clinical manifestations:* Gland obstructure, nodule *Radiographic manifestations:* Radio-opaque structure in area of salivary gland *TX:* Surgery to remove stone

Reactive Connective Tissue Hyperplasia

PYOGENIC GRANULOMA

Description: Proliferation of connective tissue; not pus producing
Location: Gingiva most common area
Clinical manifestations: Ulcerated deep red-purple lesion that bleeds easily
TX: Surgical removal if not resolved
☛ Called pregnancy tumor

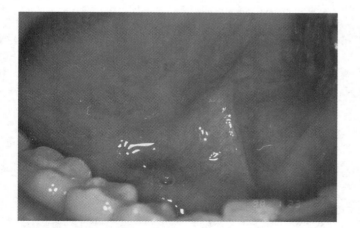

FIGURE 5-8 Ranula

GIANT CELL GRANULOMA

Description: Many multinucleated giant cells originate from periodontal ligament and is a response to injury
Location: Occurs only in jaw

PERIPHERAL GIANT CELL GRANULOMA	*Description:* Reactive hyperplasia as a result of local irritating factors *Location:* Occurs exclusively on gingiva or alveolar process anterior to molars *Clinical manifestations:* Resembles pyogenic granuloma *TX:* Surgical excision **Figure 5-9**
CENTRAL GIANT CELL GRANULOMA	*Description:* Primarily in children and young adults *Location:* Occurs within the bone of the maxilla or mandible and primarily in anterior sextants *Clinical manifestations:* Asymptomatic; divergence of the roots or teeth adjacent to lesion is common; firm to palpation *Radiographic manifestations:* Most are discovered on routine radiographs, produces radiolucency in the bone *TX:* Surgical removal

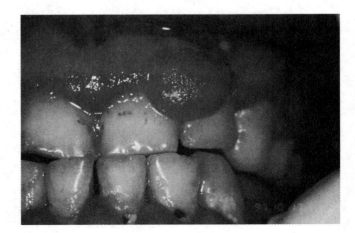

FIGURE 5-9 Peripheral Giant Cell Granuloma

EPULIS FISSURATUM

Description: Denture-induced hyperplasia caused from ill-fitting denture
Location: Along denture boarder
Clinical manifestations: Elongated folds of tissue along denture flange
TX: Surgical removal of excess tissue, new denture
Figure 5-10

PAPILLARY HYPERPLASIA

Description: Caused by removable full or partial dentures or orthodontic appliances
Location: On palate
Clinical manifestations: Erythematous papillary projections (cobblestone appearance)
TX: Surgical removal of tissue, new appliance; remove denture at night

CHRONIC HYPERPLASTIC PULPITIS (PULP POLYP)

Description: Excessive proliferation of chronically inflamed pulp tissue in children and young adults
Location: Occurs in teeth with large, open carious lesions; occurs in primary or permanent molars
Clinical manifestations: Red granulation tissue protruding from the pulp chamber fills the cavity of the tooth
TX: Extraction of tooth or endodontic treatment

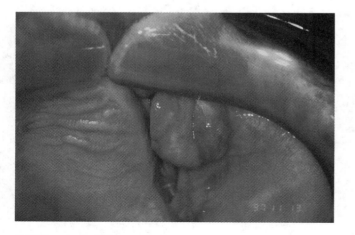

FIGURE 5-10 Epulis Fissuratum

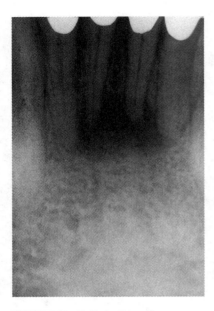

FIGURE 5-11   Radicular Cyst

Inflammatory Periapical Lesions

PERIAPICAL ABSCESS

Description: Chronic periapical inflammation with purulent exudate
Location: Root of tooth
Clinical manifestations: Radiolucency at apacies
TX: Drainage

PERIAPICAL GRANULOMA

Description: Localized mass of chronic granulation tissue
Location: Apex of nonvital root
Clinical manifestations: Asymptomatic
Radiographic manifestation: Radiolucency in well-circumscribed area
TX: Root canal/extraction

RADICULAR CYST (PERIAPICAL CYST)

Description: True cyst—pathologic cavity lined by epithelium
Location: Root of nonvital tooth
Clinical manifestations: Most are asymptomatic
Radiographic manifestations: Well-circumscribed radiolucency attached to the root of the tooth
TX: Root canal, extraction, apicoectomy
☛ Most common cyst in oral cavity
Figures 5-11 and 5-12

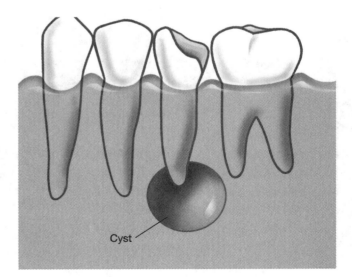

Cyst

FIGURE 5-12   Radicular Cyst

RESORPTION OF TEETH

EXTERNAL RESORPTION	*Description:* Caused by chronic inflammation or periapical granuloma *Location:* Roots of primary or permanent teeth *Clinical manifestations:* Asymptomatic *Radiographic manifestations:* Blunting of root apex, severe loss of structure *TX:* Removal of cause
INTERNAL RESORPTION	*Description:* Inflammatory response in the pulp *Location:* In root or crown of tooth *Clinical manifestations:* If coronal tooth involved → pinkish area in crown *Radiographic manifestations:* If root involvement → radiolucent area in central portion of tooth *TX:* Root canal with early diagnosis; extraction if process extends to hard tissue

ALVEOLAR OSTEITIS (DRY SOCKET)

Description: Post-op complication of an extraction; blood clot breaks down prior to healing
Location: Site of extraction
Clinical manifestations: Tooth socket appears empty, bone exposed, pain, and bad odor
TX: Irrigation, medicated dressing

Immunologic Pathology

APTHOUS ULCERS (CANKER SORES OR APTHOUS STOMATITIS)

Description:
- Painful ulcerations of unknown cause
- Recur in episodes
- Three forms: minor, major, and herpetiform; trauma is precipitating factor
- ☛ Most common ulcers in oral cavity

MINOR APHTHOUS ULCERS	*Description:* Most common *Location:* Moveable mucosal, labial, or buccal mucosal, and may extend to gingiva, tongue, and soft palate and oropharynx *Clinical manifestations:* Painful round or oval yellowish-white lesion approximately 1 cm in diameter; heals within 7–10 days *TX:* Topical corticosteroids, topical anesthetics for pain
MAJOR APTHOUS ULCERS	*Description:* Sutton's disease, periadenitis mucosal necrotica recurrens; larger and deeper than minor aphthous ulcers; reported to occur in patients with human immunodeficiency virus (HIV) infection *Location:* Moveable mucosal often in posterior part of the mouth; take several weeks to heal and cause scarring *Clinical manifestations:* Larger than 1 cm in diameter and deeper than minor apthous *TX:* Biopsy for diagnosis, topical or systemic corticosteroids, topical anesthetics for pain

HERPETIFORM APTHOUS ULCERS

Description: Acute infection resemble herpes simplex virus
Location: Anywhere in the oral cavity
Clinical manifestations: Multiple painful, tiny 1–2 mm ulcers often appear in groups
TX: Topical corticosteroids, liquid tetracycline, topical anesthetics for pain

URTICARIA AND ANGIOEDEMA
Similar lesions

URTICARIA (HIVES)	*Description:* Type I hypersensitivity *Location:* Skin *Clinical manifestations:* Multiple areas of swelling characterized by erythema and pruritus (itching) *TX:* Identify and remove cause; antihistamines

ANGIOEDEMA	*Description:* Type I hypersensitivity *Location:* Skin or mucosal *Clinical manifestations:* Diffuse swelling of tissue, no itching *TX:* Identify and remove cause, antihistamines

DERMATITIS

Description: Type IV hypersensitivity, caused by direct contact with an allergen
Location: Skin in direct contact with allergen
Clinical manifestations: Swelling, erythema, forms vesicles that will turn to crusty, scaly, white appearance
TX: Identify and remove cause, topical and systemic corticosteroids

FIXED DRUG ERUPTIONS

Description: Type III hypersensitivity, lesions that appear at same site when a drug is introduced and disappear when drug is discontinued
Location: Skin at same site each time
Clinical manifestations: Single or multiple raised reddish patches of macules on the skin that may cause pain and pruritis
TX: Identify drug and discontinue

ERYTHEMA MULTIFORME

Description: Acute explosive onset that affects the skin and mucous membranes. Most frequent in young adult males
☛ Characteristic skin lesion is "bull's eye lesion"
Location: Skin and mucous membranes
Clinical manifestations: Variety of skin lesions: macules, plaques, and bullae; oral cavity lesions are usually ulcers, crusted and bleeding lips are often seen
TX: Topical or systemic corticosteroids

LICHEN PLANUS

Description: Benign, chronic disease; characteristic pattern of interconnecting lines called striae; many drugs and chemicals may produce lesion
Location: Buccal mucosal most common, tongue, lips, floor of the mouth, and gingiva
Clinical manifestations: Interconnecting white lines called "Wickham's striae"
TX: No treatment needed

REITER'S SYNDROME

Description: Comprises a triad of arthritis, urethritis, and conjunctivitis
Location: Skin, oral mucosal, joints, conjunctiva urethra
Clinical manifestations: Arthritis, urethrites, conjunctivitis, skin and mucous membrane lesions; oral lesions are similar to aphthous ulcers, geographic tongue, erythematous lesions
TX: Aspirin, nonsteroidal anti-inflammatory drugs

Autoimmune Diseases

SJOGREN'S SYNDROME

Description: Autoimmune disease that affects the salivary and lacrimal glands, resulting in a decrease in the amount of saliva and tears
Location: Oral cavity and eyes, major and minor salivary glands
Clinical manifestations: Xerostomia → erythematous mucosa, oral discomfort, cracked and dry lips, atrophy of filiform and fungiform papillae, bilateral parotid gland enlargement, decreased lacrimal flow
TX: Nonsteroidal anti-inflammatory agents, corticosteroids, saliva and tear substitutes, good oral hygiene

SYSTEMIC LUPUS ERYTHEMATOSUS

Description: Acute and chronic inflammatory auto immune disease—predominately in women
Location: Multiple involvement

Clinical manifestations: Skin lesions—erythematous rash is most common

•– Classic "butterfly" rash over bridge of nose

Erythematous lesions on fingertips

Radiographic manifestations:

TX: Anti-inflammatory and immunosuppressive agents

•– Antibiotic premedication prior to dental treatment may be necessary

PEMPHIGUS VULGARIS

Description: Severe progressive autoimmune disease that affects the skin and mucous membranes

Location: Skin and mucous membranes

Clinical manifestations: Oral lesions—painful ulcers, vesicles, bullae

Bullae rupture → epithelium remains as gray membrane

•– Positive Nikolsky's sign

Skin lesions—erythema, vesicles, bullae, erosions, ulcers

TX: Corticosteroids, immunosuppresive drugs

Infectious Diseases: Bacterial Infections

TUBERCULOSIS

Description: Infectious chronic granutomatous disease caused by the organism *Mycobacterium tuberculosis*

Location: Lungs—bacteria may spread to other parts of the body; oral lesions are rare and occur on tongue and palate

Clinical manifestations: Oral lesions—painful, nonhealing ulcers

TX: Anti-tuberculosis agents

ACTINOMYCOSIS

Description: Infection caused by filamentous bacterium called *Actinomyces israelii*

Location: Skin and oral mucosa

Clinical manifestations: Abscesses that drain bright yellow grains called "sulfur granules"

TX: Antibiotics

SYPHILIS Description: Disease caused by spirochete *Treponema pallidum* transmitted from one person to another by direct contact, usually by sexual contact	
PRIMARY	*Location:* Oral lesions, mucous membranes *Clinical manifestations:* Chancre—highly infectious ⚷ Exhibits piled-up periphery *TX:* Antibiotics
SECONDARY	*Location:* Oral lesions, mucous membranes *Clinical manifestations:* Mucous patches—grayish-white plaques most infectious *TX:* Antibiotics
TERTIARY	*Tertiary*—Years after initial infection involve cardiovascular system and nervous system *Clinical manifestations:* Lesion called "gumma"—non-infectious *TX:* Antibiotics

ACUTE NECROTIZING ULCERATIVE GINGIVITIS (ANUG)

Description: Painful erythematous gingivitis, necrosis of the interdental papillae caused by fusiform bacillus and spirochete (*Borrelia cincentii*)
Location: Gingiva
Clinical manifestations: Gingiva is painful and erythematous with foul odor and metallic taste; cratering of interdental papilla
Systemic: Fever, cervical lymphadenopathy
TX: Antibiotics, debridement of necrotic tissues, good oral hygiene

PERICORONITIS

Description: Inflammation due to infection by bacteria of mucosal around crown of a partially erupted, impacted tooth; trauma to soft tissue flap (operculum) may also be a cause
Location: Tissue around partially erupted tooth
⚷ 3rd molar most common
Clinical manifestations: Swollen, erythematous tissue around partially erupted tooth
TX: Debridement, irrigation, antibiotics

ACUTE OSTEOMYELITIS

Description: Acute inflammation of bone and bone marrow
Location: Bone
Clinical manifestations: Jaw—result from periapical abscess
Radiographic manifestations: None
TX: Drainage, antibiotics

CHRONIC OSTEOMYELITIS

Description: Chronic inflammation of bone, perhaps from inadequate treated acute osteomyelitis
Location: Bone
Clinical manifestations: Painful swollen bone
Radiographic manifestations: Diffuse and irregular radiolucency that can eventually become radioopaque (chronic sclerosing osteomyelitis)
TX: Debridement/systemic antibiotics

Infectious Diseases: Fungal Infections

CANDIDIASIS

Description: Result of an overgrowth of yeast-like fungus *Candida albicans*
☞ Most common oral fungal infection

PSEUDOMEMBRANOUS CANDIDIASIS	*Location:* Oral mucosa *Clinical manifestations:* White curd-like material on mucosal surface, underlying mucosal is erythematous *TX:* Antifungal treatment
ERYTHEMATOUS CANDIDIASIS	*Location:* Oral mucosa *Clinical manifestations:* Erythematous painful mucosa, may be localized or generalized *TX:* Antifungal medication **Figure 5-13**
CHRONIC ATROPHIC CANDIDIASIS	*Location:* Palate and maxillary alveolar ridge *Clinical manifestations:* erythematous mucosa limited to mucosa covered by a full or partial denture *TX:* Antifungal agents ☞ Most common type affecting the mucosa, also known as denture stomatitis

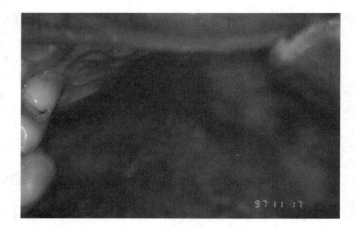

FIGURE 5-13   Erythematous Candidiasis

CHRONIC HYPER-PLASTIC CANDIDIASIS, CANDIDAL LEUKOPLA-KIA, HYPERTROPHIC CANDIDIASIS	*Location:* Oral mucosa *Clinical manifestations:* White lesions that do not wipe off *TX:* Antifungal agents
ANGULAR CHELITIS	*Description:* Candida organisms often cause angular cheilitis *Location:* Labial commissures *Clinical manifestations:* Erythema or fissures at labial commissures, frequently occurs with introral candidiasis *TX:* Antifungal agents
MEDIAN RHOMBOID GLOSSITIS	*Description:* Has been associated with candidiasis, and many lesions disappear with antifugal treatment; however, the response to antifungal agents is inconsistent and cause is unknown *Location:* Midline of the posterior dorsal tongue *Clinical manifestations:* Erythematous, rhombus-shaped flat to raised area *TX:* Antifungal agents

Infectious Diseases: Viral Infections

PAPILLOMAVIRUS INFECTION

VERRUCA VULGARIS	*Description:* Common wart; caused by papillomavirus; skin lesions are more common than oral lesions; may be trans-

	mitted from skin to oral mucosa *Location:* Intraoral—lips are most common *Clinical manifestations:* White, papillary, exophytic lesion *TX:* Surgical excision, lesions may recur
FOCAL EPITHELIAL HYPERPLASIA (HECK'S DISEASE)	*Description:* Disease caused by another human papillomavirus *Location:* Oral mucosa *Clinical manifestations:* Asymptomatic, multiple whitish–pale pink nodules *TX:* No treatment needed

HERPES SIMPLEX INFECTION

PRIMARY HERPETIC GINGIVOSTOMATITIS	*Description:* Caused by herpes simplex virus type 1, generally seen in children *Location:* Lips, gingiva, oral mucosa *Clinical manifestations:* Multiple small vesicles that form painful ulcers, swollen painful gingiva, fever, cervical lymphadenopathy *TX:* Lesions heal spontaneously in 1–2 weeks
RECURRENT HERPES SIMPLEX INFECTION	*Description:* Commonly seen on mucosa and in adults; persists in latent state; often occurs following stress, fever, fatigue, menstruation, sunlight *Location:* Common on vermilion border of the lips (herpes labialis), hard palate, and gingiva *Clinical Manifestations:* Tiny vesicles or ulcers that coalesce and form a single lesion *TX:* Lesions heal spontaneously in 1–2 weeks ☞ Herpetic Whitlow—herpes infection can cause painful infection of the fingers in dentists and dental hygienists

VARICELLA-ZOSTER VIRUS

CHICKEN POX	*Description:* Highly contagious disease mainly seen in children *Location:* Skin and mucous membranes *Clinical manifestations:* Vesicular and pustular eruptions *TX:* Self-limited disease
HERPES ZOSTER (SHINGLES)	*Description:* Occurs in adults, transmitted by contaminated droplets *Location:* Skin and mucous membranes *Clinical manifestations:* Unilateral painful vesicles along a sensory nerve *TX:* Antiviral agents, corticosteroids

COXSACKIEVIRUS

HERPANGINA	*Description:* Generally seen in young children and young adults *Location:* Soft palate *Clinical manifestations:* Vesicles, fever, malaise *TX:* Self-limited
HAND-FOOT-MOUTH DISEASE	*Description:* Commonly affects children under 5 years of age *Location:* Oral mucosa, skin—feet, hands, fingers *Clinical manifestations:* Vesicles in mouth *TX:* Self-limited

PARAMYXOVIRUS

MEASLES	*Description:* Highly contagious disease, causes systemic symptoms *Location:* Skin primarily, oral mucosa *Clinical manifestations:* Oral mucosa—Koplik's spots—erythematous macules with white, necrotic centers *TX:* Self-limited

MUMPS	*Description:* Most common in children *Location:* Salivary glands *Clinical manifestations:* Painful swelling of salivary glands *TX:* Self-limited

EPSTEIN-BARR

INFECTIOUS MONONUCLEOSIS	*Description:* Commonly occurs in adolescents and young adults *Location:* Systemic disease *Clinical manifestations:* Sore throat, fever, lymphadenopathy, malaise, fatigue, enlarged spleen *TX:* Self-limited disease
OTHER CONDITIONS	• Chronic fatigue • Burhett's lymphoma • Hairy leudoplakia

Developmental Soft Tissue Abnormalities

ANKYLOGLOSSIA

Description: Extensive adhesion of the tongue to the floor of the mouth
Location: Floor of the mouth/tongue
Clinical manifestations: Short lingual frenum
TX: Frenectomy

LINGUAL THYROID

Description: Small mass of thyroid tissue located on the tongue, resulting from failure of thyroid tissue to migrate from its developmental location
Location: Tongue
Clinical manifestations: Smooth nodular mass at the base of the tongue posterior to the circumvallate papillae near the midline
TX: Usually none, surgical removal if large

Developmental Cysts

ODONTOGENIC CYSTS Related to tooth development	
DENTIGEROUS CYST (ALSO CALLED OLLICULAR CYST)	*Description:* Forms around the crown of an unerupted or developing tooth; epithelial lining originates from the reduced enamel epithelium after the crown has completely formed and calcified *Location:* Crown of unerupted or impacted third molar (most common) *Clinical manifestations:* Can displace teeth if very large *Radiographic manifestations:* Well-defined, unilocular radiolunency around crown of unerupted or impacted teeth *TX:* Complete removal of cyst and involved tooth **Figure 5-14**
ERUPTION CYST	*Description:* Similar to dentigerous cyst *Location:* Soft tissue around the crown of an erupting tooth *Clinical manifestations:* Soft tissue around crown of an erupting tooth *TX:* No treatment needed—tooth erupts through cyst

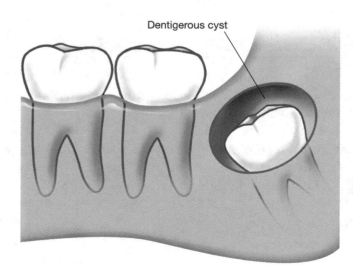

Dentigerous cyst

FIGURE 5-14 Dentigerous Cyst

PRIMORDIAL CYST	*Description:* Develops in place of a tooth; originates from remnants of enamel organ; patient history that indicates that a tooth was never present is an important diagnostic tool *Location:* Mandibular third molar area; most commonly develops in place of a tooth *Clinical manifestations:* Asymptomatic, commonly found in place of third molar or posterior to erupted third molar *Radiographic manifestations:* Well-defined, radiolucent lesion, unilocular or multilocular *TX:* Surgical removal of entire lesion **Figure 5-15**
ODONTOGENIC KERATOCYST	*Description:* Unique histologic appearance, recurring frequently; lumen is lined with epithelium 8–10 cell layers thick *Location:* Mandibular third molar region *Clinical manifestations:* Expansive lesion that can move teeth and resorb tooth *Radiographic manifestations:* Well-defined, multilocular, radiolucent unilocular lesions may also occur *TX:* Surgical excision and osseous curettage, high recurrance

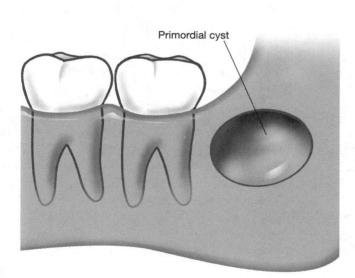

Primordial cyst

FIGURE 5-15 Primordial Cyst

LATERAL PERIO-DONTAL CYST	*Description:* Developmental *Location:* Lateral aspect of tooth usually on mandibular cuspid and premolar area *Clinical manifestations:* Asymptomatic *Radiographic manifestations:* Unilocular or multilocular radiolucent lesion located on lateral aspect of a tooth root *TX:* Surgical removal
GINGIVAL CYST	*Description:* Developmental *Location:* Soft tissue in mandibular cuspid and premolar area *Clinical manifestations:* Swelling of gingival papilla or alveolar mucosa *TX:* Surgical removal

NONODONTOGENIC CYSTS

NASOPALATINE CANAL CYST (INCISIVE CANAL CYST)	*Description:* Developmental, arises from epithelial remnants; commonly seen in adults; when in the papilla, called cyst of the palatine papilla *Location:* Nasopalatine canal or the incisive papilla *Clinical manifestations:* Asymptomatic, may have pink bulge near apecies and between roots of maxillary central incisors on the lingual surface *Radiographic manifestations:* Well-circumscribed radiolucency between maxillary central incisors *TX:* Surgical removal
MEDIAN PALATINE CYST	*Description:* A more posterior form of a nasopalatine cyst *Location:* Midline of hard palate *Clinical manifestations:* Swelling at midline of hard palate if cyst is large *Radiographic manifestations:* Unilocular radiolucency *TX:* Surgical removal Figure 5-16

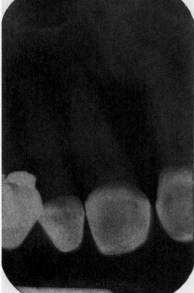

FIGURE 5-16 Median Palatine Cyst

GLOBULOMAXILLARY CYST	*Description:* Etiology unknown *Location:* Between the roots of the maxillary lateral incisor and cuspid *Clinical manifestations:* Asymptomatic—if a large enough divergence of the roots can result *Radiographic manifestations:* Well-defined pear-shaped radiolucency *TX:* Surgical removal
NASOLABIAL CYST	*Description:* Soft tissue cyst with no alveolar bone involvement; etiology unknown *Location:* Soft tissue of face at nasolabial fold *Clinical manifestations:* Swelling in nasolabial fold *TX:* Surgical removal
EPIDERMAL CYST	*Description:* Raised nodule, resembles the epithelium of skin *Location:* Skin of the face or neck *Clinical Manifestations:* Firm moveable swelling *TX:* Surgical removal
LYMPHOEPITHELIAL CYST	*Description:* Developmental cyst that arises from epithelium trapped in a lymph node during development *Location:* Major salivary glands—floor of mouth and lateral border of tongue are most common *Clinical Manifestations:* Intraoral—pinkish-yellow, raised nodule *TX:* Surgical removal

Developmental Abnormalities of the Number of Teeth

ANODONTIA

Description: Congenital lack of teeth
Location: Mandibular and maxillary arches
Clinical manifestations: Absence of all primary and permanent dentition
Radiographic manifestations: All teeth absent
TX: Prosthetic replacement

HYPODONTIA

Description: Lack of one or more teeth
Location: Any tooth in the dentition, maxillary and mandibular third molars, maxillary lateral incisors, and mandibular second premolars are most common
Clinical manifestations: Absence of one or more teeth
Radiographic manifestations: Absence of one or more teeth
TX: Prosthetic replacement, orthodontic evaluation

SUPERNUMERARY

Description: Extra teeth
Location: Maxillary and mandibular arches, maxillary most common
Clinical manifestations: One or more extra teeth, usually smaller than normal
Radiographic manifestations: One or more extra teeth
TX: Extraction
☛ Mesodens—most common supernumerary tooth located between maxillary central incisors
☛ Distomolar—second most common supernumerary tooth distal to third molar
Figure 5-17

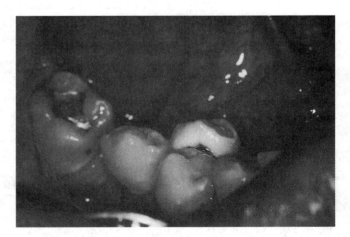

FIGURE 5-17 Supranumerary Teeth

Developmental Abnormalities in the Size of Teeth

MICRODONTIA

Description: Developmental, one or more teeth are smaller than normal
Location: Maxillary lateral incisors (peg lateral) is most common, maxillary third molars
Clinical manifestations: Tooth is smaller than normal
Radiographic manifestations: Tooth is smaller than normal
TX: Can restore tooth to resemble normal tooth

MACRODONTIA

Description: Uncommon developmental anomaly, teeth are larger than normal
Location: Any tooth
Clinical manifestations: Tooth is larger than normal
Radiographic manifestations: Tooth is larger than normal
TX: No treatment indicated

Developmental Abnormalities in the Shape of Teeth

GEMINATION

Description: Incomplete formation of two teeth, paired
Location: Primary teeth more common, anterior teeth are more commonly affected
Clinical manifestations: Large crown, appears bifed
Radiographic manifestations: Appears as single root with two crowns joined together
TX: Aesthetic problem, prosthetic treatment
☞ Gemination = neighboring tooth is present
Figure 5-18

FUSION

Description: Union of two normally separated tooth germs, can be complete or incomplete
Location: Primary teeth more common, anterior region, incisors most common
Clinical manifestations: Adjacent teeth appear fused, large crown
Radiographic manifestations: Large crown with separate fused roots
TX: Aesthetic and occlusal problems, prosthetic treatment
☞ Fused = neighboring tooth is lacking

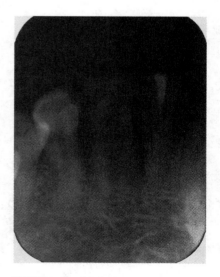

FIGURE 5-18 Gemination

CONCRESCENCE

Description: Two adjacent teeth are united by cementum only; may be caused by crowding
Location: Maxillary molars most common, adjacent supernumerary teeth, erupted, unerupted, or impacted teeth
Clinical manifestations: Cannot see clinically
Radiographic manifestations: Roots of adjacent teeth appear connected
TX: No treatment indicated, extraction of involved teeth is difficult

DILACERATION

Description: Abnormal curve or angle in the crown or root of a tooth
Location: Any tooth
Clinical manifestations: Cannot see clinically
Radiographic manifestations: Sharp bend in root of tooth
TX: No treatment required, extraction or endodontic therapy is difficult

ENAMEL PEARL

Description: Small spherical enamel projection located on a root surface
Location: Commonly found on maxillary molars, attached to cementum near the root bifurcation or trifurcation
Clinical manifestations: Cannot see clinically
Radiographic manifestations: Small sphere of enamel
TX: No treatment indicated

TALON CUSP

Description: Accessory cusp
Location: Cingulum of maxillary or mandibular permanent incisor
Clinical manifestations: Cusp that resembles an eagle's talon
Radiographic manifestations: Increased radiopacity
TX: Removal of talon cusp if it interferes with occlusion

TAURODONTISM

Description: Elongated, large pulp chambers and short roots
⚷ "Bull-like" teeth
Location: Molars of deciduous and permanent dentitions

Clinical manifestations: Normal crown
Radiographic manifestations: Abnormally short roots, pulp chamber is large and elongated
TX: No treatment indicated

DENS IN DENTE

Description: Tooth within a tooth
Location: Coronal third of the tooth, single tooth, anterior incisors most common (maxillary lateral most frequent and often peg-shaped)
Clinical manifestations: Normal shape or malformed crown with deep pit or crevice in area of cingulum, peg-shaped
Radiographic manifestations: Tooth-like structure appears within tooth
TX: Vital tooth—prophylactic restoration; nonvital tooth—endodontic treatment

Developmental Abnormalities of Tooth Structure

ENAMEL HYPOPLASIA

FEBRILE ILLNESS OR VITAMIN DEFICIENCY	*Description:* Serious disease such as measles, chicken pox, scarlet fever, or vitamin deficiency (vitamins A, C, and D) that occur during tooth development cause hypoplasia *Location:* Permanent central incisors, laterals, cuspids, first molars *Clinical manifestations:* Pitting of the enamel, one or more rows of deep pits and stains *TX:* Restorations for appearance
LOCAL INFECTION OR TRAUMA	*Description:* Occurs from infection of a deciduous tooth *Location:* Single tooth referred to as "Turner's tooth"; permanent maxillary incisor and mandibular premolars *Clinical manifestations:* Yellow to brown enamel, or severe pitting and deformity *Radiographic manifestations:* Can be identified before eruption *TX:* Restorations for appearance or improved function

FLUORIDE INGESTION	*Description:* Occurs as a result of large ingestion of concentrated fluoride *Location:* All permanent teeth *Clinical manifestations:* Mottled (irregular discoloration of enamel) discoloration of enamel *TX:* Aesthetic—Bleaching, bonding, composites, porcelain veneers, crowns
RESULT FROM CONGENITAL SYPHILIS	*Description:* Caused by congenital syphilis *Clinical manifestations:* Hutchinson's incisors—screwdriver shaped incisors; mulberry molars—berry-like cusp appearance *Location:* Permanent incisors and molars **Figure 5-19**

ENAMEL HYPOCALCIFICATION

Description: Developmental disturbance during maturation of enamel matrix
Location: Any tooth, usually middle third of crown
Clinical Manifestations: Localized chalky white spot
TX: Aesthetic, bleaching, composites, veneers, crowns

REGIONAL ODONTO-DYSPLASIA (GHOST TEETH)	*Description:* Teeth exhibit reduction of radiodensity, ghost-like appearance, very thin enamel and dentin, teeth are nonfunctional *Location:* Several teeth in a quadrant, especially maxillary primary or permanent

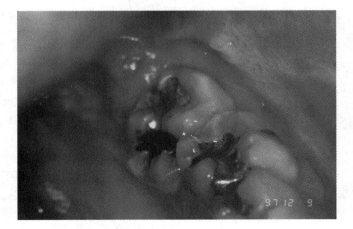

FIGURE 5-19   Mulberry Molar

Clinical manifestations: No eruption or incomplete eruption
Radiographic manifestations: Thin enamel or no enamel, large pulp chambers, reduced radiodensity
TX: Extraction

Developmental Abnormalities of Tooth Eruption

IMPACTED AND EMBEDDED TEETH

Description: Impacted—physical obstruction causes teeth not to erupt; embedded—teeth do not erupt from lack of eruptive force
Location: Most common—maxillary and mandibular third molars, maxillary cuspids
Clinical manifestations: Uneruptive teeth
Radiographic manifestations: Impacted teeth surrounded by bone
TX: Surgical removal

ANKYLOSED TEETH

Description: Deciduous teeth—bone is fused to cementum or dentin, preventing exfoliation
Location: Deciduous molars are most common
Clinical manifestations: Prevents eruption of permanent tooth or tooth erupts adjacent to ankylosed tooth
Radiographic manifestations: PDL space is lacking
TX: Extraction

Epithelial Tumors

TUMORS OF SQUAMOUS EPITHELIUM

PAPILLOMA

Description: Benign tumor
Location: Soft palate, tongue
Clinical manifestations: Small exophytic pedunculated growth composed of numerous projections that may be white or normal mucosal color
☛ "Cauliflower-like" appearance
TX: Surgical excision
Figure 5-20

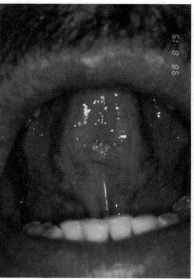

FIGURE 5-20 Papilloma

PREMALIGNANT LESIONS	
LEUKOPLAKIA	*Description:* Specific cause of lesion is unknown *Location:* Anywhere in oral cavity *Clinical manifestations:* White plaque-like lesion that cannot be rubbed off *TX:* Dependent upon histologic diagnosis
ERYTHROPLAKIA	*Description:* Describes oral mucosa that appears as a smooth, red patch; less common than leukoplakia *Location:* Anywhere in oral cavity *Clinical manifestations:* Smooth, red patch or a granular, red, and velvety patch; can also be a mixture of red and white areas called speckled leukoplakia *TX:* Dependent upon histologic diagnosis
EPITHELIAL DYSPLASIA	*Description:* Premalignant condition, cellular changes can revert to normal if stimulus is removed. *Location:* Floor of mouth, tongue, mucosa *Clinical manifestations:* Leukoplakia, erythroplakia, or speckled leukoplakia *TX:* Surgical excision ☛ Severe dysplasia involving full thickness of epithelium is called carcinoma in situ

SQUAMOUS CELL CARCINOMA	
SQUAMOUS CELL CARCINOMA, OR EPIDERMOID CARCINOMA	*Description:* Malignant tumor that can infiltrate adjacent tissues and metastasize to distant sites; invasion of tumor cells through epithelial basement membrane into underlying connective tissue *Location:* Most common on floor of mouth, tongue, lips *Clinical manifestations:* Exophytic ulcerative mass, leukoplakia, erythroplakia, speckled leukoplakia *TX:* Surgical excision, radiation therapy, chemotherapy ☛ Most common primary malignancy of the oral cavity

VERRUCOUS CARCINOMA	*Description:* Neoplastic; better prognosis than other squamous cell carcinomas *Location:* Most common vestibule, buccal mucosa *Clinical manifestations:* Slow-growing exophytic tumor with a pebbly, white, and red surface with papillary projections *TX:* Surgical excision
BASAL CELL CARCINOMA	*Description:* Malignant skin tumor associated with sun exposure *Location:* Skin and face *Clinical Manifestations:* Nonhealing ulcer characterized by rolled borders, does not occur in the oral cavity *TX:* Surgical excision, refer to dermatologist

Salivary Gland Tumors

PLEOMORPHIC ADENOMA (BENIGN MIXED TUMOR)

Description: Benign tumor that is encapsulated with a mixture of both epithelium and connective tissue.
Location: Extraoral—parotid gland; intraoral—palate, can occur wherever salivary gland tissue is present
Clinical manifestations: Slowly enlarging, nonulcerated, painless, dome-shaped mass
TX: Surgical removal
☛ Most common salivary gland neoplasm

MONOMORPHIC ADENOMA

Description: Benign encapsulated salivary gland tumor composed of a uniform pattern or epithelial cells; do not have connective tissue
Location: Most common in the upper lip, can occur anywhere salivary gland tissue is present
Clinical manifestations: Smooth-surfaced mass
TX: Surgical excision

WARTHIN'S TUMOR	*Description:* Monomorphic adenoma with two types of tissue: epithelial and lyphoid *Location:* Parotid gland often bilaterally and predominantly in adult men *Clinical manifestations:* Painless, soft, compressible mass *TX:* Surgical excision

ADENOID CYSTIC CARCINOMA

Description: Malignant tumor originating from either major or minor salivary gland tissue; microscopic appearance resembles Swiss cheese
Location: Extraoral—parotid gland; intraoral—palate
Clinical manifestations: Slow-growing ulcerative masses; pain is often present
TX: Surgical excision, radiation treatment

MUCOEPIDERMOID CARCINOMA

Description: Malignant salivary gland tumor; epidermoid cells—unencapsulated tumor with a combination of mucous cells and squamous-like epithelial cells
Location: Parotid gland—most common of major salivary glands; palate—most common of minor salivary glands
Clinical manifestations: Slow-growing masses
Radiographic manifestations: Occur occasionally intra-osseous and appear as unilocular or multilocular radiolucency
TX: Surgical excision

Odontogenic Tumors

EPITHELIAL ODONTOGENIC TUMORS

AMELOBLASTOMA	*Description:* Slow-growing aggressive tumor, encapsulated and infiltrates into surrounding tissue *Location:* Mandible more common; also maxilla *Clinical manifestations:* Slow-growing expansion of bone, asymptomatic

Radiographic manifestations: Multilocular honeycombed radiolucency
TX: Complete surgical removal

MESENCHYMAL ODONTOGENIC TUMORS

ODONTOGENIC MYXOMA	*Description:* Benign nonencapsulated infiltrating tumor, often occurs in young people 10–29 years of age *Location:* Mandible more common than maxilla *Clinical manifestations:* Asymptomatic, expansion of bone *Radiographic manifestations:* Multilocular, honeycombed radiolucency *TX:* Surgical excision
CEMENTIFYING AND OSSIFYING FIBROMA	*Description:* Benign, well-circumscribed tumor of fibrous connective tissue and rounded calcifications resembling cementum *Location:* Mandible most common *Clinical manifestations:* Asymptomatic expansion, facial asymmetry *Radiographic manifestations:* Well-defined and varies from radiolucent to radiopaque, depending on amount of calcified tissue *TX:* Surgical excision
BENIGN CEMENTO-BLASTOMA	*Description:* Cementum-producing lesion fused to the root of the tooth *Location:* Mandibular molars and premolars most common *Clinical manifestations:* Pain and localized expansion *Radiographic manifestations:* Well-defined radiopaque mass in continuity with the root; mass is surrounded by radiolucent halo *TX:* Enucleation of the tumor, removal of involved tooth

PERIAPICAL CEMENTO-OSSEOUS DYSPLASIA	*Description:* Common condition that affects periapical bone, not premalignant and is termed "dysplasia" to refer to its disordered production of cementum and bone *Location:* Anterior mandible of people over age 30 *Clinical manifestations:* Asymptomatic vital teeth *Radiographic manifestations:* Well circumscribed radiolucent lesions that mimic periapical disease, lesions become increasingly calcified with time *TX:* No treatment is indicated

MIXED ODONTOGENIC TUMORS

AMELOBLASTIC FIBROMA	*Description:* Benign, nonencapsulated tumor *Location:* Mandibular bicuspid-molar region most common *Clinical manifestations:* Asymptomatic swelling *Radiographic manifestations:* Well-defined or poorly defined unilocular or multilocular radiolucency *TX:* Surgical removal
ADENOMATOID ODONTOGENIC TUMOR	*Description:* Encapsulated benign tumor surrounded by dense fibrous connective tissue; duct-like structures are a distinctive feature, calcifications form in this tumor *Location:* 70% involve anterior maxilla and mandible *Clinical manifestations:* Asymptomatic swelling *Radiographic manifestations:* Well-defined radiolucency associated with an impacted tooth; radiopacities within the radiolucency *TX:* Enucleation

CALCIFYING ODON-TOGENIC CYST	*Description:* nonaggressive cystic lesion, ghost cell keratinization, which are round structures with clear centers *Location:* Maxilla and mandible *Radiographic manifestations:* Well-defined lesion, unilocular or multilocular radiolucency, calcifications can occur and are radiopaque within radiolucency *TX:* Enucleation
ODONTOMA	*Description:* Composed of mature enamel, dentin, cementum, and dental pulp; two types: compound and complex *Location:* Impacted or unerupted teeth, anterior maxilla, posterior mandible most common *Clinical manifestations:* Failure of permanent tooth to erupt, swelling *Radiographic manifestations:* Compound—cluster of numerous miniature teeth surrounded by radiolucent halo; complex—radiopaque mass surrounded by a thin radiolucent halo *TX:* Surgical excision ☛ Most common of odontogenic tumors

Tumors of Soft Tissue

LIPOMA

Description: Benign tumor of mature fat cells
Location: Buccal mucosa, vestibule most common
Clinical manifestations: Yellowish mass
TX: Surgical excision

Vascular Tumors

HEMANGIOMA

Description: Benign proliferation of capillaries
Location: Intraoral—tongue most common
Clinical manifestations: Deep red or blue lesions, blanch when pressure is applied
TX: Spontaneous remission

LYMPHANGIOMA

Description: Benign tumors composed of lymphatic vessels, present at birth
Location: Intraoral—tongue
Clinical manifestations: Ill-defined mass with pebbly surface
TX: Surgical excision

MALIGNANT VASCULAR TUMORS

KAPOSI'S SARCOMA

Description: Malignant vascular tumor that usually occurs in multiple sites, more aggressive form in HIV patients, also occurs in other patients with immunodeficiency
Location: Intraoral—hard palate, and gingival most common
Clinical manifestations: Purplish macules
TX: Surgical excision, radiation, chemotherapy

Tumors or Melanin-Producing Cells

MELANOCYTIC NEVI

Description: Developmental, intraoral lesions are usually benign, pigmented lesions that increase in size, or change color; may be malignant
Location: Skin or the oral cavity, intraoral—hard palate and buccal mucosa most common
Clinical manifestations: Intraoral—tan to brown macules or papules
TX: Biopsy, surgical excision

MALIGNANT MELANOMA

Description: Malignant tumor of melanocytes, exposure to the sun is the greatest causative factor
Location: Skin, intraoral lesions are uncommon, may metastasize to oral cavity
Clinical manifestations: Rapidly enlarging bluish to black mass
TX: Surgical excision, chemotherapy with surgery
☛ All melanomas are malignant

Tumors of Bone and Cartilage

OSTEOMA

Description: Benign tumor of mature, normal-appearing bone
Location: Intra-osseous
Clinical manifestations: Asymptomatic
Radiographic manifestations: Sharply defined radiopaque mass
TX: Surgical excision

OSTEOSARCOMA

Description: Malignant tumor of bone-forming tissue
Location: Mandible twice as frequent as maxilla
Clinical manifestations: Painful swelling, expansion of bone
Radiographic manifestations: Destructive radiolucent to radiopaque poorly defined lesion, asymmetric widening of periodontal ligament space
☛ "Sunburst" pattern
TX: Surgical excision, chemotherapy
☛ Most common tumor in patients under 40 years of age

Tumors of Blood

LEUKEMIA

Description: Overproduction of atypical white blood cells where normal bone marrow is replaced by immature white blood cells
Location: Gingiva
Clinical manifestations: Gingival enlargement and persistent bleeding
TX: Chemotherapy, radiation, corticosteroids

NON-HODGKIN'S LYMPHOMA

Description: Malignant tumor of lymphoid tissue
Location: Intraoral—tonsillar area most common
Clinical manifestations: Gradual enlargement of lymph nodes
TX: Radiotherapy, surgery, chemotherapy

Inherited Disorders Affecting the Gingiva and Periodontium

CYCLIC NEUTROPENIA

Description: Autosomal dominant disorder characterized by a cyclic decrease in the number of circulating neutrophils
Location: Oral mucosal and periodontium
Clinical manifestations: Severe ulcerative gingivitis, ulcers on tongue
Systemic manifestations: Fever, malaise, sore throat
Radiographic manifestations: Alveolar bone loss
TX: Antibiotics, scaling, and root planing

PAPILLON-LEFEVRE SYNDROME

Description: Autosomal recessive disease causing premature destruction of the periodontium
Location: Gingiva, periodontal ligament, palms and soles
Clinical manifestations: Mobile teeth, periodontal pockets, hyperkeratosis of hanks and soles of feet
Radiographic manifestations: Severe periodontal disease, alveolar bone loss
TX: Aggressive periodontal therapy

LABAND'S SYNDROME

Description: Autosomal dominant disease with gingival fibromatosis and sysplastic or absent nails
Location: Gingiva
Clinical manifestations: Gingival hyperplasia, abnormal nails, short fingers and toes
TX: Oral hygiene instruction, gingival surgery

Inherited Disorders Affecting the Jaw Bone and Facies

CHERUBISM

Description: Autosomal dominant disease of bilateral swelling of the face
Location: Mandible bilateral
Clinical manifestations: Bilateral enlargement of the face, increased distance between the eyes

Radiographic manifestations: Bilateral multilocular appearance radiolucencies
TX: Lesions fill in after puberty, facial deformity remains throughout life

GARDNER'S SYNDROME

Description: Autosomal dominant inheritance pattern; presence of osteomas in various bones, especially the frontal bones, mandible, and maxilla
Location: Maxilla and mandible
Clinical manifestations: Multiple osteomas of the bone, polyps of the colon, sebaceous cysts of the scalp and back
Radiographic manifestations: Odontomas and osteomas in the jaw
TX: Surgery

Blood Disorders

ANEMIA

Description: Reduction in the oxygen-carrying capacity of blood
Clinical manifestations: Skin and mucosal pallor, erythema of oral mucosal, angular cheilitis, loss of papilla (filiform, fungiform)

IRON DEFICIENCY ANEMIA	Bone marrow produces insufficient amount of iron for red blood cell development
PERNICIOUS ANEMIA	Deficiency of intrinsic factor necessary for B_{12} absorption
THALASSEMIA OR COOLEY'S ANEMIA	Inherited disorders of hemoglobin synthesis
SICKLE CELL ANEMIA	Inherited disorder predominantly in African American individuals; abnormal sickle shaped hemoglobin in red blood cells, causing a decrease in oxygen
APLASTIC ANEMIA	Bone marrow activity is severely depressed, causing a decrease in circulating blood cells.
POLYCYTHEMIA	Increased number of red blood cells

6 Pharmacology

Joe R. Anderson, PharmD, BCPS

Demetra Daskalos Logothetis, RDH, MS

➤ GENERAL PHARMACOLOGY

LATIN ABBREVIATIONS IN PRESCRIPTIONS

a	Before
a.c.	Before meals
b.i.d.	Twice daily
h	Hour
h.s.	Bedtime
o.t.c.	Over-the-counter
p.o.	By mouth
p.c.	After meals
p.r.n.	As needed
q.d.	Once a day
q.i.d.	Four times a day
q.o.d.	Every other day
q6h	Every six hours
s.l.	Sublingual
t.i.d.	Three times a day
u.d.	As directed

DRUG ACTION

DOSE-RESPONSE CURVE **Figure 6–1**	• A drug's effect on a biologic system can be measured in response to the dose of the drug given • The dose is plotted against the intensity of the effect dose-response curve, which helps determine the potency and efficacy of the drug's action
POTENCY	Amount of drug required to produce the desired therapeutic effect
THERAPEUTIC INDEX (TI)	• Ratio of the median lethal dose (LD50) to the median effective dose (ED50) • LD50 = dose of the drug required to produce death in 50% of test animals • ED50 = the dose of the drug required to produce the desired clinical effect in 50% of test animals $$TI = \frac{LD50}{ED50}$$ ☞ The higher the potency of a drug, the lower the ED50 will be
EFFICACY	Maximum response to a drug regardless of dose

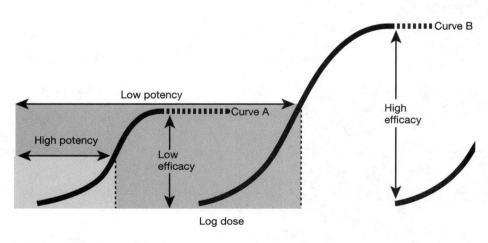

FIGURE 6-1 Dose-Response Curve

ADVERSE REACTIONS TO DRUGS

THERAPEUTIC EFFECTS	Clinically desirable actions of drugs
ADVERSE EFFECTS	Undesirable reactions of drugs ☛ Many times patients who experience side effects or an adverse reaction to a medication will confuse this with an allergic reaction; example, nausea and vomiting with a codeine derivative is often reported as an allergic reaction when in fact it is a common side effect
SIDE EFFECT	Interchangeable with adverse reaction ☛ Dose related
DRUG ALLERGY	Immunologic response to drug causing rash or anaphylaxis
IDOSYNCRATIC REACTION	Unusual drug response directly related to genetics
TOXIC REACTION	Exaggerated drug reaction
TERATOGENIC	Drug causes malformations in fetus
LOCAL EFFECTS	Drugs that cause local irritation ☛ Topical anesthetic cause tissue sloughing
DRUG INTERACTIONS	One drug alters the effect of another drug either positively or negatively

➤ PHARMACOKINETICS

What happens to the drug once it is administered into the body

ABSORPTION

Passage of a drug from its site of administration into the circulation by passing through biological membranes

PASSIVE DIFFUSION	Regulated by concentration gradient, by which drug moves from area of high concentration to area of low concentration
ACTIVE TRANSPORT	Requires energy to transport drug across concentration gradient

FACILITATED DIFFUSION	Does not move against the concentration gradient; it follows the concentration gradient
LIPID SOLUBILITY	Drugs that are lipid soluble readily pass through lipid-rich membranes ☞ Example: General anesthesia, benzodiazepines
IONIZATION	• Water-soluble drugs have difficulty crossing biological membranes • Ionized (polar) drugs are less lipid soluble and have difficulty crossing biological membranes • Nonionized (nonpolar) or uncharged molecules are lipid soluble and readily cross biological membranes • The more ionized the compound the less the drug is absorbed • The pH of the tissues at the site of administration determines the rate of drug absorption ☞ The more neutral the drug, the better it will be absorbed ☞ Example: Antacids raise pH of stomach and decrease absorption; some basic drugs are coated so that they will be absorbed in the basic environment of the small intestine
DRUG RECEPTORS	• Drug passes through biologic membranes to site of action to exert its therapeutic action • Drug must bind with receptor on cell membrane to exert its action ☞ Drug binds to specific receptor in lock and key fashion • Agonist—drug or macromolecule that binds to a receptor and causes a pharmacologic effect • Antagonist—drug that binds to a receptor and produces no effect; antagonists may produce an effect by blocking the effect produced by an agonist

DISTRIBUTION

Once drug is absorbed it is distributed throughout the body
☛ Increased blood flow = higher concentration of drug

FREE DRUG	Exerts pharmacologic effect ☛ Only free drug can cross membranes
BOUND DRUG	Reservoir for the drug
CONSTANT QUILIBRIUM	Drugs are in a constant equilibrium between bound and free drug

HALF-LIFE

Amount of time for the drug concentration to decrease by one half

SHORT HALF-LIFE	Drug is quickly removed from the body ☛ Short duration
LONG HALF-LIFE	Drug is slowly removed from the body ☛ Long duration

METABOLISM (BIOTRANSFORMATION)

LIVER	Primary site for metabolism
BIOTRANSFORMATION	Makes the drug more polar (ionized) and water soluble than its parent compound thus more readily excreted by the kidneys
MICROSOMAL ENZYME SYSTEM	• Located in smooth endoplasmic reticulum of the liver • Biological system for biotransformation • Cytochrome P450 enzyme system

EXCRETION

Drugs are excreted from the body via the kidneys, sweat, saliva, respiratory tract, gastrointestinal tract, breast milk
☛ Majority of drugs are excreted through the kidneys

ROUTES OF DRUG ADMINISTRATION

TOPICAL	Application of drugs to the surface of the body to produce a localized effect on the skin, eyes, nose, mouth, throat, rectum, or vagina ☞ Highly effective in dentistry
SUBLINGUAL	Certain drugs can be administered sublingually and absorbed into the blood through the mucous membranes of the oral cavity ☞ Example: nitroglycerine and nifedipine for management of anginal pain, and triazolam for sedation in pediatrics ☞ Advantage: bypasses the enterohepatic circulation and provides rapid absorption
INTRANASAL	Employed primarily in pediatric patients as a means of circumventing the need for injection or oral drug administration in unwilling patients
ORAL	• Drug administration by mouth • Absorption varies due to the interaction of drugs with food and gastric acid • Not suitable for use by patients who are sedated, comatose, or suffering from nausea and vomiting ☞ Most common
RECTAL	• Result in either a localized effect or a systemic effect • Useful when patients cannot take medications by mouth • Drugs absorbed from the rectum undergo relatively little first-pass metabolism in the liver ☞ Primarily in pediatric patients; advantage: rapid absorption; can be used when patient is unable to take medication orally
TRANSDERMAL	• Application of drugs to the skin for absorption into circulation • Transdermal medication, bypasses the GI tract, without the need for injection ☞ Example: motion sickness drugs, and hormone patches (can develop adverse skin reactions)

SUBCUTANEOUS	• Involves the injection of a drug beneath the skin into the subcutaneous tissues • It is useful for the administration of nonvolatile, water- or fat-soluble hypnotic and narcotic drugs
INTRAMUSCULAR	• Intramuscular administration is a parenteral technique • Suitable for drug solutions and suspensions
INHALATION (PULMONARY)	• A variety of gaseous agents may be ad ministered by inhalation to produce either sedation or general anesthesia • Nitrous oxide most frequently used in dentistry
INTRAVENOUS	• The IV route of drug administration represents the most effective method of ensuring predictable and adequate sedation • Preferred for drugs with short half-lives, and drugs whose dosage must be carefully titrated
GENERAL ANESTHESIA	• First technique of pain and anxiety control introduced into medical and dental practice

➤ AUTONOMIC PHARMACOLOGY

AUTONOMIC NERVOUS SYSTEM (ANS)

• Responsible for involuntary physiologic functions of skeletal muscles
• Originates in central nervous system (CNS), extends directly to skeletal muscle
• Two divisions: sympathetic and parasympathetic nervous system

PHYSIOLOGIC FUNCTIONS OF AUTONOMIC NERVOUS SYSTEM

☛ Produce opposite effects

SYMPATHETIC AUTONOMIC NERVOUS SYSTEM (SANS)	• Generalized and widespread action • Neurotransmitters are norepinephrine and epinephrine, which are stored in synaptic vesicles • Stimulation causes epinephrine to be released by the adrenal medulla • Action of neurotransmitters is terminated by the enzymes monoamine oxidase (MAO) and catechol-O-methyltransferase (COMT) ☛ "Fight or flight" ☛ Dominant during stress, increased activity, emergency situations
PARASYMPATHETIC AUTONOMIC NERVOUS SYSTEM (PANS)	• Discrete and generalized—vegetative responses • Acetylcholine is the released neurotransmitter from synaptic storage vesicles • Action of acetylcholine is terminated through hydrolysis by the enzyme acetylcholinesterase • Direct cholinergic agents (parasympathomimetic) act on receptors • Indirect cholinergic agents release neurotransmitter • Anticholinergic (parasympatholytic) agents prevent the action of acetylcholine, often times resulting in an opposite reaction than expected from acetylcholine ☛ Dominant when body is at rest

NEUROTRANSMITTERS

Carry messages

- Release of neurotransmitters across the synaptic cleft allows communication between nerves or between nerves and effector tissue
- Released in response to action potential
- Stored in small, membrane-bound vesicles at terminal nerve endings
- Terminated by enzymatic breakdown, and reuptake into presynaptic nerve terminal

- Drugs may prevent or enhance events of the ANS associated with action of neurotransmitters
- PANS neurotransmitter is acetylcholine (cholinergic)
- SANS neurotransmitters are norepinephrine (NE) and epinephrine (Epi)
- ☛ Both are catecholamines and help the body respond to stress

CHOLINOCEPTORS

☛ Respond to the neurotransmitter acetylcholine
☛ Classified according to whether they are stimulated by the alkaloids nicotine or musarine

MUSCARINIC M$_1$	Typical location: CNS neurons, sympathetic postganlionic neurons, some presynaptic sites
MUSCARINIC M$_2$	Typical location: myocardium, smooth muscle, some presynaptic sites
NICOTINIC	Typical location: autonomic ganglia, skeletal muscle neuromuscular end-plate, spinal cord

ADRENOCEPTORS

- Alpha-receptors (cause vasoconstriction which raises blood pressure, dilation of the pupils, constriction of sphincters in the GI tract
- Beta-receptors on the heart increase heart rate and force of contraction; beta-receptors also promote lung, vascular, and uterine smooth muscle relaxation
- ☛ Adrenoceptors respond to catecholamines (norepinephrine, epinephrine, dopamine)

ALPHA$_1$	Postsynaptic effector cells, especially smooth muscle
ALPHA$_2$	Presynaptic adrenergic nerve terminals, platelets, lipocytes, smooth muscle
BETA$_1$	Postsynaptic effector cells, especially heart; lipocytes, brain, presynaptic noradrenergic nerve terminals
BETA$_2$	Postsynaptic effector cells, especially bronchial smooth muscle, and lungs

Sympathetic and Parasympathetic Actions of Major Organs

Organ	Sympathetic Action	Parasympathetic Action
EYE (IRIS)		
Radial muscle	Alpha$_1$—contracts	——
Circular muscle	——	Muscarinic—contracts
Ciliary muscle	Beta—relaxes	Muscarinic—contracts
HEART		
Sinoatrial node	Beta$_1$—accelerates	Muscarinic—decelerates
Ectopic pacemakers	Beta$_1$—accelerates	——
Contractility	Beta$_1$—increases	Muscarinic—decreases (atria)
VASCULAR SMOOTH MUSCLE		
Skin, splanchnic	Alpha—contracts	——
vessels	Beta$_2$—relaxes	——
Skeletal muscle	Alpha—contracts	——
vessels		Muscarinic—relaxes
BRONCHIOLAR SMOOTH MUSCLE	Beta$_2$—relaxes	Muscarinic—contracts
GASTROINTESTINAL TRACT (SMOOTH MUSCLE)		
Walls	Alpha$_2$, Beta$_2$—relaxes	Muscarinic—contracts
Sphincters	Alpha$_1$—contracts	Muscarinic—relaxes
Secretion	——	Muscarinic—increases
Myenteric plexus	Alpha—inhibits	——
GENITOURINARY SMOOTH MUSCLE		
Bladder wall	Beta$_2$—relaxes	Muscarinic—contracts
Sphincter	Alpha$_1$—contracts	Muscarinic—relaxes
Uterus, pregnant	Beta$_2$—relaxes	——
	Alpha—contracts	——
Penis, seminal vesicles	Alpha—ejaculation	Muscarinic—erection
SKIN		
Pilomotor smooth	Alpha—contracts	——
muscles		
Sweat glands		
Thermoregulatory	Muscurinic—increases	——
Apocrine (stress)	Alpha—increases	——
METABOLIC FUNCTIONS		
Liver	Alpha, Beta—gluconeogenesis	——
Liver	Alpha, Beta$_2$—glycogenolysis	——
Fat cells	Alpha$_2$—inhibits lipolysis	——
	Beta$_1$—stimulates lipolysis	——
Kidney	Beta$_1$—renin release	——

☛ Actions of drugs can be predicted by receptors they block (example: beta-blockers) or by their activity or properties (example: sympathomimetics, anticholinergics)

DOPAMINE	Brain and postsynaptic effectors, especially vascular smooth muscle of the splanchnic and renal vascular beds; presynaptic receptors on nerve terminals, especially in the heart, vessels, and gastrointestinal system

Cardiovascular Agents

☛ The following doses of drugs are considered adult dosages unless specified otherwise

☛ Generic name (Brand name)

DIGOXIN (LANOXIN LANOXICAPS)	*MOA:* Inhibits Na^+/K^+ ATPase resulting in increased myocardial contractility; suppresses AV node conduction velocity, which decreases ventricular rate *Uses:* Treatment of congestive heart failure; rate control in tachyarrhythmias such as atrial fibrillation *Dose:* 0.125–0.25mg QD *Adverse effects:* Nausea, vomiting, bradycardia, heart block, visual disturbances (blurred vision, halos, etc.) ☛ May cause sensitive gag reflex resulting in difficulty taking dental impression

ANTIARRHYTHMIC AGENTS

QUINIDINE (QUINA-GLUTE; QUINIDEX)	*MOA:* Decreases myocardial excitability and conduction velocity by decreasing sodium influx during depolarization *Uses:* Restoration and maintenance of normal sinus rhythm in atrial flutter and fibrillation; ventricular tachycardia *Dose:* Sulfate: 200–600mg Q4–6H; Gluconate: 324–972mg Q8–12H *Adverse effects:* GI (bitter taste, diarrhea, nausea, vomiting, abdominal pain), hypotension, lightheadedness, skin rash, heart block ☛ Anticholinergic side effects may cause decreased saliva production

PROCAINAMIDE (PROCANBID; PRONESTYL)	*MOA:* Decreases myocardial excitability and conduction velocity by decreasing sodium influx during depolarization *Uses:* Prevention and treatment of ventricular arrhythmias; maintenance of normal sinus rhythm in atrial flutter and fibrillation *Dose:* 500mg–1g sustained release Q6H *Adverse effects*: Lupus-like syndrome; hypotension, AV block, heart block
DISOPYRAMIDE (NORPACE)	*MOA:* Decreases myocardial excitability and conduction velocity by decreasing sodium influx during depolarization *Uses:* Prevention and treatment of ventricular arrhythmias; restoration and maintenance of normal sinus rhythm in atrial flutter and fibrillation *Dose:* 150mg Q6H or 300mg Q12H *Adverse effects:* Hypotension, heart block, anticholinergic (xerostomia, blurred vision, constipation, etc.) ☞ Anticholinergic side effects may cause decreased saliva production
TOCAINIDE (TONOCARD)	*MOA:* Decreases myocardial excitability and conduction velocity *Uses:* Suppression and treatment of life-threatening arrhythmias *Dose:* 400–600mg TID *Adverse effects:* Lightheadedness, tremor, diarrhea, nausea, agranulocytosis, leukopenia
MEXILITINE (MEXITIL)	*MOA:* Slows rate of depolarization; prolongs action potential duration *Uses:* Suppression and treatment of ventricular arrhythmias *Dose:* 200–300mg Q8H *Adverse effects:* CNS (dizziness, tremor, blurred vision), hypotension, bradycardia, heart block, GI (constipation or diarrhea)

FLECAINIDE (TAMBOCOR)	*MOA:* Profound decrease in ventricular conduction velocity; prolongs action potential; marked inhibition of inward sodium currents; has local anesthetic properties *Uses:* Prevention and treatment of life-threatening ventricular arrhythmias *Dose:* 100mg Q12H *Adverse effects:* Dizziness, visual disturbances, nausea, dyspnea, proarrhythmia, heart failure
PROPAFENONE (RYTHMOL)	*MOA:* Profound decrease in ventricular conduction velocity; prolongs action potential; marked inhibition of inward sodium currents; has local anesthetic properties and beta-blocking activity *Uses:* Prevention and treatment of life-threatening ventricular arrhythmias *Dose:* 150mg Q8H *Adverse effects:* Dizziness, metallic taste, nausea, vomiting, proarrhythmia, heart failure ☛ > 10% of patients will experience dry mouth; may cause metallic taste
AMIODARONE (CORDARONE)	*MOA:* Prolongs ventricular action potential and refractoriness by inhibiting K^+ current; also has beta-blocking activity and causes vascular smooth muscle relaxation *Uses:* Life-threatening ventricular arrhythmias not controlled by other agents; restoration and maintenance of normal sinus rhythm in patients with atrial flutter and fibrillation *Dose:* 200–400mg QD *Adverse effects:* Numerous and frequent! Dizziness, phototoxicity, skin discoloration, hepatotoxicity, hypo- or hyperthyroidism, pulmonary fibrosis, tremors, neuropathy, nightmares ☛ May cause dysgeusia and abnormal salivation

SOTALOL (BETAPACE)	*MOA:* Prolongs action potential and refractory period; non-specific beta-blockade *Uses:* Life-threatening ventricular arrhythmias; restoration and maintenance of normal sinus rhythm in patients with atrial flutter and fibrillation *Dose:* 80–160mg BID-TID *Adverse effects:* Fatigue, dyspnea, chest pain, headache, nausea and vomiting; proarrhythmia ☛ Epinephrine may interact with all non-specific beta-blockers causing hypertension followed by bradycardia

ANTIHYPERTENSIVE AGENTS

ANGIOTENSIN CONVERTING ENZYME INHIBITORS (ACE INHIBITORS) • Captopril (Capoten) • Enalapril (Vasotec) • Benazepril (Lotensin) • Fosinopril (Monopril) • Lisinopril (Zestril and Prinivil) • Moexipril (Univasc) • Quinapril (Accupril) • Ramipril (Altace) • Trandolapril (Mavik)	*MOA:* Inhibits angiotensin-converting enzyme (ACE), which prevents conversion of angiotensin I to angiotensin II (a potent vasoconstrictor and stimulator of aldosterone) *Uses:* Management of hypertension and congestive heart failure *Dose:* Depends on agent *Adverse effects:* Rash, dysgeusia, insomnia, headache, hyperkalemia, dizziness, dry cough, alopecia, hypotension, blurred vision; angioedema (swelling of the lips, tongue, mouth, throat, nose) occurs in <1 % ☛ ACE-inhibitors all end with "-pril" ☛ Can cause altered taste

ANGIOTENSIN II ANTAGONISTS OR ANGIOTENSIN II RECEPTOR BLOCKERS (ARBs) • Irbesartan (Avapro) • Telomisartan (Micardis) • Candesarta (Atacand) • Losartan (Cozaar) • Valsartan (Diovan) • Eprosartan (Teveten)	*MOA:* Bind to angiotensin II AT1 receptor blocking the vasoconstrictive effects of AII and stimulation of aldosterone *Uses:* Management of hypertension *Dose:* Depends on agent *Adverse effects:* Hypotension, dizziness, hyperkalemia, nasal congestion, diarrhea, rash, angioedema; cough much less than with ACE inhibitors ☞ Angiotensin II antagonists all end with "-sartan" ☞ Can cause altered taste
BETA-ADRENEGIC BLOCKING AGENTS (BETA-BLOCKERS) **NONSELECTIVE (β_1 AND β_2)** • Nadolol (Corgard) • Penbutolol (Levatol) • Propranolol (Inderal) • Timolol (Timoptic, Blocadren) **SELECTIVE (β_1)** • Acebutolol (Sectral) • Atenolol (Tenormin) • Betaxolol (Kerlone) • Bisoprolol (Zebeta) • Esmolol (Brevibloc) • Metoprolol (Lopressor, Toprol)	*MOA:* Selective agents block cardiac β_1 receptor and decrease heart rate (inotrope), myocardial contractility (chronotrope), cardiac output, and conduction velocity; chronic administration results in decreased peripheral vascular resistance and blood pressure possibly as a result of decreased renin release; nonselective agents block both β_1 & β_2 receptors and therefore can antagonize β_2-receptor-mediated bronchodilation; those with α-blocking activity have vasodilator properties *Uses:* Angina, hypertension, cardiac arrhythmias, congestive heart failure (CHF), migraine, glaucoma *Dose:* Depends on agent *Adverse effects:* Bronchospasm, potentiate hypoglycemia, heart block, bradycardia, depression, dizziness, insomnia, fatigue, rash, decreased sexual ability ☞ Beta-blockers end with "-olol" ☞ Nonselective agents can potentiate the pressor response to epinephrine resulting in hypertension

α- AND β-BLOCKING AGENTS • Labetalol (Normodyne) • Carvedilol (Coreg)	*(see previous page)*
CALCIUM CHANNEL BLOCKERS • Verapamil (Calan, Covera-HS, Isoptin, Verelan) • Diltiazem (Cardizem, Tiazac, Dilacor) **DIHYDROPYRIDINES** • Amlodipine (Norvasc) • Isradipine (Dynacirc) • Nicardipine (Cardene, Cardene SR) • Nifedipine (Procardia, Procardia XL, Adalat CC) • Nimodipine (Nimotop) • Felodipine (Plendil) • Nisoldipine (Sular)	*MOA:* Inhibit calcium influx from extracellular sources through voltage-gated channels; this results in widespread dilatation of arteries and veins; verapamil and diltiazem slow heart rate, depress AV nodal conduction, and inhibit contractility *Uses:* Hypertension, angina, migraines, supraventricular tachycardia (verapamil and diltiazem) *Dose:* Depends on agent *Adverse effects:* Headaches, dizziness, facial flushing, hypotension, constipation (verapamil), heart block and bradycardia (verapamil and diltiazem), tachycardia (dihydropyridines) ☛ Dihydropyridines all end with "-ipine" ☛ Associated with gingival hyperplasia in about 1% of patients (particularly dihydropyridines), which is reversible with cessation of therapy
DIURETICS (THIAZIDES) • Chlorothiazide (Diuril) • Hydrochlorothiazide (Esidrix, HydroDIURIL) • Chlorthalidone (Hygroton) • Indapamide (Lozol) • Metolazone (Zaroxolyn, Diulo)	*MOA:* Block sodium chloride (NaCl) reabsorption in the distal convoluted tubule of the nephron, resulting in increased excretion of Na and water *Uses:* Hypertension, edema secondary to CHF, cirrhosis, or premenstrual tension *Dose:* Depends on agent *Adverse effects:* Hypokalemia, hypomagnesemia, hyperglycemia, photosensitivity

DIURETICS (LOOP DIURETICS) • Furosemide (Lasix) • Torsemide (Demadex) • Bumetanide (Bumex) • Ethacrynic acid (Edecrin)	*MOA:* Inhibits reabsorption of sodium and chloride in the ascending loop of Henle; results in increased excretion of water, sodium, chloride, potassium, magnesium, and calcium *Uses:* Hypertension, edema secondary to CHF, hepatic, or renal disease *Dose:* Depends on agent; usual furosemide dose 20–80 mg/day *Adverse effects:* Orthostatic hypotension, dizziness, hypokalemia, hyponatremia, hypomagnesemia, hypercalciuria, hyperuricemia, photosensitivity; high doses associated with ototoxicity
DIURETICS (POTASSIUM-SPARING) • Spironolactone (Aldactone) • Amiloride (Midamor) • Triamterene (Dyrenium)	*MOA:* Spironolactone and triamterene block aldosterone from binding in the distal renal tubule; results in increased sodium, chloride, and water excretion and conserving potassium; amiloride interferes with K^+/Na^+ exchange in distal and cortical collecting tubule through inhibition of Na^+/K^+-ATPase *Uses:* Spironolactone used for edema and ascites secondary to cirrhosis, hypertension, primary hyperaldosteronism; triamterene and amiloride used in combination with other diuretics to prevent potassium loss *Dose:* Depends on agent *Adverse effects:* Hyperkalemia, gynecomastia, abdominal pain
NITRATES • Isosorbide Dinitrate (ISDN) (Isordil) • Isosorbide Mononitrate (ISMN) (Ismo, Imdur, Monoket) • Nitroglycerin (Nitro-Bid, Nitro-Dur, Nitrodisc, Transderm-Nitro)	*MOA:* Stimulates intracellular cyclic-GMP resulting in vascular smooth muscle relaxation of both arterial and venous vasculature *Uses:* Prevention and treatment of angina pectoris, treatment of CHF *Dose:* ISDN 5–40mg Q6H except HS, ISMN 20mg BID (7 hours apart); dosed asymmetrically to avoid tolerance *Adverse effects:* Postural hypotension, headache, dizziness, lightheadedness ☞ No Viagra for patients receiving nitrates

PERIPHERAL VASODILATORS • Hydralazine (Apresoline) • Minoxidil (Loniten, Rogaine [topical])	*MOA:* Direct vasodilation of arterioles, decreasing systemic vascular resistance; hair growth is due to increased cutaneous blood flow *Uses:* Management of severe hypertension, CHF (hydralazine), treatment of male pattern baldness (minoxidil). *Dose:* Hydralazine 10–75mg QID; Minoxidil *Adverse Effects:* Palpitations, flushing, tachycardia, headache, nausea, diarrhea, hypotension, nasal congestion
ANTIADRENERGIC AGENTS (CENTRALLY ACTING) • Methyldopa (Aldomet) • Clonidine (Catapres) • Guanfacine (Tenex) • Guanabenz (Wytensin)	*MOA:* Stimulate α_2 receptors in the brainstem, which results in reduced sympathetic outflow to the periphery; results in decreased peripheral resistance and heart rate *Uses:* Hypertension (moderate to severe), alcohol and opiate withdrawal *Dose:* Depends on agent *Adverse effects:* Rebound hypertension with abrupt cessation of therapy, dry mouth, mental depression, drowsiness, constipation, hepatotoxicity (malaise, abdominal pain, nausea, vomiting), rash, nightmares, impotence, dryness of mucosa, cardiac arrhythmias ☛ Anticholinergic side effects can cause dry mouth and predispose to dental disease (caries, oral candidiasis, and peridontal disease)
ANTIADRENERGIC AGENTS (PERIPHERALLY ACTING) • Reserpine (Reserpine) • Guanethidine (Ismelin) • Guanadrel (Hylorel)	*MOA:* Deplete stores of catecholamines at the sympathetic neuroeffector junction, which decreases heart rate and arterial blood pressure *Uses:* Moderate to severe hypertension; reserpine used for agitation associated with psychotic states *Dose:* Depends on agent *Adverse effects:* Dizziness, nausea, diarrhea, nasal congestion, bradycardia, drowsiness, depression, fatigue, dry mouth, leg cramps, backache, paresthesias ☛ These agents may potentiate the activity of epinephrine or other direct-acting sympathomimetics

ALPHA₁-ADRENERGIC BLOCKERS • Prazosin (Minipress) • Terazosin (Hytrin) • Doxazosin (Cardura)	*MOA:* Competively and selectively inhibit postsynaptic alpha₁-adrenergic receptors, which results in vasodilation of veins and arterioles and a decrease in total peripheral resistance; also relaxes smooth muscle in the bladder, neck, and prostate *Uses:* Hypertension, benign prostatic hypertrophy *Dose:* Depends on agent *Adverse effects:* Orthostatic hypotension, dizziness, lightheadedness, headache, dry mouth ☛ Significant dry mouth can occur in up to 10% of patients ☛ Be careful of patient rising from dental chair due to orthostatic hypotension

AGENTS FOR HYPERTENSIVE EMERGENCIES

NITROPRUSSIDE (NITROPRESS)	*MOA:* Causes peripheral vasodilation by direct action on venous and arteriolar smooth muscle *Uses:* Management of hypertensive crises *Dose:* 0.3–0.5 mcg/kg/minute IV titrating to desired effect *Adverse effects:* Excessive hypotensive response, headache, thiocynate toxicity
DIAZOXIDE (HYPERSTAT IV)	*MOA:* Relaxes smooth muscle in the peripheral arterioles *Uses:* Emergency reduction of blood pressure *Dose:* 1–3mg/kg IV bolus; repeat dose every 15 minutes until desired BP up to a maximum of 150mg in a single injection *Adverse effects:* Hypotension, nausea, vomiting, dizziness, weakness, hyperglycemia
FENOLDOPAM (CORLOPAM)	*MOA:* Rapid-acting vasodilator; agonist to D₁-like dopamine receptors and for α₂-adrenoreceptors *Uses:* Hypertensive emergency *Dose:* Continuous IV infusion, initial dose 0.03 to 0.1 mcg/kg/minute *Adverse effects:* Hypotension, headache, nausea, and flushing

ANTIHYPERLIPIDEMIC AGENTS

BILE ACID SEQUESTRANTS • Cholestyramine (Questran) • Colestipol HCl (Colestid)	*MOA:* Forms a nonabsorbable complex with bile acids in the intestine, which inhibits enterohepatic reuptake of bile salts; this has a net result of increasing fecal loss of LDL *Uses:* Adjunct for treatment of hyper-cholesterolemia; also used for diarrhea associated with excess fecal bile acids *Dose:* Cholestyramine 4 gm 1–6 times a day; colestipol 5–30 gm in divided doses 2–4 times/day *Adverse effects:* Constipation, abdominal pain and bloating, flatulence, belching
HMG-CoA REDUCTASE INHIBITORS ("STATINS") • Cerivastatin (Baycol) • Lovastatin (Mevacor) • Simvastatin (Zocor) • Pravastatin (Pravachol) • Fluvastatin (Lescol) • Atrovastatin (Lipitor)	*MOA:* Inhibit HMG-CoA reductase, which is the enzyme representing the rate-limiting step in cholesterol synthesis; results in decreases in total and LDL cholesterol, triglycerides, and increases HDL cholesterol *Uses:* For various dyslipidemias, primary and secondary prevention of cardiovascular events *Dose:* Depends on agent *Adverse effects:* Elevated CPK levels, myopathy, rhabdomyolysis, abdominal pain, headache ☛ Erythromycin can inhibit the metabolism of "statins" with a resultant increase in risk of myopathy and rhabdomyolysis
FIBRIC ACID DERIVATIVES • Fenofibrate (Tricor) • Gemfibrozil (Lopid) • Clofibrate (Atromid-S)	*MOA:* Lowers triglyceride and increases HDL; mechanism not fully understood *Uses:* Hypertriglyceridemia *Dose:* Depends on agent *Adverse effects:* Dyspepsia, abdominal pain, cholelithiasis, taste perversion, myopathy

NICOTINIC ACID	*MOA:* Decreases total and LDL cholesterol, triglycerides, and increases HDL cholesterol; mechanism not fully understood *Uses:* Hyperlipidemia *Dose:* 500–1000mg TID *Adverse effects:* Generalized flushing with warmth, headache, nausea, bloating, abnormalities in liver function tests, hepatotoxicity ☞ Flushing avoided by slow titration and by administering ASA prior to dose

Respiratory Agents

BRONCHODILATORS

SYMPATHOMIMETICS • Levalbuterol (Xopenex) • Salmeterol (Serevent) • Albuterol (Proventil, Ventolin) • Bitolterol (Tornalate) • Isoetharine • Metaproterenol (Alupent) • Pirbuterol (Maxair) • Terbutaline (Brethine) • Isoproterenol (Isuprel, Medihaler) • Ephedrine • Epinephrine (Primatene Mist)	*MOA:* Relax bronchial smooth muscle by direct action on beta$_2$-adrenergic receptors *Uses:* Bronchodilator for reversible airway obstruction due to asthma or COPD; prevention of exercise-induced bronchospasm *Dose:* Typically 1–2 inhalations every 4 to 6 hours (albuterol) *Adverse effects:* Tachycardia, palpitations, GI upset, nervousness, insomnia, dry mouth, unusual taste

XANTHINE DERIVATIVES • Theophylline (Slo-Phyllin, Theolair, Theo-24, Theo-Dur, Uniphyl) • Aminophylline (Phyllocontin)	*MOA:* Directly relax the smooth muscle of the bronchi and pulmonary blood vessels, stimulate the CNS, increase gastric acid secretion, reduce lower esophogeal sphincter tone, and inhibit uterine contraction *Uses:* Relief and prevention of bronchial asthma and reversible bronchospasm associated with chronic bronchitis and emphysema *Dose:* Depends on agent and formulation *Adverse effects:* Theophylline toxicity (nausea, vomiting, diarrhea, irritability), palpitations, tachycardia, irritability, insomnia ⚷ Caffeine can potentiate the effects; epinepherine will increase heart rate
ANTICHOLINERGICS • Ipratropium	*MOA:* Anticholinergics prevent increases in intracellular cyclic GMP caused by interaction of acetycholine with the muscarinic receptor on bronchial smooth muscle, which then leads to bronchodilation *Uses:* Bronchospasm associated with COPD, chronic bronchitis, and emphysema *Dose:* 2 puffs QID Adverse Effects: Dry mouth; systemic effects rare ⚷ Dry mouth in > 10% of patients

LEUKOTRIENE RECEPTOR ANTAGONISTS

• Zafirlukast (Accolate) • Montelukast (Singulair)	*MOA:* Selective and competitive antagonists of leukotriene (LT) receptors (LTC_4, LTD_4, LTE_4); LTs have been correlated with the pathophysiology of asthma, causing airway edema, smooth muscle contraction, altered cellular activity associated with the inflammatory process *Uses:* Prophylaxis and chronic treatment of asthma *Dose:* Zafirlukast: 20mg BID 1 hour before or 2 hours after meals; montelukast: 10mg QD in the evening *Adverse effects:* Headache, nausea, diarrhea; drug interactions with zafirulukast

	☛ Erythromycin inhibits the bioavail-ability of zafirlukast
• Zileuton (Zyflo)	*MOA:* Inhibits 5-lipoxygenase, thus inhibiting the formation of leukotrienes *Uses:* Prophylaxis and chronic treatment of asthma *Dose:* 600mg QID *Adverse effects:* Hepatoxicity requires close monitoring of ALT, drug interactions, headache, dyspepsia, nausea, abdominal pain

CORTICOSTEROIDS

INHALED • Beclomethasone (Beclovent, Vanceril) • Budesonide (Pulmicort) • Flunisolide (AeroBid) • Fluticasone (Flovent) • Triamcinolone (Azmacort)	*MOA:* Glucocorticoid activity; glucocorticoids may decrease the number and activity of inflammatory cells, inhibit bronchoconstrictor mechanisms, produce direct smooth muscle relaxation, and decrease airway hyperresponsiveness *Uses:* Maintenance and prophylactic treatment of asthma *Dose:* Depends on agent *Adverse effects:* Localized fungal infections in the oropharynx; depressed immune function; pharyngitis, coughing, dryness of nose, mouth, and throat; loss of taste and smell ☛ Oral fungal infections
INTRANASAL • Flunisolide (Nasalide, Nasarel) • Beclomethasone (Beconase, Vancenase) • Triamcinolone (Nasocort) • Budesonide (Rhinocort) • Fluticasone (Flonase) • Mometasone (Nasonex)	*MOA:* Glucocorticoid activity; inhibitory activity against cells involved in allergic and nonallergic inflammation *Uses:* Management of symptoms of seasonal or perennial allergic rhinitis and nonallergic perennial rhinitis *Dose:* Depends on agent *Adverse effects:* HPA suppression (rare), localized fungal infections of the nose and pharynx; immunosuppression, nasal irritation, burning, dryness

MAST CELL STABILIZERS

• Cromolyn (Intal, Nasalcrom) • Nedocromil (Tilade)	*MOA:* Inhibit the degranulation of mast cells, thus inhibiting the release of histamine *Uses:* Prophylaxis of bronchial asthma; prevention of exercise-induced bronchospasm (cromolyn), allergic rhinitis (cromolyn) *Dose:* 2 puffs QID (asthma) *Adverse effects:* Hoarseness, cough, unpleasant taste

NASAL DECONGESTANTS

• Phenylpropanolamine (Removed from market) • Pseudoephedrine (Afrin, Sudafed) • Phenylephrine (Neo-Synephrine, Sinex) • Epinephrine (Adrenalin) • Ephedrine (Pretz-D) • Naphazoline (Privine) • Oxymetazoline (Afrin, Afrin Children's) • Tetrahydrozoline (Tyzine) • Xylometazoline (Otrivin)	*MOA:* Stimulate α-adrenergic receptors of vascular smooth muscle causing vasoconstriction, pressor effects, nasal decongestion; topical agents have less systemic effects; additional α-effects include contraction of the GI and urinary sphincters, mydriasis and decreased pancreatic beta cell secretion; also stimulate β-receptors, causing bronchial relaxation *Uses:* Temporary relief of nasal congestion due to the common cold, hay fever, or other upper respiratory allergies, and nasal congestion associated with sinusitis; may also be used adjunctively for middle ear infections by decreasing Eustachian tube congestion *Dose:* Depends on agent; topical agents should be used for no longer than 3 to 5 days *Adverse effects:* Arrhythmias, palpitations, tachycardia, transient hypertension, anxiety, tenseness, restlessness, dizziness, tremor, insomnia; topical agents can cause burning, stinging, and rebound congestion ☛ Use with caution with local anesthetic/vasoconstrictor, as the combination could cause a pressor response ☛ Found in various OTC products; typically marketed as "nondrowsy" or "daytime"

ANTIHISTAMINE

NON-SELECTIVE	
• Brompheniramine (Dimetane) • Chlorpheniramine (Chlor-Trimeton) • Dexchlorphenira-mine (Polaramine) • Clemastine (Tavist) • Diphenhydramine (Benadryl) • Tripelennamine (PBZ) • Promethazine (Phenergan) • Hydroxyzine (Atarax, Vistaril) • Azatadine (Optimine) • Cyproheptadine (Periactin) • Phenindamine (Nolahist) • Azelastine (Astelin)	*MOA:* Reversible competitive antagonists of histamine (H_1) receptors; blocks histamine effects both centrally and peripherally resulting in inhibition of respiratory, vascular, and GI smooth muscle contraction, and decreased capillary permeability (reducing wheal, flare, and itch response) *Uses:* For the relief of immediate-type hypersensitivity reactions; some of these agents are used as sedatives, antiemetics, antitussives, antiparkinson agents, and for motion sickness *Dose:* Depends on agent *Adverse effects:* Nonselective agents have sedative properties and thus may cause drowsiness and altered mental status; anticholinergic activity may cause urinary retention, constipation, increased intraocular pressure, drying of oral and nasal mucosa, and hypotension ☛ Chronic use of antihistamines can result in decreased salivary flow, which may contribute to periodontal disease
SELECTIVE	
• Cetrizine (Zyrtec) • Astemizole (Hismanal) • Fexofenadine (Allegra) • Loratadine (Claritin)	*MOA:* Selectively block H_1 receptors peripherally; therefore are associated with less sedation *Uses:* Relief of nasal and non-nasal symptoms of seasonal allergic rhinitis *Dose:* Depends on agent *Adverse effects:* Headache, somnolence, fatigue ☛ Dry mouth

NON-NARCOTIC ANTITUSSIVES

DEXTROMETHORPHAN (ROBITUSSIN-DM, DELSYM)	*MOA:* d-isomer of codeine; lacks analgesic and addictive properties; has suppressant effect on cough center in the medulla *Uses:* To control nonproductive cough *Dose:* 10–30mg every 4 to 8 hours *Adverse effects:* Sedation, nausea, dizziness, constipation

BENZONATATE (TESSALON PERLES)	*MOA:* Related to tetracaine; anesthetizes stretch receptors in respiratory passages, lungs, and pleura, reducing the cough reflex *Uses:* Symptomatic relief of cough *Dose:* 100mg TID *Adverse effects:* Sedation, headache, mild dizziness

EXPECTORANTS

GUAIFENESIN (RO-BITUSSIN, HUMIBID, ORGANIDIN)	*MOA:* Increases the output of respiratory tract fluid by reducing adhesiveness and viscosity of mucus; making nonproductive coughs more productive *Uses:* Symptomatic relief of respiratory conditions characterized by dry, nonproductive cough *Dose:* 100–400mg every 4 hours *Adverse effects:* Nausea, vomiting, dizziness, headache
IODINATED GLYCEROL (IOPHEN)	*MOA:* Increases respiratory tract secretions by decreasing mucus viscosity *Uses:* Expectorant used for adjunctive treatment of bronchitis, bronchial asthma, pulmonary emphysema, cystic fibrosis, or chronic sinusitis *Dose:* 60mg QID *Adverse effects:* Diarrhea, nausea, vomiting

Gastrointestinal Agents

SUCRALFATE (CARAFATE)	*MOA:* Forms an ulcer-adherant complex, which covers the ulcer and protects it against gastric acid *Uses:* Short-term treatment of duodenal ulcer; also has been used for GERD; suspension used for oral and esophageal ulcers due to cancer treatment *Dose:* 1g QID *Adverse effects:* Constipation; numerous drug interactions

MISOPROSTOL (CYTOTEC)	*MOA:* A prostaglandin (E$_1$) analog; decreases gastric acid secretion and increases bicarbonate and mucus production *Uses:* For the prevention of NSAID-induced gastric ulcers *Dose:* 200mcg QID with food *Adverse effects:* Diarrhea, abdominal pain, headache, flatulence

HISTAMINE H$_2$ ANTAGONISTS

• Cimetidine (Tagamet) • Ranitidine (Zantac) • Nizatidine (Axid) • Famotidine (Pepcid)	*MOA:* Reversible, competitive blockers of histamine at the H$_2$ receptor, mainly in the gastric parietal cell; they block gastric acid secretion induced by histamine, muscarinic agonists, and gastrin, thereby increasing gastric pH *Uses:* Used for the treatment and maintenance of gastric and duodenal ulcers, and GERD *Dose:* Depends on agent *Adverse effects:* Gynecomastia (cimetidine), hepatoxicity (nizatidine, IV ranitidine), dizziness, constipation; numerous drug interactions with cimetidine ☛ End with "tidine"

PROTON PUMP INHIBITORS

• Omeprazole (Prilosec) • Lansoprazole (Prevacid)	*MOA:* Suppresses gastric acid secretion by inhibiting the parietal cell H+/K+ ATP pump *Uses:* Eradication of *H. pylori* in patients with duodenal ulcer disease; short-term treatment of severe erosive esophagitis and symptomatic GERD not responsive to usual treatment *Dose:* Omeprazole—20mg QD *Adverse effects:* Headache, rash, diarrhea

ANTACIDS

• Magnesia (Milk of Magnesia) • Aluminum Hydroxide (Amphogel, AlternaGEL) • Calcium Carbonate (Tums, Mylanta, Maalox) • Magnesium Oxide (Mag-Ox) • Magaldrate (Riopan) • Sodium Bicarbonate • Sodium Citrate	*MOA:* Neutralize gastric acidity, resulting in an increase in the gastric and duodenal pH *Uses:* Heartburn, GERD, treatment and maintenance of duodenal ulcer *Dose:* Depends on agent *Adverse effects:* Aluminum products inhibit gastric emptying and are associated with constipation, osteomalacia and hypophosphatemia; magnesium products may act as a GI cathartic and cause diarrhea; hypermagnesemia in renal failure ☛ Will inactivate tetracycline derivatives—drug interaction

ANTICHOLINERGICS/ANTISPASMODICS

BELLADONNA ALKALOIDS • L-Hyoscyamine (Levsin, Levbid) • Atropine • Scopolamine (Scopace) • Belladonna	*MOA:* GI anticholinergics are used to decrease smooth muscle tone (motility) in GI, biliary, and urinary tracts; inhibit (Ach) at postganglionic parasympathetic neuroeffector sites *Uses:* Diarrhea, irritable bowel syndrome, ulcerative colitis, diverticulitis, neurogenic bladder, motion sickness, adjunctive treatment of peptic ulcer ☛ Atropine can be used pre-operatively to decrease salivation in dentistry for patients with excessive salivation to keep a dry field *Dose:* Depends on agent *Adverse effects:* C/I in patients with narrow angle glaucoma, GI obstructive disease, myasthenia gravis; dry skin, constipation, dry nose and throat, decreased sweating; CNS confusion, depression, and excitation ☛ Dry mouth

QUATERNARY ANTICHOLINERGICS • Methscopolamine (Pamine) • Glycopyrrolate (Robinul) • Propantheline (Pro-Banthine)	*MOA:* GI anticholinergics are used to decrease smooth muscle tone (motility) in GI, biliary, and urinary tracts; inhibit the muscarinic actions of acetylcholine at postganglionic parasympathetic neuroeffector sites; quaternary compounds do not cross the blood–brain barrier and therefore lack significant CNS side effects *Uses:* Adjunctive treatment of peptic ulcer disease; inhibit salivation and excessive secretions of the respiratory tract preoperatively *Dose:* Depends on agent *Adverse effects:* Dry skin, constipation, dry nose and throat, decreased sweating ☞ Dry mouth
ANTISPASMODIC • Dicyclomine (Bentyl)	*MOA:* Blocks the action of Ach at parasympathetic sites in smooth muscle, secretory glands, and the CNS *Uses:* Treatment of functional disturbances of GI motility such as irritable bowel syndrome *Dose:* 20mg QID *Adverse effects:* Dry skin, constipation, dry nose and throat, decreased sweating ☞ Dry mouth

INFLAMMATORY BOWEL DISEASE AGENTS

• Mesalamine (Asacol, Pentasa, Rowasa) • Olsalazine (Dipentum) • Sulfasalazine (Azulfidine)	*MOA:* Converted in the colon by bacteria to 5-ASA (5-aminosalicylic acid), which possesses antiinflammatory properties; inhibits local production of cyclooxygenase, thus inhibiting prostaglandin synthesis; this results in decreased production of inflammatory mediators such as leukotrienes *Uses:* Inflammatory bowel disease *Dose:* Depends on agent *Adverse effects:* Headache, malaise, abdominal pain, cramps, flatulence, gas

LAXATIVES

SALINE LAXATIVES • Epsom Salt • Milk of Magnesia • Citrate of Magnesia • Sodium Phosphates (Fleet Phospho-soda)	*MOA:* Attract/retain water in intestinal lumen, increasing intraluminal pressure and cholyecystokinin release; affect large and small intestine *Uses:* Short-term treatment of constipation; evacuation of colon for rectal and bowel examination *Dose:* Depends on agent *Adverse effects:* May alter fluid and electrolyte balance ☛ Onset of action 0.5–3 hours, except sodium phosphate 0.03–0.25 hours
IRRITANTS OR STIMULANTS • Cascara Sagrada • Sennosides (Ex-Lax) • Senna (Senokot, Fletcher's Castoria) • Castor Oil/ Purge • Bisacodyl (Dulcolax, Correctol)	*MOA:* Direct action on intestinal mucosa; stimulate myenteric plexus; alter water and electrolyte secretion; effect colon; mineral oil has activity in the small intestine *Uses:* Short-term treatment of constipation *Dose:* Depends on agent *Adverse effects:* Abdominal cramps, nausea, diarrhea; may alter fluid and electrolyte balance; cathartic colon from chronic use ☛ Onset 6–10 hours; bisacodyl suppositories 0.25–1 hour; castor oil 2–6 hours
BULK-PRODUCING • Methycellulose (Citrucel, Unifiber) • Polycarbophil (Fibercon, Mitrolan) • Psyllium (Metamucil, Perdiem)	*MOA:* Holds water in stool; mechanical distention; active in small and large intestine *Uses:* Short-term treatment of constipation; useful for patients with constipation or diarrhea secondary to irritable bowel syndrome; psyllium can be used to lower cholesterol *Dose:* Depends on agent *Adverse effects:* Diarrhea, constipation, abdominal cramps ☛ Onset: 12–24 hours, up to 72 hours

| MISCELLANEOUS
• Mineral oil
• Docusate (Colace, Peri-colace, Surfak)
• Glycerin
• Lactulose (Cephulac, Enulo) | *MOA:* Mineral oil retards colonic absorption of fecal water and softens stool; docusate has detergent activity, promoting mixture of fat and water to soften stool; lactulose is osmotically active, drawing water into the stool
Uses: Short-term treatment of constipation; useful for patients who should avoid straining (post-MI, painful anorectal conditions) and patients receiving opiates for pain management
Dose: Depends on agent
Adverse effects: Diarrhea, abdominal cramps
• Onset: mineral oil 6–8 hours; docusate 24–72 hours; glycerin suppository 0.25–0.5 hours; lactulose 24–48 hours |

ANTIDIARRHEALS

| DIPHENOXYLATE AND ATROPINE (LOMOTIL, LONOX) | *MOA:* Inhibits GI motility and GI propulsion
Uses: Treatment of diarrhea
Dose: 15–20mg of diphenoxylate in 3–4 divided doses
Adverse effects: Drowsiness, dizziness, dry mouth, blurred vision, urinary retention
• Up to 10% will complain of dry mouth |
| LOPERAMIDE (IMODIUM) | *MOA:* Inhibits peristalsis and prolongs transit time enhancing fluid and electrolyte movement through intestinal mucosa
Uses: Control and symptomatic relief of acute nonspecific diarrhea and chronic diarrhea secondary to inflammatory bowel disease
Dose: 4mg initially, then 2mg after each unformed stool, NTE 16mg/day
Adverse effects: Rare; constipation, dry mouth, drowsiness |

BISMUTH SUBSALICYCYLATE (PEPTO-BISMOL)	*MOA:* Antisecretory and antimicrobial effects and may have some anti-inflammatory effects *Uses:* Control of diarrhea, including traveler's diarrhea, within 24 hours; has been used to prevent traveler's diarrhea (2 tablets QID) *Dose:* 2 tablets or 30 mL, repeat every 30 minutes to 1 hour as needed, NTE 8 doses/24 hours *Adverse effects:* May turn stool gray-black color; darkening of tongue

GI STIMULANTS

METOCLOPRAMIDE (REGLAN)	*MOA:* Blocks dopamine receptors in the chemoreceptor trigger zone of the CNS; enhances response to Ach of tissue in upper GI tract, causing enhanced motility and accelerated gastric emptying *Uses:* Symptomatic treatment of diabetic gastric stasis, GERD, prevention of nausea associated with chemotherapy *Dose:* 10mg QID *Adverse effects:* Drowsiness, diarrhea, weakness, dry mouth, extrapyramidal reactions (particularly elderly)
CISAPRIDE (PROPULSID)	*MOA:* GI prokinetic agent by enhancement of Ach release at the myenteric plexus; increases lower esophageal sphincter pressure and lower esophageal peristalsis; accelerates gastric emptying *Uses:* Treatment of GERD, gastroparesis, refractory constipation, and nonulcer dyspepsia *Dose:* 10mg QID *Adverse effects:* Diarrhea, GI cramping, dry mouth, nausea ☛ Contraindicated in patients taking clarithromycin, erythromycin, ketoconazole, itraconazole, and fluconazole; these drugs inhibit cisapride metabolism and have resulted in QT prolongation and torsades de pointe

☞ Manufacturer Janssen voluntarily removed Cisapride from market

Endocrine Agents

SEX HORMONES

ESTROGENS	
• Estrone • Estradiol (Estrace, Vivelle, Climara, Estraderm) • Conjugated Estrogens (Premarin) • Ethinyl Estradiol (Estinyl) • Esterified Estrogens (Estratab, Menest) • Estropipate (Ogen, Ortho-Est)	*MOA:* The 3 significant female estrogens are 17 β-estradiol, estrone, and estriol. Estradiol is 12 times more potent than estrone and 80 times more potent than estriol. Estrogen is important for female reproduction and secondary sex characteristics. Estrogen replacement therapy (ERT) is the most effective single modality for prevention of osteoporosis, and is associated with a decreased incidence of CHD in post-menopausal women without a previous history of CHD *Uses:* Used as a component of combination contraceptives or as hormone replacement therapy; benefits include relief of moderate–severe vasomotor symptoms, decreased risk of osteoporosis, and cardiovascular disease *Dose:* Depends on agent and patient response *Adverse effects:* May increase the risk of endometrial, breast, cervical, vaginal, and liver cancer; increased risk of gallbladder disease. Headache, peripheral edema, enlargement of breasts, breast tenderness, nausea, bloating
SERMs • Raloxifene (Evista)	*MOA:* Selective estrogen receptor modulator (SERM); has estrogen-like effects on bone and on lipid metabolism, but is also an estrogen antagonist and lacks estrogen-like effects in uterine and breast tissue *Uses:* Osteoporosis prevention in post-menopausal women *Dose:* 60mg QD *Adverse effects:* Contraindicated in women with history of thromboembolism due to an increased risk with raloxifene; hot flashes and leg cramps

PROGESTINS
- Progesterone (Prometrium)
- Medroxyproges-terone (Cycrin, Provera)
- Norethindrone (Aygestin)
- Megestrol (Megace)

MOA: Natural steroid hormone that induces secretory changes in the endometrium, promotes mammary gland development, relaxes uterine smooth muscle, blocks follicular maturation and ovulation, and maintains pregnancy
Uses: Contraception and to prevent endometrial hyperplasia in postmenopausal women receiving ERT
Dose: Depends on agent
Adverse effects: Edema, breakthrough bleeding, spotting, muscle weakness
⚷ Progestins may predispose the patient to gingival bleeding

COMBINATION PRODUCTS

- Estrogen/ progesterone (Prempro, Premphase)
- Estrogen/ methyltestosterone (Estratest)

MOA: Estrogen and progesterone hormone replacement therapy
Uses: Postmenopausal hormone replacement therapy
Dose: 1 of each tablet every day
Adverse effects: Same as those listed individually for progesterone and estrogen

CONTRACEPTIVES

MONOPHASIC
- Mestranol & norethindrone (Genora 1/50, Norethin 1/50, Ortho-Novum 1/50)
- Ethinyl estradiol, norethindrone, & norgestrol (Ovcon 50, Demulen 1/50, Ovral)

MOA: Combination oral contraceptives (OCs) inhibit ovulation by suppressing the gonadotropins, follicle-stimulating hormone (FSH) and luteinizing hormone (LH); alters cervical mucus, which inhibits sperm penetration, and likelihood of implantation
Uses: For the prevention of pregnancy
Dose: Monophasic-fixed dosage of estrogen and progestin throughout the cycle; biphasic amount of estrogen remains the same for the first 21 days of the cycle; decreased progestin:estrogen

- Ethinyl estradiol & norethindrone (Necon 1/35, Ortho-Novum 1/35, Modicon, Ovcon-35, Loestrin)
- Ethinyl estradiol & norgestimate (Ortho-Cyclen)
- Ethinyl estradiol & ethynodiol (Demulen 1/35, Zovia 1/35)
- Ethinyl estradiol & norgestrol (Lo/Ovral)
- Ethinyl estradiol & desogestrel (Desogen, Ortho-Cept)
- Ethinyl estradiol & levonorgestrol (Levlen, Levora, Nordette, Alesse, Levlite)

BIPHASIC
- Norethindrone & ethinyl estradiol (Jenest-28, Nelova 10/11, Ortho-Novum 10/11)
- Desogesterol & Ethinyl estradiol (Mircette)

TRIPHASIC
- Norethindrone & ethinyl estradiol (Tri-Norinyl, Ortho-Novum 7/7/7)
- Ethinyl estradiol & levonorgestrol (Tri-levlen, Triphasil)
- Ethinyl estradiol norgestimate (Ortho Tri-cyclen)

ratio in first half of cycle (allowing endometrial proliferation) and increased ratio in second half of cycle (providing adequate secretory development)
Adverse effects: Increased risk of thromboembolic events (smoking increases risk); increased risk of gallbladder disease; adverse effects associated with estrogen excess: nausea, bloating, headaches, breast fullness and tenderness, edema; progestin excess: weight gain, fatigue, acne, hair loss, depression
☞ Decreased effect of oral contraceptives when co-administered with oral antibiotics; patients should be warned to use supplemental methods of birth control

BISPHOSPHONATES

• Alendronate (Fosamax) • Etidronate (Didronel) • Pamidronate (Aredia) • Tiludronate (Skelid) • Risedronate (Actonel)	*MOA:* Inhibit bone resorption via actions on osteoclasts *Uses:* Treatment and prevention of osteoporosis; Paget's disease of the bone; hypercalcemia of malignancy *Dose:* Depends on agent; pamidronate only available in IV formulation *Adverse effects:* Headache, rash, abdominal pain, diarrhea, arthralgias, esophagitis ulcer
• Calcitonin-Salmon (Calcimar, Miacalcin)	*MOA:* Directly inhibits osteoclastic bone resorption; promotes the renal excretion of calcium, phosphate, sodium, magnesium, and potassium *Uses:* Treatment of Paget's disease of bone; prevention of postmenopausal osteroporosis; treatment of hypercalcemia *Dose:* 200 IU nasally every day *Adverse effects:* Facial flushing, nausea, diarrhea, anorexia, rhinitis and nasal irritation; risk of systemic allergic reaction

ANTIDIABETIC AGENTS

RAPID-ACTING INSULIN • Regular (Novulin-R, Humulin-R) • Semilente • Lispro (Humalog) **INTERMEDIATE-ACTING INSULIN** • Isophane (NPH) (Novulin-N, Humulin-N) • Insulin Zinc (Lente) (Novulin-L, Humulin-L) • NPH & Regular (Humulin 70/30)	*MOA:* Lower blood glucose levels by stimulating peripheral glucose uptake, especially by skeletal muscle and fat and by inhibiting hepatic glucose production *Uses:* For the treatment of Type 1 and Type 2 diabetes mellitus *Dose:* Depends on agent and patient response *Adverse effects:* Hypoglycemia and hypokalemia ☛ Monitor for stress-induced hypoglycemia (particularly Type I diabetics)

LONG-ACTING INSULIN
- Protamine Zinc (PZI) (Humulin-U)
- Extended Zinc (Ultralente)

SULFONYLUREAS • Chlorpropamide (Diabinese) • Tolazamide (Tolinase) • Tolbutamide (Orinase) • Glipizide (Glucotrol, Glucotrol XL) • Glimepirid (Amaryl) • Glyburide (Glynase PresTab, DiaBeta, Micronase)	*MOA:* Increases pancreatic beta cell release of insulin in response to glucose *Uses:* For the treatment of Type 2 diabetes *Dose:* Depends on the agent *Adverse effects:* Hypoglycemia, disulfiram-like syndrome with alcohol; syndrome of inappropriate secretion of antidiuretic hormone ☞ Monitor for stress-induced hypoglycemia
ALPHA-GLUCOSIDASE INHIBITORS • Acarbose (Precose) • Miglitol (Glyset)	*MOA:* Competitive, reversible inhibition of pancreatic and intestinal alpha-glucosidase enzymes; these enzymes are responsible for hydrolysis of complex starches to simple sugars; inhibition of these enzymes results in delayed glucose absorption *Uses:* For the treatment of Type 2 diabetes *Dose:* Acarbose, 25mg tid; Miglitol, 50–100mg TID with meals *Adverse effects:* Flatulence, abdominal pain, elevated hepatic transaminase levels ☞ Can contribute to hypoglycemia when used in combination with insulin or sulfonylureas; if hypoglycemia occurs, administer dextrose or D-glucose; table sugar's (sucrose) absorption is inhibited by the alpha-glucosidase inhibitors

BIGUANIDE • Metformin (Glucophage)	*MOA:* Decreases hepatic glucose production, decreases intestinal absorption of glucose and improves insulin sensitivity *Uses:* For the treatment of Type 2 diabetes *Dose:* 500–1000mg BID with meals *Adverse effects:* Anorexia, nausea, vomiting, diarrhea, bloating, metallic taste, altered liver enzymes
MEGLITINIDES • Repaglinide (Prandin)	*MOA:* A nonsulfonylurea hypoglycemic agent that works by a similar mechanism; stimulates release of insulin from the pancreas; insulin release is glucose-dependent and diminishes at low glucose concentrations; rapidly eliminated from the bloodstream (short half-life) *Uses:* For the treatment of Type 2 diabetes *Dose:* 0.5–4mg 15–30 minutes before meals *Adverse effects:* Hypoglycemia, headache
THIAZOLIDINEDIONES • Troglitazone (Rezulin) • Rosiglitazone (Avandia) • Pioglitazone (Actos)	*MOA:* Decrease hepatic gluconeogenesis and increase insulin-dependent muscle glucose uptake *Uses:* For the treatment of Type 2 diabetes *Dose:* Depends on agent *Adverse effects:* Headache, pain, peripheral edema, infection, elevated hepatic transaminase levels ⚬⇁ Troglitazone removed from the market

ADRENOCORTICAL STEROIDS

GLUCOCORTICOIDS • Betamethasone (Celestone) • Dexamethasone (Decadron) • Hydrocortison (Cortef, Solu-Cortef)	*MOA:* Decrease inflammation by suppressing migration of white blood cells and reversing capillary permeability; suppress the immune system; suppress adrenal function at high doses *Uses:* Treatment of a variety of conditions including adrenocortical insufficiency, hypercalcemia, rheumatic and

• Methylpred-nisolone (Medrol, Solu-Medrol) • Prednisolone (Prelone, Pediapred) • Prednisone (Ora-sone, Deltasone) • Triamcinolone (Aristocort, Kenacor)	collagen disorders, organ transplantation, neoplastic diseases, respiratory disorders *Dose:* Depends on agent *Adverse effects:* Increased appetite, insomnia, nervousness, infections, impaired wound healing, sodium and fluid retention, peptic ulcer, hyperglycemia ☛ Corticosteroids are used to treat a variety of oral diseases of allergic, inflammatory, or autoimmune origin
MINERALCORTICOID • Fludrocortisone (Florinef)	*MOA:* Adrenal cortical steroid with high mineralcorticoid and glucocorticoid activity; mineralcorticoids act on the renal distal tubule to enhance the reabsorption of sodium; they also increase urinary excretion of potassium and hydrogen ions *Uses:* Replacement therapy for primary and secondary adrenocortical insufficiency in Addison's disease *Dose:* Adult dose, 0.1–0.2mg/day; children's dose, 0.05–0.1mg/day *Adverse effects:* Edema, hypertension, congestive heart failure

THYROID HORMONES

DESICCATED THYROID (ARMOUR THYROID)	*MOA:* Dessicated thyroid is derived from beef and pork and consists of T_4 and T_3 hormone; although natural, synthetic thyroid supplementation is preferred due to uniform standardization of potency; the principle effect of thyroid hormone is to increase the metabolic rate of body tissues; influences growth and maturation of various tissues *Uses:* Hypothyroidism *Dose:* 30–120mg QD *Adverse effects:* Related to therapeutic overdosage and include palpitations, tachycardia, angina, tremors, headache, nervousness, insomnia

LEVOTHYROXINE (T$_4$) (LEVOTHROID, SYNTHROID, LEVOXYL)	*MOA:* Synthetic thyroid hormone replacement; T$_4$ is converted to the active form of thyroid hormone T$_3$ *Uses:* Hypothyroidism *Dose:* 0.05–0.2mg QD *Adverse effects:* Related to therapeutic overdosage and include palpitations, tachycardia, angina, tremors, headache, nervousness, insomnia
LIOTHYRONINE (T$_3$) (CYTOMEL)	*MOA:* Synthetic T$_3$ hormone replacement *Uses:* Hypothyroidism *Dose:* 25–75mcg QD *Adverse effects:* Related to therapeutic overdosage and include palpitations, tachycardia, angina, tremors, headache, nervousness, insomnia
LIOTRIX (T$_4$ & T$_3$) (THYROLAR)	*MOA:* A synthetic mixture of T$_4$ and T$_3$ in a 4 to 1 ratio *Uses:* Hypothyroidism *Dose:* 1/4 to 2 grains per day *Adverse effects:* Related to therapeutic overdosage and include palpitations, tachycardia, angina, tremors, headache, nervousness, insomnia
ANTITHYROID AGENTS • Propylthiouracil (PTU) • Methimazole (Tapazole)	*MOA:* Inhibit the synthesis of thyroid hormones; they do not inactivate existing T$_4$ and T$_3$; PTU partially inhibits peripheral conversion of T$_4$ to T$_3$ *Uses:* Hyperthyroidism *Dose:* PTU, 50mg Q8H; Methimazole, 5mg Q8H *Adverse effects:* Skin rash, fever, leukopenia, jaundice

Central Nervous System Agents

CNS STIMULANTS

CAFFEINE (NODOZ, CAFFEDRINE, VIVARIN)	*MOA:* Potent CNS stimulant; cortical effects are milder and of shorter duration than amphetamines; stimulates medullary, vagal, vasomotor, and respiratory centers

	Uses: Fatigue, drowsiness, respiratory depression *Dose:* 100–200mg Q3-4H as needed *Adverse effects:* Tachycardia, palpitations, insomnia, restlessness, nervousness, tinnitus ☞ Epinephrine/vasoconstrictors potentiate effect
AMPHETAMINES • Amphetamine • Amphetamine mixtures (Adderall) • Dextroamphetamine (Dexedrine, Dextrostat)	*MOA:* Sympathomimetic amines with CNS stimulant activity; CNS effects are mediated by release of norepinephrine from central noradrenergic neurons *Uses:* Narcolepsy, attention-deficit disorder, weight loss *Dose:* Depends on agent *Adverse effects:* False feeling of well-being, nervousness, restlessness, insomnia, tachycardia, palpitations, blood pressure elevation ☞ Use vasoconstrictors with caution; use local anesthetic without vasoconstrictors in patients who present with high blood pressure
METHYLPHENIDATE (RITALIN)	*MOA:* Mild CNS stimulant with action similar to amphetamines *Uses:* Attention-deficit disorder, narcolepsy *Dose:* 10–60mg per day in divided doses 2 or 3 times a day *Adverse effects:* Tachycardia, nervousness, insomnia, anorexia, blood pressure elevation ☞ Use vasoconstrictors with caution; use local anesthetic without vasoconstrictors in patients who present with high blood pressure
PEMOLINE (CYLERT)	*MOA:* CNS stimulant with activity similar to amphetamines and methylphenidate *Uses:* Attention-deficit disorder *Dose:* 56.25–75mg QD *Adverse effects:* Insomnia, anorexia, weight loss, skin rash ☞ Has minimal sympathomimetic activity; can be used with vasoconstrictors

ANOREXIANTS • Diethylpropion (Tenuate) • Phentermine (Fastin, Zantryl, Adipex-P)	*MOA:* Non-amphetamine anorexiants; indirect-acting sympathomimeticamines; exact mechanism unknown but thought to directly stimulate the satiety center in the hypothalamic and limbic regions *Uses:* Treatment of exogenous obesity *Dose:* Diethylpropion, 25mg TID; Phentermine, 8mg TID before meals *Adverse effects:* Hypertension, euphoria, nervousness, insomnia, tachycardia, palpitations ☛ Use vasoconstrictors with caution; use local anesthetic without vasoconstrictors in patients who present with high blood pressure
• Sibutramine (Meridia)	*MOA:* Produces its therapeutic effects by inhibiting norepinephrine, serotonin, and dopamine reuptake *Uses:* Obesity treatment *Dose:* 10–15mg QD *Adverse effects:* Hypertension, tachycardia, palpitation, headache, dry mouth, insomnia, skin rash ☛ Use vasoconstrictors with caution; use local anesthetic without vasoconstrictors in patients who present with high blood pressure

ANALGESIC AGENTS

NARCOTIC AGONIST • Codeine • Hydrocodone APAP, Hydroco-done ASA (Vicodin, Lortab, Lorcet) • Hydromorphone (Dilaudid) • Levorphanol (Levo-Dromoran) • Morphine (MS Contin, Oramorph, Roxanol)	*MOA:* Narcotic analgesics are classified as agonist, agonist-antagonists, or partial agonists based on their activity at opioid receptors; five major receptors are known: mu, kappa, sigma, delta, and epsilon; actions of analgesics can be determined by their activity at 3 receptors: mu, kappa, and delta; when occupied by agonist, mu receptors mediate morphine-like supraspinal analgesia, euphoria, respiratory and physical depression, miosis, and reduced GI motility; kappa receptors mediate spinal analgesia and miosis; the delta receptors mediate dysphoria, and respiratory and

• Oxycodone, Oxycodone APAP, OxycodoneASA (Roxicodone, Percocet, Roxicet, Percodan) • Oxymorphone (Numorphan) • Alfentanil (Alfenta) • Fentanyl (Sublimaze, Actiq, Duragesic) • Meperidine (Demerol) • Sufentanil (Sufenta) • Methadone (Dolophine) • Propoxyphene (Darvon-N)	vasomotor stimulation caused by drugs with antagonist activity *Uses:* Analgesia/anesthesia *Dose:* Depends on agent *Adverse effects:* Lightheadedness, dizziness, sedation, nausea, vomiting, constipation, respiratory depression with high doses. ☞ May cause dry mouth ☞ Drugs combined with APAP should not exceed a total daily dose of 4 g of APAP or single dose of 1 g of APAP
NARCOTIC AGONIST-ANTAGONIST • Buprenorphine (Buprenex) • Butorphanol (Stadol) • Nalbuphine (Nubain) • Pentazocine (Talwin, Talwin NX)	*MOA:* Narcotic agonist-antagonist analgesics compete with other substances at the mu receptor; there are two types: (1) those that are antagonists at the mu receptor and (2) partial agonists that have limited agonist activity at the mu receptor; agonist-analgesics are potent analgesic agents with a lower abuse potential than pure agonists *Uses:* Relief of moderate to severe pain *Dose:* Depends on agent *Adverse effects:* Lightheadedness, dizziness, sedation, nausea, vomiting, constipation, respiratory depression at high dose
TRAMADOL (ULTRAM)	*MOA:* Centrally acting synthetic analgesic compound that is not related to opiates; analgesia results from binding to mu-opioid receptors and inhibition of norepinephrine and serotonin reuptake *Uses:* Moderate to severe pain *Dose:* 50–100mg Q4-6H *Adverse effects:* Lightheadedness, dizziness, sedation, nausea, vomiting, constipation

ACETAMINOPHEN (TYLENOL)	*MOA:* Reduces fever through direct action on hypothalamic heat-regulating centers; inhibits the synthesis of prostaglandins in the CNS and peripherally blocks pain impulse generation; does not inhibit peripheral prostaglandin synthesis *Uses:* Analgesis/antipyretic *Dose:* Adults, 325–650mg Q4-6H; children (< 12y), 10–15mg/kg/dose Q4-6H *Adverse effects:* Can cause hepatoxicity if overdosed; chronic dosing of 5–8gm over several weeks or 3–4gm over 1 year have resulted in liver damage
SALICYLATES • Aspirin • Diflunisal (Dolobid) • Magnesium salicylate • Choline magnesium trisalate (Trilisate) • Salsalate (Disalcid)	*MOA:* Have analgesic, antipyretic, and anti-inflammatory effects; lower body temperature through vasodilation of peripheral vessels; anti-inflammatory and analgesia result from inhibition of prostaglandin (PG) synthesis; aspirin (ASA) differs from other salicylates in that it is a more potent inhibitor of PG synthesis and irreversibly inhibits platelet aggregation *Uses:* Mild–moderate pain, fever, inflammatory conditions; ASA is used to lower the risk of cerebrovascular and cardiovascular events *Dose:* Depends on agent *Adverse effects:* Nausea, vomiting, dyspepsia, epigastric discomfort, heartburn, gastric ulceration ☛ Avoid aspirin for 1 week prior to surgery because of the possibility of bleeding; use ASA with caution in patients with asthma due to the possibility of aspirin allergy that can cause wheezing and bronchoconstriction (incidence of allergy is 0.2%)
NONSTEROIDAL ANTI-INFLAMMATORY AGENTS (NSAIDs) • Fenoprofen (Nalfon)	*MOA:* NSAIDs have analgesic and antipyretic activities; mechanism is believed to be inhibition of cyclooxygenase activity and prostaglandin synthesis; reversible inhibition of platelet aggregation

- Flurbiprofen (Ansaid)
- Ibuprofen (Motrin, Advil)
- Ketoprofen (Orudis, Oruvail)
- Naproxen (Anaprox, Naprosyn, Aleve)
- Oxaprozin (Daypro)
- Diclofenac (Voltaren)
- Etodolac (Lodine)
- Indomethacin (Indocin)
- Ketorolac (Toradol)
- Nabumetone (Relafen)
- Sulindac (Clinoril)
- Tolmetin (Tolectin)
- Piroxicam (Feldene)

Uses: Management of pain and swelling, inflammatory diseases

Dose: Depends on agent

Adverse effects: Nausea, vomiting, abdominal pain, dyspepsia, heartburn, gastric ulceration

☛ Can promote bleeding; use with caution, if at all, in patients receiving anticoagulation therapy with warfarin; do not give to patients in whom aspirin, iodides, or other NSAIDs have induced symptoms of asthma, rhinitis, urticaria, nasal polyps, angioedema, bronchospasm, or other allergic symptoms

MIGRAINE AGENTS

5-HT₁ RECEPTOR AGONISTS

- Naratriptan (Amerge)
- Rizatriptan (Maxalt)
- Sumatriptan (Imitrex)
- Zolmitriptan (Zomig)

MOA: Migraines are thought to be due to vasodilation of cranial blood vessels; 5-HT$_1$ agonists cause cranial vessel constriction and inhibit pro-inflammatory neuropeptide release; rizatriptan and zolmitriptan cross the blood–brain barrier and inhibit central activity on the trigemino-vascular system

Uses: Migraine treatment, cluster headache (sumatriptan injection only)

Dose: Depends on agent

Adverse effects: Dizziness, hot flashes, injection site reactions, tightness in chest, burning sensation, drowsiness, headache, increased blood pressure (rizatriptan)

METHYSERGIDE (SANSERT)	*MOA:* Semisynthetic ergot derivative; inhibits or blocks the effects of serotonin; serotonin is central neurohumoral agent and is known as a "headache substance" acting directly or indirectly to lower pain threshold; serotonin is also a potent vasoconstrictor; methysergide may displace serotonin on receptor pressor sites on the walls of cranial arteries during a migraine attack, preserving the vasoconstriction caused by serotonin *Uses:* Prevention or reduction of vascular headache *Dose:* 4–8mg daily with meals *Adverse effects:* Retroperitoneal and pleuropulmonary fibrosis may occur if treated for long-term; postural hypotension, peripheral ischemia, insomnia, nausea, vomiting, abdominal pain, diarrhea
DIHYDROERGOTAMINE (MIGRANAL, D.H.E. 45)	*MOA:* Ergot alkaloid alpha-adrenergic blocker directly stimulates vascular smooth muscle to vasoconstrict peripheral and cerebral vessels *Uses:* Abort or prevent vascular headache *Dose:* 1mg IM may repeat hourly to a max dose of 3mg *Adverse effects:* Localized edema, peripheral vascular effects, drowsiness, dizziness, diarrhea, nausea, vomiting, paresthesia. ☞ > 10% of patients experience dry mouth
• Ergotamine (Ergomar) • Ergotamine & caffeine (Cafergot, Ercaf, Wigraine)	*MOA:* Partial agonist and/or antagonist activity against tryptaminergic, dopaminergic and alpha-adrenergic receptors depending upon their site; causes constriction of peripheral and cranial blood vessels and depression of central vasomotor centers *Uses:* Abort or prevent vascular headache

	Dose: Cafergot, 2 tablets at onset, then 1 tablet every 30 minutes as needed. NTE 6 tablets per attack *Adverse effects:* Tachycardia, bradycardia, arterial spasm, claudication, rebound headache, localized edema, drowsiness, dizziness, nausea, vomiting, diarrhea ☞ > 10% of patients experience dry mouth
ISOMETHEPTENE, DICHLORALPHENAZONE & ACETAMINOPHEN (MIDRIN)	*MOA:* Isometheptene has sympathomimetic properties and acts by constricting dilated cranial and cerebral arterioles *Uses:* Relief of migraine and tension headache *Dose:* 2 capsules immediately, then 1 capsule every 60 minutes until relieved. NTE 5 capsules in a 12-hour period *Adverse effects:* Drowsiness, dizziness, skin rash

ANTIEMETIC/ANTIVERTIGO AGENTS

ANTIDOPAMINERGICS • Metoclopramide (Reglan) • Prochloperazine (Compazine) • Promethazine (Phenergan) • Thiethylperazine (Torecan)	*MOA:* Block dopamine receptors in chemoreceptor trigger zone of the CNS *Uses:* Management of nausea and vomiting *Dose:* Depends on agent *Adverse effects:* Drowsiness, thickening of bronchial secretions, extrapyramidal reactions (akathisia) in elderly, anticholinergic side effects (memory loss, confusion, dry mouth, urinary retention); hypotension when administered parenterally due to alpha-receptor blockade; tardive dyskinesia may occur (particularly in elderly) and is dose and duration dependent ☞ > 10% of patients experience dry mouth

ANTICHOLINERGICS • Dimenhydrinate (Dramamine) • Meclizine (Antivert, Dramamine II) • Scopolamine (Scopace, Transderm-Scop) • Trimethobenzamide (Tigan)	*MOA:* Block the action of acetylcholine at parasympathetic sites in smooth muscle, secretory glands, and the CNS; central anticholinergic action by blocking the chemoreceptor trigger zone (meclizine and dimenhyrinate); decreases excitability and conduction of the middle ear labyrinth (meclizine and dimenhydrinate); dry secretions and antagonize histamine and serotonin *Uses:* Preoperative to reduce secretions (scopolamine); prevention and treatment of nausea and vomiting from motion; management of vertigo (meclizine and dimenhydrinate) *Dose:* Depends on agent *Adverse effects:* Drowsiness, thickening of bronchial secretions, dry mouth, blurred vision ☛ > 10% of patients experience dry mouth
5-HT₃ RECEPTOR ANTAGONISTS • Dolasetron (Anzemet) • Granisetron (Kytril) • Ondansetron (Zofran)	*MOA:* Selective inhibition of peripheral and central type 3 serotinergic (5-HT$_3$) receptors; 5-HT$_3$ receptors play a major role in acute emesis but only a minor role in delayed nausea and vomiting *Uses:* Prophylaxis and treatment of chemotherapy-related emesis; generally used for patient's refractory to standard antiemetic therapy receiving moderate to highly emetogenic chemotherapy *Dose:* Depends on agent *Adverse effects:* Headache, constipation, diarrhea
DRONABINOL (MARINOL)	*MOA:* Not well defined, probably inhibits the vomiting center in the medulla oblongata *Uses:* Alternative when conventional antiemetics fail to relieve the nausea and vomiting associated with chemotherapy; also used for AIDS-related anorexia *Dose:* 5mg/m^2 1–3 hours before chemotherapy, then Q2-4H post-chemotherapy for a total of 4–6 doses/day

Adverse effects: Drowsiness, dizziness, detachment, anxiety, difficulty concentrating, mood change, increased appetite

ANTIANXIETY

| BENZODIAZEPINES
• Alprazolam (Xanax)
• Clorazepate (Tranxene)
• Chlodiazepoxide (Librium)
• Diazepam (Valium)
• Lorazepam (Ativan)
• Oxazepam (Serax)
• Midazolam (Versed) | *MOA:* Potentiate the effects of gamma-aminobutyrate (GABA) and other inhibitory transmitters by binding to specific benzodiazepine receptor sites; benzodiazepines cause muscle relaxation, ataxia, have anticonvulsant and anxiolytic properties
Uses: For the management of anxiety disorders; additionally some benzodiazepines are useful as hypnotics, anticonvulsants, and muscle relaxants; midazolam, an injectable short-acting agent, is used for induction of general anesthesia, preoperative sedation, conscious sedation, and to supplement nitrous oxide for short surgical procedures
Dose: Depends on agent
Adverse effects: Drowsiness, ataxia, amnesia, slurred speech, lightheadedness
• > 10% of patients experience dry mouth or changes in salivation |
| MISCELLANEOUS
• Buspirone (Buspar)

(*cont.*) | *MOA:* Mechanism is unknown; does not have significant affinity for benzodiazepine receptors or facilitate GABA binding; does have high affinity for serotonin receptors and moderate affinity for brain D_2-dopamine receptors and appears to act as a presynaptic dopamine agonist
Uses: Management of anxiety disorders; full benefits not seen for 3–4 weeks
Dose: 5mg TID
Adverse effects: Dizziness, lightheadedness, headache, restlessness, nausea |

• Doxepin (Sinequan)	*MOA:* A tricyclic antidepressant with antianxiety effects; increases synaptic concentration of serotonin and/or norepinephrine in the CNS by inhibition of their reuptake by presynaptic neurons *Uses:* Treatment of depression and treatment of anxiety disorders *Dose:* 75–150mg QHS *Adverse effects:* Sedation, drowsiness, dizziness, headache, constipation, increased appetite, nausea, unpleasant taste, weight gain ☛ > 10% experience dry mouth; increased risk of caries as a result of decreased salivation
• Hydroxyzine (Atarax, Vistaril)	*MOA:* Induces a calming effect in anxious, tense, psychoneurotic adults and children *Uses:* Symptomatic relief of anxiety and tension associated with psychoneurosis and as an adjunct for organic disease states in which anxiety is manifest (prior to dental procedures, in acute emotional problems, in alcoholism, allergic conditions) *Dose:* 50–100mg QID *Adverse effects:* Slight-moderate drowsiness, thickening of bronchial secretions ☛ 1–10% experience dry mouth; increased risk of caries as a result of decreased salivation
• Meprobamate (Equanil, Miltown)	*MOA:* Effects multiple sites in the CNS; inhibits multineuronal spinal reflexes; has mild tranquilizing properties; has some anticonvulsant and muscle relaxant properties *Uses:* Management of anxiety disorders; useful for the treatment of muscle spasm associated with acute temporomandibular joint pain *Dose:* 400mg TID-QID; sustained release, 400–800mg BID *Adverse effects:* Drowsiness, clumsiness, ataxia, loss of motor coordination ☛ < 1% experience stomatitis

ANTIDEPRESSANTS

TRICYCLIC ANTIDE-PRESSANTS (TCAs)

- Amitriptyline (Elavil)
- Amoxapine (Asendin)
- Clomipramine (Anafranil)
- Desipramine (Norpramin)
- Doxepin (Sinequan)
- Imipramine (Tofranil)
- Nortriptyline (Pamelor)
- Protriptyline (Vivactil)
- Trimipramine (Surmontil)

TETRACYCLIC

- Maprotiline (Ludiomil)
- Mirtazapine (Remeron)

MOA: Block amine pump (block presynaptic reuptake of norepinephrine and serotonin), have peripheral and central anticholinergic action

Uses: Relief of symptoms of depression; treatment of anxiety and panic disorder; treatment of premenstrual symptoms

Dose: Depends on agent

Adverse effects: Sedation and anticholinergic effects (dry mouth, blurred vision, mydriasis, constipation, urinary retention), unpleasant taste, weight gain; hypotension, arrhythmias, tachycardia, sudden death; sexual dysfunction

☛ > 10% experience dry mouth; increased risk of caries by reducing salivation and salivary buffer capacity; increased pressor response when norepinephrine or epinephrine are used in combination with tricyclic antidepressants

SEROTONIN REUPTAKE INHIBITORS (SSRIs)

- Citalopram (Celexa)
- Fluoxetine (Prozac)
- Fluvoxamine (Luvox)
- Paroxetine (Paxil)
- Sertraline (Zoloft)

MOA: Potent and selective inhibitors of serotonin reuptake by presynaptic neurons within the central nervous system; weak inhibitors of norepinephrine and dopamine reuptake

Uses: Treatment of depression, obsessive–compulsive disorder, bulimia nervosa, panic disorder, and generalized anxiety disorder

Dose: Depends on agent

Adverse effects: Nausea, insomnia, nervousness, headache, anxiety, somnolence, tremor, impotence

☛ > 10% experience dry mouth

MISCELLANEOUS ANTIDEPRESSANTS

VENLAFAXINE (EFFEXOR, EFFEXOR XR)	*MOA:* Strong inhibitor of neuronal serotonin and norepinephrine reuptake and weak inhibitor of dopamine reuptake; does not inhibit monoamine oxidase *Uses:* Treatment of depression and generalized anxiety disorder *Dose:* 75–225mg in divided doses two to three times daily; sustained release product administered as single daily dose *Adverse effects:* Headache, somnolence, dizziness, insomnia, nervousness, nausea, constipation, neck pain, weakness, sweating, elevated blood pressure, tachycardia, palpitations ☛ > 10% experience significant dry mouth; increased risk of caries as a result of decreased salivation
NEFAZODONE (SERZONE)	*MOA:* Inhibits neuronal uptake of norepinephrine and serotonin; antagonizes central serotonin (5-HT$_2$) receptors and alpha$_1$-receptors *Uses:* Treatment of depression *Dose:* 100mg BID (range 300–600mg in two divided doses) *Adverse effects:* Headache, drowsiness, insomnia, agitation, dizziness, confusion, nausea, tremor ☛ > 10% experience significant dry mouth; increased risk of caries as a result of decreased salivation
TRAZODONE (DESYREL)	*MOA:* Inhibits reuptake of serotonin and norepinephrine by the presynaptic neurons *Uses:* Treatment of depression; often used to treat insomnia in conjuction with SSRIs *Dose:* 50mg TID, increased by 50mg/day every 3–7 days; maximum dose 600mg/day *Adverse effects:* Dizziness, headache, confusion, nausea, bad taste, muscle tremors ☛ > 10% experience significant dry mouth; increased risk of caries as a result of decreased salivation

| **BUPROPION (WELLBUTRIN)** | *MOA:* Mechanism not known; has minimal reuptake inhibition. Inhibits reuptake of dopamine to slight extent; does not inhibit monoamine oxidase
Uses: Treatment of depression; an aid for smoking cessation
Dose: 150mg QD to max of 150mg BID with at least an 8-hour interval between doses
Adverse effects: Agitation, insomnia, fever, headache, psychosis, confusion, anxiety, restlessness, dizziness, seizures, chills, akathisia, nausea, vomiting, constipation, weight loss, impotence; dose-dependent risk of seizures (> 300mg/day)
☛ > 10% experience dry mouth; increased risk of caries as a result of decreased salivation |
| **MONOAMINE OXIDASE INHIBITORS (MAOIs)**
• Phenelzine (Nardil)
• Tranylcypromine (Parnate)
• Isocarboxazid (Marplan) | *MOA:* Monoamine oxidase (MAO) in an enzyme responsible for metabolism of biogenic amines (norepinephrine, epinephrine, dopamine, serotonin); MAO-A metabolizes epinephrine, norepinephrine, dopamine, tyramine, and serotonin; MAO-B metabolizes dopamine, tyramine, benzylamine and phenylethylamine; MAOIs inhibit both MAO-A and -B, which causes an increase in these amines
Uses: Treatment of atypical depression and depression unresponsive to other antidepressant therapy
Dose: Depends on agent
Adverse effects: Orthostatic hypotension
☛ Avoid use of vasoconstrictor due to possibility of hypertension when combined; orthostatic hypotension occurs in > 10%; avoid use of meperidine (Demerol) with these agents |

ANTIPSYCHOTIC AGENTS

TYPICAL ANTIPSYCHOTIC AGENTS
PHENOTHIAZINES
- Chlorpromazine (Thorazine)
- Fluphenazine (Prolixin)
- Mesoridazine (Serentil)
- Perphenazine (Trilafon)
- Prochlorperazine (Compazine)
- Promazine (Sparine)
- Trifluoperazine (Stelazine)
- Thioridazine (Mellaril)

THIOXANTHENES
- Thiothixene (Navane)

PHENYLBUTYLPIPER-ADINES
- Haloperidol (Haldol)

DIHYDROINDOLONES
- Loxapine (Loxitane)

DIBENZEPINE
- Molindone (Moban)

ATYPICAL ANTIPSYCHOTIC AGENTS
- Clozapine (Clozaril)
- Olanzapine (Zyprexa)
- Quetiapine (Seroquel)
- Risperidone (Risperidal)

MOA: Dopamine receptor antagonists; greater affinity for D_2 vs. D_1 receptors; the agents vary in their selectivity among the cortical dopamine tracts; blockade of nigrostriatal tract results in movement disorders, mesolimbic results in relief of hallucinations and delusions, mesocortical results in relief of psychosis and worsening of negative symptoms, and the tuberoinfundibular tract results in prolactin release; they also bind with varying affinities to cholinergic, alpha$_1$-adrenergic, and histamine receptors

Uses: Management of the manifestations of psychotic disorders

Dose: Depends on agent

Adverse effects: Varies according to affinity to various receptors; D_2 blockade results in extrapyramidal side effects (EPS) such as tardive dyskinesia, pseudoparkinsonism, akathisia, dystonia; anticholinergic side effects such as dry mouth, urinary retention, constipation, drowsiness, fatigue, sinus tachycardia; anti-alpha$_1$-adrenergic effects such as orthostatic hypotension and reflex tachycardia

☛ Significant orthostatic hypotension may occur; greater than 10% experience dry mouth; EPS of the TMJ are possible

MOA: Considered atypical because they have a decreased ability to induce EPS; may be beneficial for patients resistant to typical agents and may be more effective at relieving negative symptoms; compared to typical antipsychotic agents, atypical agents have increased affinity for serotonin 5-HT$_2$ receptors compared with D_2 receptors; antagonize one or more types of dopamine receptors (D_1, D_2, D_4, D_5); atypicals have selectivity for limbic dopamine receptors; they also have vary-

ing degrees of antagonism at one or more serotonin receptors (5-HT$_2$, 5-HT$_6$, 5-HT$_7$); antagonize alpha$_1$-adrenergic receptors
Uses: Management of the manifestations of psychotic disorders
Dose: Depends on agent
Adverse Effects: Headache, somnolence, insomnia, agitation, dizziness, xerostomia, constipation, hypotension

• Lithium

MOA: Lithium is a monovalent cation, which alters sodium transport in nerve and muscle cells; affects the synthesis, storage, release, and reputake of central monoamine neurotransmitters such as norepinephrine, serotonin, dopamine, acetylcholine, and gamma-aminobutyrate (GABA); antimanic effects may be the result of increases in norepinephrine reuptake and increased serotonin receptor sensitivity
Uses: For the treatment of manic episodes of manic-depressive illness (bipolar disorder); maintenance therapy prevents or decreases frequency of manic episodes
Dose: 300mg TID-QID adjusted to maintain serum level between 0.6 to 1.2 mEq/L
Adverse effects: Polydipsia, nausea, diarrhea, impaired taste, trembling, tremor
☛ Avoid concomitant use of NSAIDs as they may precipitate lithium toxicity

CHOLINESTERASE INHIBITORS

TACRINE (COGNEX)

MOA: Elevates Ach concentrations in the cortical areas by slowing the metabolism of Ach released by intact cholinergic neurons
Uses: Treatment of mild to moderate dementia of Alzheimer's type
Dose: 10mg–40mg QID
Adverse effects: Cholinergic (diarrhea, nausea, abdominal discomfort)

DONEPEZIL (ARICEPT)	*MOA:* Reversibly inhibits acetylcholinesterase, leading to increased Ach concentrations *Uses:* Treatment of mild to moderate dementia of the Alzheimer's type *Dose:* 5mg po QHS *Adverse effects:* Headache, nausea, diarrhea

SEDATIVES AND HYPNOTICS

ZOLPIDEM (AMBIEN)	*MOA:* Binds to benzodiazepine receptors (omega-1), causing hypnotic and anxiolytic activity that is similar to benzodiazepines; has reduced effects on skeletal muscle and seizure threshold *Uses:* Short-term treatment of insomnia *Dose:* 5–10mg po QHS *Adverse effects:* Headache, drowsiness, dizziness, myalgia, nausea, diarrhea
BENZODIAZEPINES • Flurazepam (Dalmane) • Temazepam (Restoril) • Triazolam (Halcion) • Quazepam (Doral)	*MOA:* Depresses all levels of CNS likely through increased action of gamma-aminobutyric acid (GABA), which is an inhibitory neurotransmitter *Uses:* Short-term treatment of insomnia *Dose:* Depends on agent *Adverse effects:* Tachycardia, chest pain, drowsiness, fatigue, lightheadedness, memory impairment, depression, headache, rash, decreased libido, constipation, decreased salivation, nausea, vomiting, diarrhea, blurred vision, sweating ⊶ > 10% experience dry mouth; increased risk of caries as a result of decreased salivation
CHLORAL HYDRATE	*MOA:* Central Nervous System depressant through unknown mechanism *Uses:* Sedative/hypnotic *Dose:* Children 50–75mg/kg/dose 30–60 minutes prior to procedure; do not exceed dose of 1000mg *Adverse effects:* Nausea, vomiting, diarrhea

ANTICONVULSANTS

PHENOBARBITAL	*MOA:* Interferes with transmission of impulses from the thalamus to the cortex of the brain *Uses:* Management of generalized tonic-clonic (grand mal) and partial seizures; neonatal seizures, febrile seizures in children *Dose:* Adults, 1–3mg/kg/day or 50–100 mg 2–3 times a day; Children (1–5 yrs), 6–8 mg/kg/d in divided doses, (5–12 yrs) 4–6 mg/kg/d in 1–2 divided doses *Adverse effects:* Hypotension, cardiac arrhythmias, bradycardia, dizziness, drowsiness, lethargy, impaired judgement
• Phenytoin (Dilantin) • Fosphenytoin (Cerebyx)	*MOA:* Inhibits seizure activity in the motor cortex; inhibitory activity likely a result of increasing efflux of sodium ions from neurons, which stabilizes the hyperexcitability threshold *Uses:* Management of generalized tonic-clonic (grand mal), simple partial, and complex partial seizures *Dose:* Adults, 300mg/day or 5–6 mg/kg/d *Adverse effects:* Mental confusion, slurred speech, dizziness, drowsiness, constipation, nausea, vomiting, trembling; numerous drug interactions ☛ Gingival hyperplasia occurs frequently and during the first 6 months of treatment; a program of professional cleaning should begin during the first 10 days of treatment

CLONAZEPAM (KLONOPIN)	*MOA:* Suppresses the spike-and-wave discharge in absence seizures by depressing nerve transmission in the motor *Uses:* Used alone or as adjunctive therapy for Lennox-Gastaut syndrome, akinetic and myoclonic seizures. Can be used in patients with refractory absence (petit mal) seizures *Dose:* Children (< 10 yrs), 0.1–0.2 mg/kg/ day in divided doses TID; adults, 0.5mg TID; NTE 20 mg/day *Adverse effects:* Somnolence, ataxia, fatigue, amnesia, lightheadedness, rash, constipation, diarrhea, nausea, vomiting
LAMOTRIGINE (LAMICTAL)	*MOA:* Inhibits release of the excitatory amino acid glutamate and inhibits voltage-sensitive sodium channels, which stabilizes neuronal membranes *Uses:* Adjunctive therapy in the treatment of partial seizures in adults and as adjunctive therapy in children and adults with Lennox-Gastaut syndrome; may be used in adults with generalized tonic-clonic, typical and atypical absence, myoclonic seizures *Dose:* Children, 2–15 mg/kg/d in divided doses BID; adults, 100–400 mg/d; in 1–2 divided doses *Adverse effects:* Serious rashes (including Stevens-Johnson syndrome), which occur more often in children and during first 2–8 weeks of therapy; also dizziness, sedation, ataxia
CARBAMAZEPINE (TEGRETOL)	*MOA:* Exact mechanism unknown but appears to be a result of reducing polysynaptic responses and blocking post-tetanic potentiation *Uses:* Management of partial seizures with complex symptoms; also used for treatment of generalized tonic-clonic seizures; mixed seizure patterns, or other partial or generalized seizures; additionally used for treatment of trigeminal neuralgia, restless legs syndrome, psychiatric disorders, diabetic neuropathy

Dose: Adults, 800–1200 mg/d in divided doses TID-QID
Adverse effects: Rash, sedation, dizziness, fatigue, slurred speech, clumsiness, confusion; numerous drug interactions
☞ Used for treatment of trigeminal neuralgia; some patients may experience sore throats or mouth ulcers

FELBAMATE (FELBATOL)	*MOA:* Mechanism unknown but has weak inhibitory effects on GABA-receptor and benzodiazepine-receptor binding *Uses:* Not for first-line use; used as adjunctive therapy for partial seizure and Lennox-Gastaut syndrome *Dose:* 2400–3600 mg/d in divided doses TID-QID *Adverse effects:* Aplastic anemia, liver toxicity and failure; fatigue, dizziness, nausea, diarrhea, cough
GABAPENTIN (NEURONTIN)	*MOA:* Mechanism unknown but has anticonvulsant properties similar to other anticonvulsants *Uses:* Adjunctive treatment for drug-refractory partial and secondarily generalized seizures in adults *Dose:* 900–1800 mg/d in divided doses Q8H *Adverse effects:* Somnolence, dizziness, ataxia
VALPROIC ACID (DEPAKENE, DEPAKOTE)	*MOA:* Increases brain levels of GABA (inhibitory neurotransmitter) *Uses:* Treatment of simple and complex absence seizures, myoclonic and generalized tonic-clonic seizures *Dose:* 30–60 mg/kg/d in divided doses BID-TID *Adverse effects:* Change in menstrual cycle, abdominal cramps, anorexia, diarrhea, nausea, numerous drug interactions

TOPIRAMATE (TOPAMAX)	*MOA:* Exact mechanism unknown, but thought to be due to GABA potentiation, sodium channel blockade, and/or blocking glutamate activity *Uses:* Adjunctive therapy for partial onset seizures in adults *Dose:* 200 mg BID *Adverse effects:* Fatigue, dizziness, ataxia, somnolence, memory difficulties, speech problems, nausea, paresthesia, tremor 🔑 10% of patients experience dry mouth
TIAGABINE (GABITRIL)	*MOA:* Unknown, but thought to be due to increased activity of GABA *Uses:* Adjunctive therapy for partial seizures *Dose:* 4–32 mg/d in divided doses BID-QID *Adverse effects:* Dizziness, headache, somnolence, memory disturbance, ataxia, tremors

ANTIPARKINSON AGENTS

ANTICHOLINERGICS • Benztropine (Cogentin) • Trihexyphenidyl (Artane)	*MOA:* Suppress central cholinergic activity and may inhibit the reuptake and storage of dopamine, thereby prolonging the action of dopamine *Uses:* Used as adjunctive therapy for the treatment of Parkinson's disease *Dose:* Benztropine, 1–2 mg/d in divided doses BID-QID; trihexyphenidyl, 6–10 mg/d in divided doses TID with meals *Adverse effects:* Dry skin, constipation, dry nose, throat, decreased sweating, constipation 🔑 > 10% experience significant dry mouth, prolonged xerostomia may contribute to the development of caries, peridontal disease, oral candidiasis and discomfort

SKELETAL MUSCLE RELAXANTS

BACLOFEN (LIORESAL)	*MOA:* Inhibits both monosynaptic and polysynaptic reflexes at the spinal level; may have GABA-ergic activity *Uses:* Treatment of reversible spasticity associated with multiple sclerosis or spinal cord lesions; also used but not indicated for the treatment of trigeminal neuralgia, intractable hiccups, bladder spasticity *Dose:* 40–80 mg/d in divided doses TID *Adverse effects:* Drowsiness, vertigo, dizziness, insomnia, slurred speech, ataxia, weakness
CARISOPRODOL (SOMA)	*MOA:* Exact mechanism unknown but may be due to central depressant actions *Uses:* Skeletal muscle relaxant, used for treatment of muscle spasm associated with temporomandibular joint (TMJ) pain *Dose:* 350mg TID-QID *Adverse effects:* Drowsiness ☛ Useful for muscle spasm from TMJ pain
CHLORZOXAZONE (PARAFON FORTE DSC)	*MOA:* Acts on spinal cord and subcortical levels by depressing polysynaptic reflexes *Uses:* Treatment of muscle spasm *Dose:* 250–500mg TID-QID *Adverse effects:* Drowsiness ☛ Useful for muscle spasm from TMJ pain
CYCLOBENZAPRINE (FLEXARIL)	*MOA:* Centrally acting skeletal muscle relaxant related to tricyclic antidepressants; reduces tonic somatic motor activity influencing both alpha and gamma motor neurons *Uses:* Treatment of muscle spasm *Dose:* 10mg BID-QID *Adverse effects:* Drowsiness, dizziness, lightheadedness ☛ Useful for muscle spasm from TMJ pain; >10% of patients have dry mouth

METAXALONE (SKELAXIN)	*MOA:* Central nervous system depression *Uses:* Relief of discomfort associated with acute painful musculoskeletal conditions *Dose:* 800 mg TID-QID *Adverse effects:* Somnolence, dizziness, headache, nausea, vomiting
METHOCARBAMOL (ROBAXIN)	*MOA:* Reduces transmission of impulses from the spinal cord to skeletal muscle *Uses:* Treatment of muscle spasm *Dose:* 500–750mg TID-QID *Adverse effects:* Drowsiness, dizziness, lightheadedness ☛ Useful for muscle spasm from TMJ pain
ORPHENADRINE (NORFLEX)	*MOA:* Indirect muscle relaxant thought to work due to central anticholinergic activity *Uses:* Treatment of muscle spasm *Dose:* 100mg BID *Adverse effects:* Drowsiness, dizziness, lurred vision ☛ Decreases normal salivary flow
TIZANIDINE (ZANAFLEX)	*MOA:* An alpha$_2$-adrenergic agonist, which decreases excitatory input to alpha motor neurons; effects are greatest on polysynaptic pathways *Uses*: Acute and intermittent management of increased muscle tone associated with spasticity *Dose:* 2–4 mg TID *Adverse effects:* Hypotension, sedation, somnolence, xerostomia ☛ > 10% of patients experience significant dry mouth

DOPAMINERGICS

AMANTADINE (SYMMETREL)	*MOA:* Releases dopamine from intact dopaminergic terminals in the substantia nigra

Uses: Symptomatic and adjunctive treatment of parkinsonism; also used for prophylaxis and treatment of influenza A viral infections and for drug-induced extrapyramidal symptoms
Dose: 100mg BID
Adverse effects: Orthostatic hypotension; peripheral edema; dry nose, throat, and mouth; constipation
☛ > 10% experience significant dry mouth, prolonged xerostomia may contribute to the development of caries, periodontal disease, oral candidiasis and discomfort

| BROMOCRIPTINE (PARLODEL) | *MOA:* A dopamine agonist, it stimulates the dopamine receptors in the corpus striatum
Uses: Used with levodopa/carbidopa for the treatment of parkinsonism or used in place of levodopa in patients allergic or unresponsive
Dose: 30–90 mg/d in divided doses TID
Adverse effects: Hypotension, mental depression, confusion, hallucinations, nausea, constipation, anorexia, nasal congestion |
| CARBIDOPA, LEVODOPA (SINEMET) | *MOA:* Levodopa crosses the blood–brain barrier into the CNS and is converted to dopamine in the striatal regions of the brain; carbidopa prevents the peripheral breakdown of levodopa, thereby increasing levels of levodopa in the brain
Uses: Treatment of parkinsonian syndrome
Dose: 25/100 mg BID-QID increased as needed to a maximum of 200/2000 mg/d
Adverse effects: Orthostatic hypotension, palpitations, cardiac arrhythmias, confusion, nightmares, dizziness, anxiety, nausea, vomiting, anorexia, constipation, dry mouth
☛ Patients may have significant orthostatic hypotension, so care should be taken when assisting patient from dental chair |

PERGOLIDE (PERMAX)	*MOA:* Centrally acting dopamine agonist *Uses:* Adjunctive treatment to levodopa/carbidopa in the management of Parkinson's disease *Dose:* 2–3 mg/day divided TID *Adverse effects:* Dizziness, somnolence, insomnia, confusion, hallucinations, anxiety, dystonia, nausea, constipation, rhinitis ☛ > 10% experience significant dry mouth, prolonged xerostomia may contribute to the development of caries, periodontal disease, oral candidiasis, and discomfort
SELEGILINE (ELDEPRYL, CARBEX)	*MOA:* Inhibits monoamine oxidase (MAO) type-B, which reduces the metabolism of dopamine *Uses:* Adjunctive therapy for the treatment of parkinsonian patients in whom levodopa/carbidopa therapy is failing *Dose:* 5 mg BID with breakfast and lunch *Adverse effects:* Mood changes, dyskinesias, dizziness, nausea, vomiting, abdominal pain ☛ > 10% experience significant dry mouth, prolonged xerostomia may contribute to the development of caries, periodontal disease, oral candidiasis, and discomfort
TOLCAPONE (TASMAR)	*MOA:* Selective and reversible inhibitor of catechol-o-methyltransferase, which reduces the metabolism of dopamine *Uses:* Adjunct to levodopa/carbidopa for the treatment of signs and symptoms of Parkinson's disease *Dose:* 100–200 mg TID *Adverse effects:* Orthostatic hypotension, excessive dreaming, headache, dizziness, somnolence, confusion, nausea, diarrhea, dystonia ☛ Patients may have significant orthostatic hypotension, so care should be taken when assisting patient from dental chair

PRAMIPEXOLE (MIRAPEX)	*MOA:* Pre- and postsynaptic D-2 receptor agonist with preferential affinity for D-2$_3$-receptor subtypes *Uses:* Treatment of signs and symptoms of Parkinson's disease *Dose:* 1.5–4.5 mg in divided doses TID ☛ Patients may have significant orthostatic hypotension, so care should be taken when assisting patient from dental chair
ROPINIROLE (REQUIP)	*MOA:* Stimulation of postsynaptic D-2-type receptors in the caudate-putamen area of the brain *Uses:* Treatment of Parkinson's disease in patients with early disease not receiving levodopa or patients with advanced disease on concomitant levodopa *Dose:* 3–24 mg/day in divided doses TID *Adverse effects:* Somnolence, dizziness, headache, nausea, dyspepsia, and confusion ☛ Patients may have significant orthostatic hypotension, so care should be taken when assisting patient from dental chair; < 2% of patients experience dry mouth

Hematological Agents

HEMATOPOIETIC AGENTS

RECOMBINANT HUMAN Erythropoietin (Epogen)	*MOA:* Induces erythropoiesis through stimulation of erythroid progenitor cells; this results in an increase in reticulocytes (within 10 days) and ultimately an increase in the hemoglobin and hematocrit (within 2–6 weeks) *Uses:* Anemia associated with end-stage renal disease; anemia related to therapy with AZT-treated HIV-infected patients; anemia in cancer patients receiving chemotherapy; anemia of prematurity *Dose:* 50–100 units/kg SQ or IV 3 times/week *Adverse effects:* Hypertension, chest pain, edema

FILGRASTIM (G-CSF) Neupogen	*MOA:* Stimulates the production, maturation, and activation of neutrophils *Uses:* To reduce the duration of neutropenia and the associated risk of infection *Dose:* 5 mcg/kg/d *Adverse effects:* Neutropenic fever, alopecia, nausea, vomiting, diarrhea, mucositis, bone pain, splenomegaly
SARGAMOSTIM (GM-CSF) Leukine	*MOA:* Stimulates production, differentiation and functional activity neutrophils, eosinophils, monocytes, and macrophages *Uses:* Acceleration of myeloid recovery, or bone marrow transplant failure or engraftment delay, and induction chemotherapy in acute myelogenous leukemia *Dose:* 250 mcg/m^2/day IV *Adverse effects:* Tachycardia, neutropenic fever, alopecia, nausea, vomiting, diarrhea, mucositis, skeletal pain
ANTIPLATELET AGENTS • Cilostazol (Pletal) • Clopidogrel (Plavix) • Ticlopidine (Ticlid)	*MOA:* Inhibit the binding of the ADP to its platelet receptor and the subsequent ADP-mediated activation GPIIb/IIIa complex, thereby inhibiting platelet aggregation *Uses:* Used for the reduction of atherosclerotic events in patients with atherosclerosis documented by recent stroke, recent MI, or established peripheral arterial disease (clopidogrel and ticlopidine); used for intermittent claudication (cilostazol) *Dose:* Cilostazol, 100mg BID; clopidogrel, 75mg QD; ticlopidine, 250mg BID *Adverse effects:* Skin rash, diarrhea, nausea, vomiting, GI pain, neutropenia (ticlopidine) ☞ If patient undergoes oral surgery, these agents should be discontinued 7 days prior to minimize the risk of bleeding; concomitant use with NSAIDs increases the risk of GI bleeding

| **DIPYRIDAMOLE (PERSANTINE)** | *MOA:* Inhibits platelet adhesion by inhibiting red blood cell uptake of adenosine, an inhibitor of platelet reactivity; inhibits phosphodiesterase which leads to increased cAMP within platelets and inhibits formation of thromboxane A_2; following IV administration, dipyridamole decreases systemic and coronary arterial resistance; results in worsened regional myocardial perfusion distal to partial occlusion of coronary arteries
Uses: Adjunct of coumadin for prevention of thromboembolism postcardiac valve replacement; used to maintain patency of grafts after coronary artery bypass surgery
Dose: 75–400 mg/day divided TID-QID
Adverse effects: May exacerbate angina, dizziness, hypotension, hypertension, tachycardia, headache |

ANTICOAGULANTS

| **LOW MOLECULAR WEIGHT HEPARINS**
• Ardeparin (Normiflo)
• Dalteparin (Fragmin)
• Enoxaparin (Lovenox) | *MOA:* These agents have antithrombotic activity through inhibition of Factor Xa and thrombin by binding to and accelerating antithrombin III activity; main activity is due to inhibition of Factor Xa
Uses: Used for prophylaxis or treatment of thromboembolic complications following surgery or ischemic complications of unstable angina and MI
Dose: Depends on agent
Adverse effects: Bruising, bleeding, thrombocytopenia |

HEPARIN	*MOA:* In combination with antithrombin III, inhibits conversion of prothrombin to thrombin and subsequent conversion of fibrinogen to fibrin; in addition inactivates activated coagulation factors IX, X, XI, and XII *Uses:* Prophylaxis and treatment of thromboembolic disorders *Dose:* Given IV for treatment; SQ for prophylaxis; dose varies depending on indication and route of administration *Adverse effects:* Bruising, bleeding from gums, hemorrhage, thrombocytopenia
WARFARIN (COUMADIN)	*MOA:* Interferes with the synthesis of vitamin K-dependent coagulation factors (II, VII, IX, X) *Uses:* Prophylaxis and treatment of venous thrombosis, pulmonary embolis, nd thromboembolic disorders *Dose:* Varies *Adverse effects:* Bleeding, bruising, bleeding gums ☛ Bleeding from gingival tissue may be an early sign of overanticoagulation with warfarin
HEMOSTATICS • Aminocaproic acid (Amicar) • Tranexamic acid (Cyklokapron)	*MOA:* Inhibits fibrinolysis through inhibition of plaminogen activator substances (tranexamic acid is 10x more potent) *Uses:* Treatment of excessive bleeding from fibrinolysis *Dose:* Aminocaproic acid, 5 gm PO or IV, followed by 1–1.25 gm hourly Tranexamic acid, 20–25 mg/kg Q8H *Adverse effects:* Hypotension, dizziness, nausea, diarrhea, vomiting, cramps, nasal congestion, myopathy ☛ Tranexamic acid mouthwashes have been used to prevent oral bleeding in hemophilia patients and patients receiving oral anticoagulation therapy

Anti-Infectives

ANTIBIOTICS—PENICILLINS

NATURAL
- Penicillin G (Wycillin) (Penicillin G procaine)
- Penicillin V (Veetids, Pen Vee K)

PENICILLINASE-RESISTANT
- Cloxacillin (Cloxapen)
- Dicloxacillin (Dynapen, Cycill, Pathocil)
- Nafcillin (Unipen, Nallpen)
- Oxacillin (Bactocill)

AMINOPENICILLINS
- Amoxicillin (Amoxil, Trimox, Wymox)
- Amoxicillin; potassium clavulanate (Augmentin)
- Ampicillin (Principen, Omnipen)
- Ampicillin (Sulbactam, Unasyn)
- Bacampicillin (Spectrobid)

EXTENDED-SPECTRUM
- Carbenicillin (Geocillin)
- Mezlocillin (Mezlin)
- Piperacillin (Pipracil)

(cont.)

MOA: Penicillins inhibit the biosynthesis of cell wall mucopeptide, which results in cell death; they are bacteriocidal against susceptible organisms

Uses: For the treatment of mildly to moderately severe infections caused by penicillin-sensitive microoganisms

Dose: Depends on agent

Adverse effects: Nausea, vomiting, diarrhea, vaginitis, oral candidiasis, rash, hypersensitivity reactions

☞ Penicillin V Potassium (K) is the antibiotic of choice for the treatment of common orofacial infections caused by aerobic gram-positive cocci and some anaerobes

☞ Amoxicillin is used as a standard prophylactic regimen for dental patients who are at risk (patients with cardiac valve abnormalities or replacement)

☞ Amoxicillin/Clavunate is used for treatment of orofacial infections due to beta-lactamase-producing staphylococci and bacteroides

- Piperacillin (tazobactam sodium/ Zosyn)
- Ticarcillin (Ticar)
- Ticarcillin/ potassium clavulanate (Timentin)

(*see previous page*)

ANTIBIOTICS—CEPHALOSPORINS

FIRST GENERATION
- Cefadroxil (Duricef)
- Cefazolin (Ancef, Kefzol)
- Cephalexin (Keflex, Biocef, Keftab)
- Cephapirin (Cefadyl)
- Cephradine (Velosef)

SECOND GENERATION
- Cefaclor (Ceclor)
- Cefmetazole (Zefazone)
- Cefonicid (Monocid)
- Cefotetan (Cefotan)
- Cefoxitin (Mefoxin)
- Cefprozil (Cefzil)
- Cefuroxime (Ceftin, Zinacef, Kefurox)
- Loracarbef (Lorabid)

THIRD GENERATION
- Cefdinir (Omnicef)

MOA: Structurally and pharmacologically similar to penicillins; groups (generations) are based on antibacterial spectrum; progression from first to third generation reveals broadening gram-negative coverage and loss of activity against gram-positive organisms, greater coverage against resistant organisms, and greater cost

Uses: For the treatment of mildly to moderately severe infections caused by cephalosporin-sensitive microoganisms

Dose: Depends on agent

Adverse effects: Cross-allergenicity with penicillin (administer with caution), nausea, diarrhea

☞ Cross-allergenicity with penicillin is 5–8%; if patient has a Type I hypersensitivity reaction (urticaria or anaphylaxis) to penicillin, the incidence of cross-allergenicity increases to 20%

☞ Cephalexin can be used as an alternative antibiotic in patients allergic to penicillin (provided they have not had an immediate, local, or systemic IgE-mediated anaphylactic allergic reaction to penicillin) for treatment of orofacial infection caused by aerobic gram-positive bacteria and anaerobes

• Cefepime (Maxipime) • Cefixime (Suprax) • Cefoperazone (Cefobid) • Cefotaxime (Claforan) • Cefpodoxime (Vantin) • Ceftazidime (Fortaz) • Ceftibuten (Cedax) • Ceftizoxime (Ceftizox) • Ceftriaxone (Rocephin)	
FLUOROQUINOLONES • Ciprofloxacin (Cipro) • Enoxacin (Penetrex) • Grepafloxacin (Raxar) • Levofloxacin (Levaquin) • Lomefloxacin (Maxaquin) • Norfloxacin (Noroxin) • Ofloxacin (Floxin) • Sparfloxacin (Zagam)	*MOA:* Synthetic, broad spectrum (gram-positive and gram-negative organisms) antibacterial agents; bactericidal through inhibition of DNA gyrase, which is needed for synthesis of bacterial DNA *Uses:* Treatment of lower respiratory, skin, bone and joint, and urinary tract infections, infectious diarrhea, typhoid fever, sexually transmitted diseases (uncomplicated cervical and urethral gonorrhea due to *N. gonorrhoeae*) *Dose:* Depends on agent *Adverse effects:* Headache, nausea, vomiting, diarrhea, tremor, insomnia, increased transaminases 🔑 Fluoroquinolones end with "-floxacin" (except enoxacin)

TETRACYCLINES • Tetracycline (Sumycin, Panmycin) • Demeclocycline (Declomycin) • Doxycycline (Vibramycin, Oryx, Monodox) • Minocycline (Dynacin, Minocin, Vectrin)	*MOA:* Inhibit bacterial protein synthesis by binding with the 30S and possibly 50S ribosomal subunit of susceptible bacteria; they are bacteriostatic with activity against gram-positive and gram-negative organisms *Uses:* For the treatment of mildly to moderately severe infections caused by microoganisms with demonstrated susceptibility *Dose:* Depends on agent, route of administration, and indication *Adverse effects:* Nausea, vomiting, diarrhea, photosensitivity, lightheadedness, and dizziness (minocycline) ☛ Tetracyclines end with "-cycline" ☛ Tetracyclines are contraindicated in pregnant women and children < 8 years of age due to the risk of permanent discoloration (yellow-gray-brown) of deciduous and permanent teeth ☛ Avoid concomitant administration with antacids, dairy products, or iron-containing products due to binding and decreased bioavailability of the tetracycline
MACROLIDES • Azithromycin (Zithromax) • Clarithromycin (Biaxin) • Dirithromycin (Dynabac) • Erythromycin (E-mycin, Ery-tab, Eryc, EryPed, Ilosone, EES) • Troleandomycin (Tao)	*MOA:* Reversibly bind to the P site of the 50S ribosomal subunit of susceptible bacteria and inhibits RNA-dependent protein synthesis; they are bacteriostatic or bacteriocidal depending on factors such as drug concentration *Uses:* For the treatment of mildly to moderately severe infections caused by microoganisms with demonstrated susceptibility *Dose:* Depends on agent, route of administration, and indication *Adverse effects:* Abdominal pain, cramping, nausea, vomiting, oral candidiasis, headache ☛ Macrolides are useful as an alternative antibiotic for treatment of orofacial infections in patients allergic to penicillin

AMINOGLYCOSIDES • Streptomycin • Kanamycin • Gentamicin • Tobramycin • Amikacin • Netilimicin • Neomycin	*MOA:* Bacteriocidal antibiotics used primarily in the treatment of gram-negative infections; irreversibly bind to 30S subunit of bacterial ribosomes blocking protein synthesis and causing cell death *Uses:* Treatment of serious gram-negative infections caused by susceptible organisms; oral neomycin used as a bowel prep for GI surgery *Dose:* Depends on agent *Adverse effects:* Nephrotoxicity and ototoxicity, neurotoxicity (vertigo, ataxia)
METRONIDAZOLE (FLAGYL)	*MOA:* Active against anaerobic bacteria and protozoa; it is reduced to a product that interacts with DNA causing strand breakage and inhibition of protein synthesis with subsequent cell death *Uses:* For the treatment of anaerobic, intra-abdominal, skin, gynecologic, CNS, and lower respiratory infections, endocarditis; has been used for treatment of antibiotic-associated pseudomembranous colitis, treatment of *Helicobacter pylori,* Crohn's disease, and hepatic encephalopathy; also used topically for bacterial vaginosis and acne rosacea; used in the treatment of oral soft tissue infections due to anaerobic bacteria including all anaerobic cocci, anaerobic gram-negative bacilli, and gram-positive spore forming bacilli; also used in combination with either amoxicillin, augmentin, or ciprofloxacin in the treatment of periodontitis with the presence of *Actinobacillus actinomycetemcomitans* (AA) *Dose:* Depends on route of administration and indication *Adverse effects:* Dizziness, headache, nausea, diarrhea, loss of appetite, vomiting; less than 1% will experience dry mouth and metallic taste ☛ Avoid concurrent alcohol ingestion

CLINDAMYCIN (CLEOCIN)	*MOA:* Binds to 50S subunit of bacterial ribosomes and suppress protein biosynthesis *Uses:* Treatment of serious infections due to susceptible strains of streptococci, pneumococci, staphylococci, and anaerobic organisms *Dose:* 150–450mg Q6H *Adverse effects:* Pseudomembranous colitis (discontinue immediately if patient has severe persistent diarrhea and cramping), nausea, vomiting, esophagitis, metallic taste, glossitis, rash ☛ Alternate antibiotic in penicillin-allergic patients for prevention of bacterial endocarditis in patients undergoing dental procedures
SULFONAMIDES • Sulfadiazine • Sulfisoxazole • Sulfamethoxazole • Sulfamethoxazole/ Trimethoprim (TMP-SMZ) (Bactrim, Bactrim DS, Septra, Cotrim) • Sulfamethizole	*MOA:* Bacteriostatic through antagonism of para-aminobenzoic acid (PABA), which is essential in the synthesis of folic acid; sulfonamides have a broad antibacterial spectrum, which includes both gram-positive and gram-negative organisms; trimethoprim blocks the production of tetrahydrofolic acid from dihydrofolic acid by binding to and reversibly inhibiting dihydrofolate reductase *Uses:* Used for treatment of urinary tract infections, *pneumocystis carinii* pneumonia, otitis media, chronic bronchitis, travelers' diarrhea, prostatitis, nocardiosis, toxoplasmosis *Dose:* Depends on agent, route of administration, and indication *Adverse effects:* Photosensitivity, allergic reactions ☛ Fever, dizziness, headache, itching, skin rash, photosensitivity, anorexia, nausea, vomiting, diarrhea
VANCOMYCIN (VANCOCIN)	*MOA:* Inhibits cell-wall biosynthesis by altering bacterial–cell–membrane permeability and RNA synthesis; active only against gram-positive bacteria

Uses: For serious or severe infections not treatable with other antimicrobials; oral vancomycin is only useful for treatment of antibiotic-associated pseudo-membranous colitis produced by *C. difficle*
Dose: 1 gm IV Q12H; also used as 1 gm 1 hour prior to dental surgery
Adverse effects: Hypotension and flushing of face and upper body

ANTIFUNGALS

FLUCYTOSINE (ANCOBON)	*MOA:* Active against *Candida* and *Cryptococcus;* penetrates fungal cells and is converted to fluorouracil, which competes with uracil and interferes with fungal RNA and protein synthesis *Uses:* Adjunctive treatment of susceptible fungal infections in combination with amphotericin B, fluconazole, or itraconazole *Dose:* 50–150 mg/kg/d in divided doses Q6H *Adverse effects:* Skin rash, abdominal pain, diarrhea, loss of appetite, nausea, vomiting
GRISEOFULVIN (GRIS-PEG, FULVICIN)	*MOA:* Inhibits fungal cell wall mitosis, binds to keratin, making it resistant to fungal invasion *Uses:* Treatment of tinea infections of the skin, hair, and nails *Dose:* Microsize, 500–1000 mg/day; ultramicrosize, 330–375–750 mg/day *Adverse effects:* Skin rash, urticaria, nausea, vomiting, oral thrush
AMPHOTERICIN B	*MOA:* Binds to ergosterol-altering cell membrane permeability in susceptible fungi and causing leakage of cell components with subsequent cell death *Uses:* Treatment of severe fungal infections and meningitis caused by susceptible organisms *Dose:* 0.25 mg/kg IV × 1, then 1–1.5 mg/kg/dose IV QOD *Adverse effects:* Fever, chills, headache, malaise, hypokalemia, hypomagnesemia, anorexia, anemia, nephrotoxicity

NYSTATIN (MYCOSTATIN, NILSTAT)	*MOA:* Binds to sterols in the cell membrane of the fungus, which alters membrane permeability, allowing leakage of intracellular components *Uses:* Treatment of oral candidiasis *Dose:* 500,000–1,000,000 units TID *Adverse effects:* Nausea, vomiting, diarrhea, abdominal pain ☛ Available as a suspension (swish and swallow) or an oral troche for treatment of oral candidiasis
IMIDAZOLES • Ketoconazole • Fluconazole • Itraconazole	*MOA:* Impair the synthesis of ergosterol, the main sterol of fungal cell membranes, which allows increased cellular permeability and leakage of intracellular components *Uses:* Ketoconazole treatment of candidiasis (oral and systemic), blastomycosis, coccidioidomycosis, histoplasmosis, chromomycosis and paracoccidioidomycosis, onychomycosis; fluconazole treatment of oral candidiasis, candidal urinary tract infections, peritonitis, candidemia, cryptococcal meningitis; itraconazole treatment of blastomycosis, histoplasmosis, aspergillosis, onychomycosis, candidiasis *Dose:* Depends on agent and indication *Adverse effects:* Nausea, vomiting, diarrhea, hepatoxicity (ketoconazole and itraconazole) ☛ Can be used for treatment of oropharyngeal and esophogeal candidiasis
TERBINAFINE	*MOA:* Inhibits squalene epoxidase, a key enzyme in sterol biosynthesis in fungi, resulting in deficiency of ergosterol in cell wall and subsequent cell death *Uses:* Treatment of onychomycosis of the toenail or fingernail due to dermatophytes *Dose:* Fingernail, 250 mg/day for 6 weeks; toenail, 250 mg/day for 12 weeks *Adverse effects:* Headache, nausea, diarrhea, abnormal taste, rash, liver enzyme elevation

ANTITUBERCULOSAL AGENTS

ISONIAZID	*MOA:* Active against actively growing tubercle bacilli; bactericidal through interference with lipid and nucleic acid biosynthesis in growing organisms *Uses:* Prevention and treatment of tuberculosis *Dose:* Treatment, 5 mg/kg/day; prevention, 300 mg/day *Adverse effects:* Loss of appetite, nausea, vomiting, stomach pain, hepatitis, peripheral neuritis, weakness
RIFAMPIN	*MOA:* Inhibits DNA-dependent RNA polymerase, which blocks RNA transcription *Uses:* Treatment of tuberculosis, asymptomatic *Neisseria meningitidis* carriers *Dose:* 600 mg QD *Adverse effects:* Diarrhea, stomach cramps, discoloration (reddish-orange) of feces, saliva, sputum, urine, sweat, and tears, elevation of liver enzymes
RIFABUTIN	*MOA:* Inhibits DNA-dependent RNA polymerase, which blocks RNA transcription *Uses:* Prevention of disseminated *Mycobacterium avium* complex *Dose:* 300 mg QD *Adverse effects:* Rash, discoloration (brownish-orange) of urine, feces, saliva, sputum, perspiration, tears, and skin; neutropenia
ETHAMBUTOL	*MOA:* Inhibits the synthesis of one or more metabolites, causing impaired cell metabolism, inhibition of multiplication, and cell death *Uses:* Combination treatment of tuberculosis *Dose:* 15 mg/kg QD *Adverse effects:* Headache, hyperuricemia, nausea, anorexia, optic neuritis

ANTIVIRAL AGENTS

ACYCLOVIR (ZOVIRAX)	*MOA:* A synthetic purine nucleoside analog with activity against Herpes simplex virus (HSV) Types 1 and 2, varicella-zoster, Epstein-Barr, and cytomegalovirus; acyclovir is selectively taken up and converted to triphosphate form by infected cells; acyclovir triphosphate interferes with HSV DNA polymerase and inhibits viral DNA replication *Uses:* Treatment of initial and recurrent episodes of genital herpes, mucosal and cutaneous HSV-1 and HSV-2, and varicella-zoster (shingles) infections *Dose:* Depends on route of administration and indication *Adverse effects:* Headache, diarrhea, rash, nausea, vomiting
FAMCICLOVIR (FAMVIR)	*MOA:* Undergoes rapid biotransformation to active form, penciclovir, which has activity against HSV-1 and HSV-2, and varicella-zoster; penciclovir is converted to the triphosphate form, which inhibits HSV-2 polymerase, which results in inhibition of herpes viral DNA synthesis and replication *Uses:* Management of acute herpes zoster (shingles) and treatment of recurrent mucocutaneous herpes simplex infections *Dose:* Zoster, 500 mg PO Q8H × 7 days; recurrent herpes simplex, 125 mg PO BID × 5 days *Adverse effects:* Headache, nausea, diarrhea
VALACYCLOVIR (VALTREX)	*MOA:* Rapidly converted to acyclovir with a similar mechanism of action as acyclovir *Uses:* Treatment of herpes zoster and episodic treatment of recurrent genital herpes *Dose:* Zoster, 1 gm PO TID × 7 days; genital herpes, 500 mg PO BID × 5 days *Adverse effects:* Nausea, headache

AMANTADINE (SYMMETREL)	*MOA:* Blocks the uncoating of influenza A virus, preventing penetration of virus into host *Uses:* Prophylaxis and treatment of influenza A viral infection *Dose:* 100 mg PO BID *Adverse effects:* Dry mouth, hypotension, nausea, dizziness, lightheadedness, insomnia ☛ > 10% experience significant dry mouth
RIMANTADINE (FLUMADINE)	*MOA:* Blocks the uncoating of influenza A virus preventing penetration of virus into host; is 2- to 8-fold more potent than amantadine *Uses:* Prophylaxis and treatment of influenza A viral infection *Dose:* 100 mg PO BID × 7 days post initial symptoms *Adverse effects:* Nausea, vomiting, fatigue, insomnia, nervousness, headache, dry mouth
ZANAMIVIR (RELENZA)	*MOA:* Inhibits influenza virus neraminidase the enzyme necessary for viral replication *Uses:* Treatment of uncomplicated acute illness due to influenza virus *Dose:* 2 inhalations by mouth Q12H × 5 days *Adverse effects:* Well tolerated

ANTIRETROVIRAL AGENTS

PROTEASE INHIBITORS • Saquinavir (Invirase, Fortovase) • Ritonavir (Norvir) • Indinavir (Crixivan) • Nelfinavir (Viracept) • Amprenavir (Agenerase)	*MOA:* Inhibit human immunodeficiency virus (HIV) protease; HIV protease cleaves protein precursors to generate functional proteins in HIV-infected cells; results in formation of immature noninfectious viral particles *Uses:* In combination with antiretroviral agent for the treatment of HIV infection *Dose:* Depends on agent *Adverse effects:* Diarrhea, abdominal discomfort, nausea, taste perversion, headache, hypertriglyceridemia, hyperglycemia, hypercholesterolemia

NUCLEOSIDE REVERSE TRANSCRIPTASE INHIBITORS	MOA, Uses, Dose, Adverse effects
NUCLEOSIDE REVERSE TRANSCRIPTASE INHIBITORS • Didanosine (ddI) (Videx) • Lamivudine (3TC) (Epivir) • Stavudine (d4T) (Zerit) • Zalcitabine (ddC) (Hivid) • Zidovudine (AZT) (Retrovir) • Abacavir (Ziagen)	*MOA:* Converted to nucleoside triphosphate, which interferes with the HIV-RNA-dependent DNA polymerase (reverse transcriptase) by competing with the natural nucleoside triphosphate for binding to active site of the enzyme; once incorporated into the growing chains of DNA, the DNA chain is terminated *Uses:* For the treatment of HIV-infected adults; typically these agents are used in combination *Dose:* Depends on agent *Adverse effects:* Headache, insomnia, nausea, neutropenia, leukopenia, oral ulcers (Zalcitabine), irritability, nausea, diarrhea, peripheral neuropathy (Didanosine, Stavudine, and Lamivudine)
NON-NUCLEOSIDE REVERSE TRANSCRIPTASE INHIBITORS • Nevirapine (Viramune) • Delavirdine (Rescriptor) • Efavirenz (Sustiva)	*MOA:* Bind directly to reverse transcriptase and block RNA-dependent and DNA-dependent DNA polymerase activities *Uses:* In combination with nucleoside analogs for the treatment of HIV-1 infected adults *Dose:* Depends on agent *Adverse effects:* Severe rash (Nevirapine), headache, drowsiness, dizziness, insomnia, abnormal dreaming, hallucinations, confusion, drug fever, diarrhea, nausea, increased liver enzymes, increased serum cholesterol 🔑 Dry mouth and taste disturbance in < 2% of patients treated with efavirenz

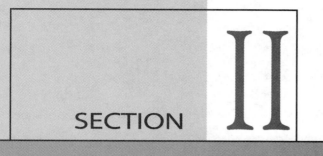

SECTION **II**

Provision of Clinical Dental Hygiene Services

➤ Assessing Patient Characteristics

➤ Obtaining and Interpreting Radiographs

➤ Planning and Managing Dental Hygiene Care

➤ Performing Periodontal Procedures

➤ Reassessment and Maintenance

➤ Using Preventive Agents

➤ Providing Supportive Treatment

7 Assessing Patient Characteristics

Demetra Daskalos Logothetis, RDH, MS

➤ **MEDICAL AND DENTAL HISTORY**

Medical History

STATUS OF PATIENT'S GENERAL HEALTH

- Patient's feeling of his/her general health
- Identification of disabilities
- Identification of medical conditions
- Indication of how patient will handle dental appointment

MEDICAL EXAMINATIONS

Is patient currently under the care of a physician?
- Dates and reason for most frequent examinations
- Laboratory tests and results
- New prescriptions and refill prescriptions
- Anticipated surgeries
- Medical consult may be necessary
- Immediate dental treatment may be needed prior to surgery (e.g., transplant or heart surgery)
- Reason for prescriptions

SERIOUS ILLNESSES, HOSPITALIZATION, SURGERIES

- Seek information regarding any medical conditions that might be of significance to planned dental treatment
- Course of healing: normal, abnormal

MEDICATIONS PRESCRIBED BY PHYSICIAN AND OVER THE COUNTER MEDICATIONS

- Relation to dental care
- Drug interactions
- Patient's regularity of taking medication
- ☛ List all drugs by name and dosage

HISTORY OF ALLERGIC REACTIONS

- Penicillin or other antibiotics
- Local anesthetics
- Sulfa drugs
- Barbiturates, sedatives
- Aspirin, ibuprofen
- Iodine (☛ Betadine contains iodine)
- Codeine or other narcotics
- Latex (☛ *must* use latex-free products when providing treatment)

☛ A patient exhibiting a positive allergic reaction indicates an absolute contraindication to administering these drugs, or using these products

MEDICAL CONDITIONS

BLEEDING PROBLEMS	• Bleeding associated with previous dental appointments • Anticoagulant medications • Coagulation problems • Aspirin use • Review laboratory test for bleeding time ☛ May need special measures for treatment and medical consultation
BLOOD TRANSFUSION	Risk of communicable diseases
DAMAGED HEART VALVE, ARTIFICIAL HEART VALVES, HEART MURMUR, RHEUMATIC FEVER, OR PROSTHETIC DEVICES (JOINTS, VALVES)	• Evaluate need for premedication • Determine type of valve or murmur • Medical consult indicated prior to treatment

CARDIOVASCULAR DISEASE (HEART TROUBLE, HEART ATTACK, ANGINA, HIGH BLOOD PRESSURE, HARDENING OF THE ARTERIES, STROKE)	• Chest pain • Shortness of breath • Ankles swell • Congenital heart defects • Pacemaker ☛ Minimize stress and premedicate if necessary ☛ Review prescribed medications ☛ Has patient been taking prescribed medication? ☛ Monitor vital signs ☛ Anesthesia—limit epinephrine to .04 mg
HYPERTENSION	• Monitor vital signs • Postural hypotension (raise chair slowly) • Review patient medications: 　• Diuretics 　• Antiadrenergic agents 　• Vasodilators 　• Calcium channel-blocking agents • Anesthesia—limit epinephrine to .04 mg
ANGINA PECTORIS	Prevent stress, morning appointments ☛ Prepare for symptoms: have amyl nitrite, nitroglycerin ready
HEART DISEASE	• History of disease • Physician consultation • Monitor vital signs • Short frequent appointments • Pacemakers—check use of ultrasonics • Review medications: 　• Glycosides (digitalis) 　• Anticoagulants 　• Antiarrhythmic drugs
ASTHMA OR HAY FEVER	☛ Prilocaine local anesthetic metabolized primarily in the lungs
FAINTING SPELLS, SEIZURES, EPILEPSY, OR CONVULSIONS	• May indicate presence of abnormal anxiety, fear, seizures, or orthostatic hypotension • Stress may provoke a seizure even in well-controlled epileptics ☛ Stress reduction procedures indicated

DIABETES	• Uncontrolled; requires antibiotic pre-medication • Undiagnosed: excessive thirst, change in appetite, and urination ☛ Periodontal disease accelerated ☛ Short morning appointments ☛ Prepare for emergency: insulin; apple juice, frosting
HEPATITIS, YELLOW JAUNDICE, CIRRHOSIS, OR LIVER DISEASE	• History of disease • Present disease; communicability • Jaundice history • Clarification of type of hepatitis ☛ Precautions against percutaneous injury ☛ Impaired drug metabolism; reduce the amount of amide local anesthetic if liver disease is present, or choose to administer prilocaine
AIDS OR HIV INFECTION	• Oral manifestations • Risk group identification • Wide variety of infections and complications and drugs ☛ Precautions against percutaneous injury
THYROID PROBLEMS (GOITER)	• Hyperthyroidism • Hypothyroidism

RESPIRATORY PROBLEMS, EMPHYSEMA, BRONCHITIS, BLACK LUNG, ETC.	• Breathing problems
	• Persistent cough
	• Precipitation of asthmatic attack
	• Review medications
	  • Antihistamines
	  • Bronchial dilator
	  • Expectorant
	  • Decongestant
	  • Steroid
	☛ Consider position of dental chair
	☛ Air-powder polisher contraindicated
	☛ Nitrous oxide contraindicated

KIDNEY TROUBLE	• Many drugs are nephrotoxic • Monitor vital signs • Bleeding tendency • Poor healing • Susceptibility to infection ☛ Stress reduction protocol

TUBERCULOSIS OR POSITIVE TB SKIN TEST	• Active or passive
	• Duration of disease
	• Medical consult regarding status
	• Chest x-ray results
	• Review medications
	  • Isoniazid
	  • Rifampin
	  • Pyrazinamide
	☛ Postpone dental treatment until status is known

SWOLLEN GLANDS IN NECK	Check during oral cancer exam and refer to physician if necessary
LOW BLOOD OR ANEMIA	Presence of methemoglobinemia, either congenital or idiopathic, represents a relative contraindication to the administration of articaine and prilocaine local anesthetics
GONORRHEA, SYPHILIS, HERPES, OR OTHER SIMILAR DISEASES	• Oral and pharyngeal lesions may be indicators of disease • Herpes lesion can be transmitted readily—postpone routine care when oral lesions are present

PROBLEMS WITH MENTAL HEALTH OR NERVES	• Emotional problems hinder oral care
	• Limited stress tolerance
	• Review medications
	  • Antipsychotic drugs
	  • Antianxiety drugs
	  • Antidepressants
	  • Tranquilizers
	☛ Drug interactions between tricyclic antidepressants and epinephrine, and monoamine oxidase inhibitors and epinephrine
	☛ Epinephrine containing local anesthetics should be administered in the smallest effective dose (.04 mg)

CANCER	• Head and neck radiation effects on oral cavity and salivary glands • Update treatment prior to surgery and radiation therapy • Fluoride treatment • Bleeding and increased infection with poor healing • Dental caries preventive measures • Xerostomia

ALCOHOL USE/ RECOVERING ALCOHOLIC	• Frequency, amount • Avoid all alcohol-containing mouth rinses • Excessive use: effect on anesthesia metabolism; increased healing time

WOMEN'S ISSUES

PREGNANCY OR PLANNING TO BECOME PREGNANT	• Month, due date • Possible oral manifestations • Patient comfort • Frequent appointments ☞ Radiographs contraindicated
ORAL CONTRA-CEPTIVES	Antibiotic treatment decreases the effectiveness of oral contraceptives

Dental History

CHIEF COMPLAINT

Get a sense of how the patient feels in his/her own words

PAIN OR DISCOMFORT	• Requirements for immediate treatment • Requirements for pain control

DENTAL HISTORY

DATE OF LAST TREATMENT	Patient's knowledge concerning regular dental care, regularity of visits
ORAL HYGIENE	Patient's knowledge, home care

PREVIOUS TREATMENT

PERIODONTAL	• History of acute infections • Surgery: post-treatment healing
ORTHODONTIC	• Age during treatment • Habit corrections • Oral hygiene—patient education on decalcification and importance of fluoride
ENDODONTIC	• Etiology • Endodontic evaluation

PROSTHODONTIC	• Types of prostheses • Extent of restorations • Implants • ☛ Oral hygiene care for prostheses

ANESTHETICS USED

- Local, general, conscience sedation, topical
- Adverse reactions
- Determine choice of anesthetic

ATTITUDE TOWARD DENTAL HEALTH AND TREATMENT

PSYCHOLOGICAL ATTITUDE	Bad dental experience, cooperation antici-pated, need for psychosedation during treatment

RADIATION HISTORY

- Type, number, dates of both medical and dental radiographs
- Therapeutic radiation

☛ Amount of exposure: limitations

☛ Xerostomia considerations

INJURIES TO FACE OR TEETH

- Causes and extent of treatment
- Fractured teeth
- Dental anxiety

☛ Limitations opening mouth

☛ Spousal/child abuse suspected and legal requirements of reporting

TEMPOROMANDIBULAR JOINT

- History
- Discomfort
- Previous treatment

☛ Opening the mouth: dislocation, accessibility

HABITS

- Clenching, bruxism
- Mouth breathing
- Biting objects
- Thumb sucking
- Cheek biting or lip biting

☛ Patient awareness of habit, and evaluation of need for oral appliance

TOBACCO USE

Form and frequency of tobacco use

☛ Patient education regarding effects on oral tissues

☛ Tobacco cessation program

☛ Dental staining

☛ Soft tissue changes

☛ Nicotine stomatitis

FLUORIDES

Systemic, topical, drinking water

PERSONAL DAILY ORAL HYGIENE ROUTINE

- Toothbrushing and flossing frequency and procedures
- Additional devices and frequency

American Heart Association Guidelines for Premedication

CARDIAC CONDITIONS CONSIDERED FOR PROPHYLAXIS

HIGH RISK CATEGORY	<ul><li>Prosthetic cardiac valves</li><li>Previous bacterial endocarditis</li><li>Complex cyanotic congenital heart disease</li><li>Surgically constructed systemic pulmonary shunts</li></ul>

MODERATE RISK CATEGORY	• Most other congenital cardiac malformations • Acquired valvular dysfunction (e.g., rheumatic heart disease) • Hypertrophic cardiomyopathy • Mitral valve prolapse with regurgitation and/or thickened leaflets

NEGLIGIBLE RISK: NO ANTIBIOTIC PROPHYLAXIS RECOMMENDED

- Isolated secundum atrial septal defect
- Surgical repair of atrial septal defect, ventricular septal defect, or patent ductus arteriosus of more than six months' duration
- Previous coronary artery bypass graft surgery
- Physiological or functional heart murmur
- Previous Kawasaki disease without valvular dysfunction
- Previous rheumatic fever without valvular dysfunction
- Cardiac pacemakers
- Implanted defibrillators

DENTAL PROCEDURES CONSIDERED FOR ANTIBIOTIC PROPHYLAXIS IN SUSCEPTIBLE PATIENTS

HIGH RISK CATEGORY	• Dental extractions • Periodontal procedures including surgery, scaling, root planing, and probing • Dental implant placement, reimplantation of teeth • Endodontic instrumentation or surgery beyond the tooth apex • Subgingival placement of antibiotic fibers or strips • Initial placement of orthodontic bands but not brackets • Intraligamentary local anesthetic injection • Prophylactic cleaning of teeth or implants with anticipated bleeding

Antibiotic Prophylactic Regimens

STANDARD PROPHYLAXIS	
AMOXICILLIN	Adults, 2.0 grams; children, 50 mg/kg orally one hour before procedure

PATIENT WHO CANNOT USE ORAL MEDICATIONS	
AMPICILLIN	Adults, 2.0 grams IM or IV; children, 50 mg/kg IM or IV within 30 minutes before procedure

PATIENTS ALLERGIC TO PENICILLIN	
CLINDAMYCIN	Adults, 600 mg; children, 20 mg/kg orally one hour before procedure
CEPHALEXIN OR CEFADROXIL	Adults, 2.0 g; children, 50 mg/kg orally one hour before procedure
AXITHROMYCIN OR CLARITHROMYCIN	Adults, 500 mg; children, 15 mg/kg orally one hour before procedure

ALLERGIC TO PENICILLIN AND UNABLE TO TAKE ORAL MEDICATIONS	
CLINDAMYCIN	Adults, 600 mg; children, 15 mg/kg IV one hour before procedure
CEFAZOLIN	Adults, 1.0 g; children, 25 mg/kg IM or IV within 30 minutes before procedure

Vital Signs

BODY TEMPERATURE	
NORMAL ADULT	37.0°C (98.6°F) Normal range 35.5° to 37.5°C (96.0°F to 99.5°F) ⚷ Over 70 years of age: the average temperature is slightly lower

NORMAL CHILD	• First year: 37.3°C (99.1°F) • Fourth year: 37.5°C (99.4°F) • Fifth year: 37°C (98.6°F) • Twelfth year: 36.7°C (98.0°F)

FACTORS THAT ALTER BODY TEMPERATURE

TIME OF DAY	Highest in late afternoon and early evening; lowest during sleep and early morning
PATHOLOGIC STATES	Infection, dehydration, hyperthyroidism, myocardial infarction, or tissue injury from trauma

METHODS OF DETERMINING TEMPERATURE

ORAL	Most common, indicated when patient can follow directions, and has no mouth injuries or problems breathing through nose
RECTAL	When oral thermometer is contraindicated
EXTERNAL	Axillary and groin positions; least accurate

PROCEDURE FOR BODY TEMPERATURE

PATIENT PREPARATION	Explain procedure
PREPARE THERMOMETER	• Hold by the stem, never by the bulb • Check that reading is below 35.6°C (96°F), shake down mercury if not below this level
TAKE THE TEMPERATURE	• Place bulb under patient's tongue • Have patient hold gently between lips and breathe through the nose • Remove after 3 minutes • Hold thermometer by the stem and read at eye level • Retake if reading is unusually high or low

PULSE

NORMAL PULSE, ADULT	Range is 60 to 100 beats per minute (bpm) ☛ No absolute normal
NORMAL PULSE, CHILDREN	• In utero: 150 bpm • At birth: 130 bpm • Second year: 105 bpm • Fourth year: 90 bpm • Tenth year: 70 bpm

FACTORS THAT INFLUENCE THE PULSE RATE

INCREASED PULSE	• Exercise • Stimulants • Eating • Some forms of heart disease
DECREASED PULSE	• Sleep • Depressants • Fasting

PROCEDURE FOR TAKING PULSE

SITES	• Radial pulse: most common; radial artery at the wrist • Temporal artery: on the side of the head in front of the ear **Figure 7-1**
PREPARE THE PATIENT	• Explain procedure • Locate radial pulse **Figure 7-2**
COUNT	Count for 1 minute
RHYTHM	Regular, regularly irregular, or irregularly irregular
VOLUME AND STRENGTH	Full, strong, poor, weak, or thready
RECORD	Date, pulse rate, and other characteristics

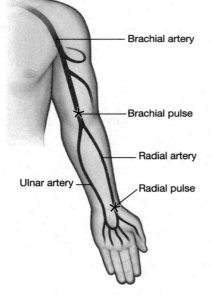

Brachial artery
Brachial pulse
Radial artery
Ulnar artery
Radial pulse

FIGURE 7-1   Radial Pulse

RESPIRATION

NORMAL, ADULT	Range is 14–20 per minute
NORMAL, CHILDREN	• First year: 30 per minute • Second year: 25 per minute • Eighth year: 20 per minute • Fifteenth year: 18 per minute

FACTORS THAT INFLUENCE RESPIRATION RATE

INCREASED RESPIRATION	• Work • Exercise • Excitement • Nervousness • Strong emotions • Pain • Hemorrhage • Shock
DECREASED RESPIRATION	• Sleep • Certain drugs • Pulmonary insufficiency

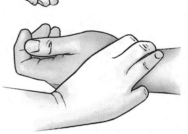

FIGURE 7-2 Location of Radial Pulse

PROCEDURE

DETERMINE RATE	• Count respirations (number of times chest rises) immediately following pulse count for 1 minute • Maintain fingers over radial pulse so patient is unaware
OBSERVE DEPTH	• Shallow • Normal • Deep
OBSERVE RHYTHM	• Regular • Irregular
OBSERVE QUALITY	• Strong • Easy • Weak • Labored (noisy)
OBSERVE SOUNDS	Deviant sounds during inspiration, expiration, or both
RECORD	All findings

BLOOD PRESSURE

Force exerted by the blood on the blood vessel walls

SYSTOLIC PRESSURE	Highest pressure caused by ventricular contractions ☞ Normal adult systolic is less than 130 mmHg
DIASTOLIC PRESSURE	Lowest pressure and is the effect of ventricular relaxation ☞ Normal adult diastolic is less than 85 mmHg
PULSE PRESSURE	Difference between the systolic and diastolic pressures ☞ Normal is less than 45 mmHg
NORMAL AVERAGE BLOOD PRESSURE IN CHILDREN	• 3 years: 108/70 • 6 years: 114/74 • 12 years: 122/78

FACTORS THAT INFLUENCE BLOOD PRESSURE

INCREASE BLOOD PRESSURE	• Exercise • Eating • Stimulants • Stress
DECREASE BLOOD PRESSURE	• Fasting • Rest • Depressants

BLOOD PRESSURE PROCEDURE

PREPARE PATIENT	• Explain procedure • Use either arm • Take pressure on bare arm
APPLY CUFF	• Apply deflated cuff to patient's arm • Place inflatable bladder directly over the brachial artery • Fasten cuff evenly and snugly • Locate brachial artery pulse—1 inch below the antecubital fossa and place stethoscope endpiece • Position stethoscope earpieces in ears **Figure 7-3**

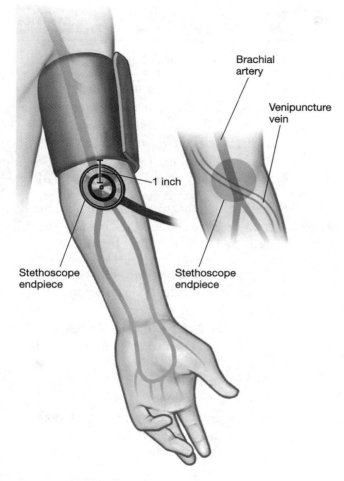

FIGURE 7-3 Application of Blood Pressure Cuff

LOCATE RADIAL PULSE	Hold fingers on the pulse
INFLATE CUFF	• Close needle valve • Pump to inflate cuff until radial pulse stops and pump 20–30 mmHg beyond where the radial pulse was no longer felt
DEFLATE CUFF	Release air lock slowly and listen for first sound (systolic pressure) and last sound (diastolic pressure)
RECORD	Record pressure as fraction

DENTAL TREATMENT CONSIDERATIONS FOR PATIENTS WITH HYPERTENSION

< 140/< 90	Routine dental management
140–160 / 90–95	• Recheck blood pressure prior to dental therapy for three consecutive appointments; if all exceed these guidelines, medical consultation is indicated • Routine dental management • Stress reduction protocol if indicated
160–200 / 95–111	• Recheck blood pressure in five minutes • If still elevated, medical consultation is indicated before further treatment
>200 / > 115	• Recheck blood pressure in five minutes • Immediate medical consultation if still elevated • No dental therapy, routine or emergency, until elevated blood pressure is corrected • Emergency therapy with drugs (analgesics, antibiotics) • Refer to hospital if immediate dental therapy indicated

➤ HEAD AND NECK EXAMINATION

METHODS OF EXAMINATION

DIRECT OBSERVATION	• Patient position • Optimum lighting • Retraction for accessibility
DIGITAL PALPATATION	Single finger ☛ Example: presence of torum mandibularis **Figure 7-4**
BIDIGITAL PALPATATION	Finger and thumb ☛ Example: palpation of the lips **Figure 7-5**
BIMANUAL PALPATATION	Finger or fingers and thumb from each hand applied simultaneously ☛ Example: palpate floor of the mouth **Figure 7-6**

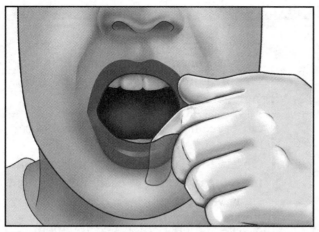

Digital palpation—Use index finger. Example—detect the presence of exostosis on the border of the mandible.

FIGURE 7-4

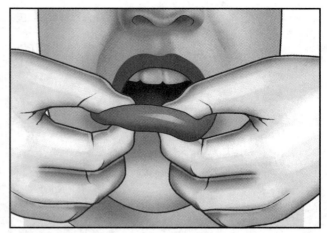

Bidigital palpation—Use finger and thumb of same hand. Example—palpate the lips.

FIGURE 7-5

BILATERAL PALPATATION	Two hands used at same time to examine corresponding structures on opposite sides of the body 🔑 Example: palpate submandibular lymph nodes **Figure 7-7**

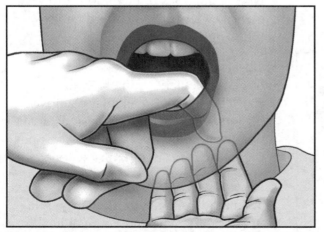

Bimanual palpation—Use finger(s) and/or thumb from each hand. Example—palpate floor of mouth.

FIGURE 7-6

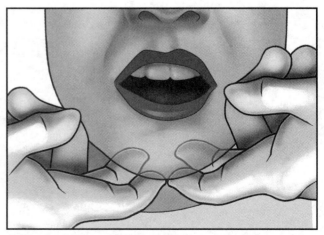

Bilateral palpation—Use both hands at same time to examine corresponding structures on opposite sides of body. Example—examine submental nodes.

FIGURE 7-7

SEQUENCE OF EXAMINATION

OVERALL APPRAISAL OF THE PATIENT	Observe and note abnormalities of posture, gait, general health status; hair and scalp, breathing, state of fatigue, voice, cough, and hoarseness
FACE	• Observe and note expression and possible evidence of fear • Observe facial twitching, paralysis; jaw movements during speech, injuries, and signs of abuse
SKIN	Observe and note color, texture, blemishes, traumatic lesions, eruptions, swellings, or growths
EYES	Observe and note size of pupils as well as color of sclera; eyeglasses, protruding eyeballs
NODES	• Palpate preauricular, occipital, submental/submaxillary, cervical chain, supraclavicular: note indurations, area of tenderness • Interview patient as to history of recent illness or tenderness in the area of concern **Figure 7-8**
TMJ	• Observe and palpate area while patient is opening and closing mouth • Note limitations or deviations of movement; tenderness, sensitivity, noises (clicking, popping, crepitus)
LIPS	• Observe closed, then open • Look for deviations in color, texture, size, shape; cracks, angular cheilosis; blisters, ulcers; traumatic lesions, irritation from lip biting; limitations of opening, muscle elasticity, muscle tone; evidence of mouth breathing; induration
BREATH ODOR	Note malodors indicating severity, relation to oral hygiene and gingival health

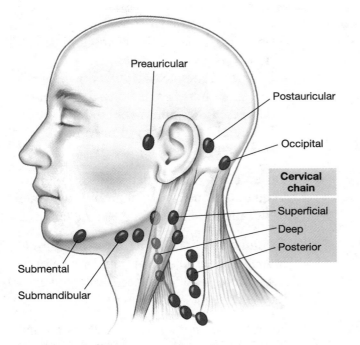

FIGURE 7-8 Nodes Palpated during Head and Neck Examination

INTRA-ORAL EXAMINATION

LABIAL AND BUCCAL MUCOSA	• Systematically examine the vestibule, mucobuccal fold, frena, and opening of Stenson's duct, buccal mucosa • Observe and note deviations from normal in color, size, texture, and contour • Note abrasions, traumatic lesions, cheekbite; effects of tobacco use; ulcers, growths; moistness of surfaces; relation of frena to free gingiva; areas of induration
TONGUE	• Examine the dorsal ventral surface; lateral borders; base of tongue (retracted) • Observe and note deviations from normal in shape; color, size, texture, consistency; fissures, papilla; coating; lesions—elevated, depressed, flat; indurations

FLOOR OF THE MOUTH	• Examine ventral surface of tongue, duct openings, mucosa, frena and tongue action • Observe and note deviations from normal in varicosities; lesions—elevated, depressed, flat, traumatic; indurations; limitation of freedom of movement, frena (ankyloglossia)
SALIVA	Observe and note deviations from normal in quantity; quality (thick, ropy); evidence of dry mouth; lip wetting; tongue coating
HARD PALATE	Examine and note deviations from normal in height, contour, color; appearance of rugae; tori, growths, ulcers, lesions; surface texture
SOFT PALATE AND UVULA	Examine and note deviations from normal in color, size, shape; petechiae, lesions, ulcers, growths
TONSILLAR REGION AND THROAT	Examine and note deviations from normal in tonsils (color, size, shape, surface texture); lesions; trauma

DESCRIPTION OF OBSERVATIONS

SIZE	• Record length and width, height of lesion in mm (measure with perio probe) • Elevated lesions may be significant
COLOR	Red, pink, white, and red and white are the most common; also may be blue, purple, gray, yellow, black, or brown
SURFACE TEXTURE	• May be smooth or irregular • Texture may be papillary, verrucous (wart-like), fissured, corrugated, or crusted
CONSISTENCY	Lesions may be soft, spongy, resilient, hard, or indurated
HISTORY	Note the length of time the lesion has been present, and whether lesion comes and goes

Morphologic Categories

BLISTERFORM	Contain fluid and are usually soft and transparent • Vesicles: less than 1 cm in diameter • Pustules: contains pus • Bullae: greater than 1 cm in diameter
NONBLISTERFORM	• Solid and do not contain fluid • Nonblisterform also characterized by base of attachment • Sessile: wide base • Pedunculated: attached by narrow stalk or pedicle • Papules: solid tissue less than 5mm in diameter • Nodules: solid tissue less than 1 cm in diameter • Tumors: solid tissue greater than 2 cm in diameter • Plaques: slightly raised, long, flat top

On same level as normal skin or mucosa; may be single or multiple; may be regular or irregular in form
☛ Macule—nonpalpable lesion of abnormal color

Below level of skin or mucosa; outline may be regular or irregular; border may be flat or raised; depth described as superficial or deep (greater than 3 mm is deep)

ULCERS	• Loss of continuity with epithelium; extends beyond surface of epithelium • Center often gray to yellow with red border
EROSIONS	Shallow, depressed lesions that follow rupture of vesicle or bulla, that do not extend through epithelium

DESCRIPTIVE TERMS

CONFLUENT	Originally separate but subsequently blended together
CRUST	Hard, scab-like surface formed from coagulation of blood
DISCRETE	Separate; not blended
ERYTHEMA	Areas of marked redness
EXOPHYTIC	Outward in growth
INDURATED	Hard
PAPILLARY	Nipplelike growths
PATECHIAE	Red-purple discoloration (spots) less than 0.5 cm in diameter
SESSILE	Lesion attached by a broad base
TORUS	Bony growth
VERRUCOUS	Wart-like surface

APPEARANCE OF EARLY CANCER

WHITE AREAS	Leukoplakia: vary from filmy, barely visible, to heavy, thick, keratinized tissue
RED AREAS	Erythroplakia: bright red patches
ULCERS	Flat or raised margins
MASSES	Ulcerated, or elevated, some may be found only by palpation
PIGMENTATION	Brown or black

➤ PERIODONTAL EVALUATION

The Gingiva

GINGIVAL TISSUES

COLOR	Pink vs. darker pink, various shades of red, and/or bluish (erythematous, cyanotic)

SHAPE	Overall scalloped appearance Margins: Flat and knife-like margins vs. rolled, red, and/or clefted Papilla: Flat and pyramidal papilla that fill the interdental spaces vs. blunted, cratered, or bulbous papilla
CONSISTENCY AND TONE	Firm and dense vs. soft, spongy, edematous, and easily retractable ☛ During acute disease phases, edematous changes are typical; however, a denser, firm tissue change called "fibrous" frequently is the result of longstanding, chronic disease processes
BLEEDING	No bleeding vs. bleeding upon probing or presence of spontaneous bleeding ☛ Indicates presence of inflammation
EXUDATE	Fluid accumulation escaped from blood vessels into surrounding tissues ☛ Result of inflammation
SIZE	Not enlarged vs. enlarged
POSITION	Epithelial attachment at level of CEJ, no recession vs. apical migration of epithelial attachment and/or recession

TERMINOLOGY TO UTILIZE IN QUANTIFYING TISSUE CHANGES

LOCALIZED	Involvement only around a tooth or group of teeth
GENERALIZED	Involvement around all or nearly all teeth
MARGINAL	Change confined to free or marginal gingiva (localized or generalized, as well as slight, moderate, or severe)
PAPILLARY	Change involves papilla, but not the rest of the free gingiva around a tooth ☛ Localized or generalized as well as slight, moderate, or severe

DIFFUSE	• Attached gingiva is involved as well as free gingiva • Usually confined to small segments (localized), but not necessarily ☛ In addition to the distribution, the condition must be quantified as slight, moderate, or severe

Healthy versus Diseased Descriptions Associated with the Periodontium

COLOR	
HEALTHY	Uniform pale pink
DISEASE	• Various degrees of darker pink to red • Increased blood flow due to increased capillary permeability (initial phase of inflammatory process) • Inflammation may initially involve only the papilla, then spread to the margin, then extend to the attached gingiva ☛ If tissue changes extend to the MGJ, alveolar mucosal becomes involved

SIZE	
HEALTHY	Flat, free gingival margin closely adapted to tooth or gently rounded
DISEASE	• Initial rolling of free gingiva • More involvement exhibited by enlarged margins and bulbous papilla • Poor adaptation of tissue to tooth • Exudate and spontaneous bleeding may be present • Fibrotic tissue (tends to be firm and dense, yet possibly still pink) indicative of chronic disease

SHAPE	
HEALTHY	• Overall scalloped appearance • Margins flat and pyramidal, filling interdental spaces in areas of adequate contact

DISEASE	• Ranges from slight loss of scalloped contour to total loss of contour • Papilla may be blunted or cratered (not filling interdental spaces) • Papilla may become bulbous—note that although interdental space may be filled, shape is not ideal; also note recession, clefting, festooning **Figure 7-9**

CONSISTENCY

HEALTHY	Firm, resilient, and firmly attached
DISEASE	• Acute: edematous to some degree • Chronic: edema possible, yet long-standing disease likely to manifest fibrous connective tissue repair process fibrosis, so tissues are termed "fibrotic" • Can have ongoing chronic inflammation with acute inflammatory process concurrently (not mutually exclusive) ⚷ Presence or absence of stippling is least indicator of health/disease

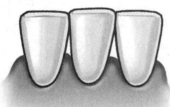

A Blunted papilla

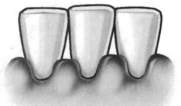

B Bulbous papilla

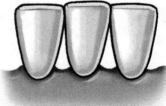

C Cratered papilla

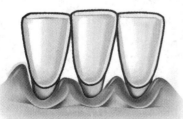

D Rolled "McCall's" festoons

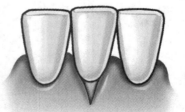

E V-shaped Stillman's cleft

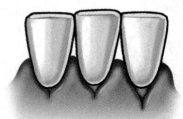

F Stilt-like Stillman's cleft

FIGURE 7-9 Diseased Gingiva

POSITION OF CEJ	
HEALTHY	• Fully-erupted: margin 1–2 mm • CEJ: at or slightly below enamel counter

DISEASE	• Enlarged gingiva: margin coronal to CEJ (yields deeper PPD reading)
	  • GM–CEJ reading will be a negative number
	• Recession: margin apical to normal
	  • Root surface exposed
	  • GM–CEJ reading positive

POSITION OF JUNCTIONAL EPITHELIUM	
HEALTHY	• During eruption: along the enamel surface • Fully erupted tooth: the junctional epithelium is at CEJ
DISEASE	Position, determined by use of periodontal probe, is on the root surface **Figure 7-10** **Figure 7-11**

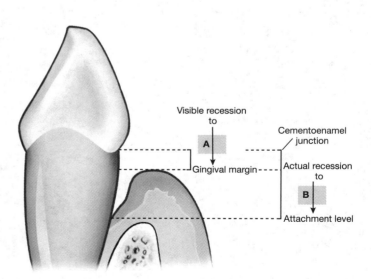

FIGURE 7-10 Gingival Recession: A) Visible—measured from CEJ to Gingival Margin; B) Actual—Measured from CEJ to Base of Pocket

BLEEDING

HEALTHY	No spontaneous bleeding upon probing
DISEASE	• Spontaneous bleeding and/or bleeding upon probing • Bleeding upon probing: bleeding near margin in acute conditions; bleeding deep in pocket in chronic conditions

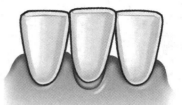

A Wide shallow recession

EXUDATE

HEALTHY	• No exudate on pressure
DISEASE	• White fluid, pus visible on digital pressure • Amount not related to depth of pocket associated with acute phase of inflammation

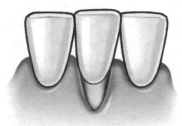

B Wide, deep, with narrow attached gingiva

Gingival versus Periodontal Pockets

Figure 7-12

GINGIVAL POCKET (PSEUDOPOCKET)

DEFINITION	• Gingival enlargement forms pocket without apical migration of junctional epithelium • Gingival tissues have moved coronally • ☞ Can be reversed to health by plaque control regimen • ☞ Always suprabony

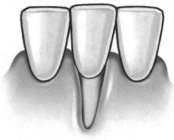

C Narrow, deep, with no attached gingiva

FIGURE 7-11 Types of Recesion

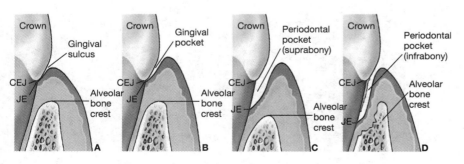

FIGURE 7-12 Types of Pockets: A) Healthy; B) Gingivitis; C) Suprabony; D) Infrabony

CAUSES	• Swelling or edema due to plaque
	• Certain drugs
	• Drug examples
	  • Phenytoid: seizures
	  • Cyclosporin: immunosuppressant
	  • Nifedipine: angina and ventricular arrhythmia

PERIODONTAL POCKET

DEFINITION	Pocket formed by plaque, causing an apical migration of the junctional epithelium
CAUSES	• Inflammation • Alveolar bone resorption
SUPRABONY	Junctional epithelium has migrated below the CEJ but remains coronal to the crest of the alveolar bone
INFRABONY	Junctional epithelium has migrated apical to the crest of the alveolar bone

Furcation Involvement
Figure 7-13

FURCATION CLASSIFICATIONS

CLASS I	Beginning involvement ☛ Probe can slightly enter the furcation area

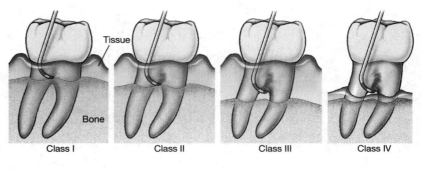

Class I   Class II   Class III   Class IV

FIGURE 7-13 Furcation Classifications

CLASS II	Moderate involvement ☞ Probe can enter the furcation area, but cannot pass through the roots
CLASS III	Severe involvement ☞ Probe can pass through the entire furcation
CLASS IV	Severe involvement ☞ Probe can pass through the entire furcation ☞ Gingival recession allows furcation to be clinically visible

Determining Attachment Level—Mucogingival Problems

ABBREVIATIONS

- AL: attachment level
- LOA: loss of attachment
- PPD: periodontal probing depth (from sulcus/pocket depth to gingival margin)
- GM–CEJ: From gingival margin (GM) to cementoenamel junction (CEJ)

LOSS OF ATTACHMENT (LOA)
Figure 7–14

LOA occurs as the junctional epithelium migrates away from the CEJ and toward the apex of the tooth. To determine AL, the clinician must assess and record two measurements in millimeters (mm) with a periodontal probe:

- PPD
- GM–CEJ

☞ Best indicator of damage to periodontium

MEASURING AL WHEN RECESSION IS VISIBLE	1. Measure the PPD and record the number 2. Measure the GM–CEJ (you will be measuring the amount of root visible, which is recession; this is the only time that the GM–CEJ number will be positive); record this number 3. Add the PPD number and the GM–CEJ number together and record the number on the dental chart

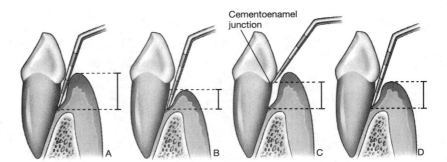

FIGURE 7-14   Loss of Attachment: A) PPD—Measure from Gingival Sulcus to GM; B) Recession—Measure from GM to CEJ; C) GM covers CEJ—Locate CEJ, Measure Distance to CEJ, then Subtract from Probing Depth; D) GM is at CEJ—Measure from GM to CEJ

MEASURING AL WHEN THE CEJ IS COVERED BY GINGIVA	1. Measure the PPD and record the number in the dental chart 2. Next, slide the probe along the tooth surface into the sulcus/pocket until the CEJ is felt; record this measurement number (meaning a negative number) on the dental chart; if the CEJ cannot be detected with the probe, the CEJ location can be estimated based on normal dental anatomy 3. Add the PPD number to GM–CEJ number (which will be a negative number) together and record this number on the dental chart if it is a positive number; if PPD + GM–CEJ = zero (0), record it on dental chart ☞ This can occur when the tissue is healthy *or* hyperplastic
MEASURING FREE GINGIVAL MARGIN WHEN LEVEL/EQUAL WITH THE CEJ	1. Measure the PPD and record the number on the dental chart 2. Record a zero (0) for the GM–CEJ on the dental chart 3. Add the PPD number and the GM–CEJ number (which will be zero) together; record this as a positive number on the dental chart

MUCOGINGIVAL PROBLEMS

Mucogingival problems involve the amount of attached gingiva
Two factors are assessed:
- PPD
- GM to the mucogingival junction

MEASURING ATTACHED GINGIVA	1. Measure the total gingiva by laying the probe over the surface of the gingiva, measure from the GM to the mucogingival junction, referred to as total attached gingiva 2. Measure the pocket depth 3. Subtract the PPD from the total attached gingiva
ADEQUATE ATTACHMENT	Most researchers consider 1 mm of truly attached gingiva to be an adequate zone of attached gingiva
MUCOGINGIVAL DEFECT (MGD)	Areas having less than 1 mm of attached gingiva, but the base of the PPD is at or above the mucogingival junction with no bleeding present
MUCOGINGIVAL INVOLVEMENT (MGI)	Areas with no attached gingiva present, the PPD will be present below the mucogingival junction

Tooth Mobility

TOOTH MOBILITY CLASSIFICATIONS

CLASS I	Tooth can be moved up to 1 mm
CLASS II	Tooth can be moved more than 1 mm ☞ Tooth is not depressible in the socket
CLASS III	Tooth can be moved in any direction ☞ Tooth is depressible in the socket

American Dental Association and Academy of Periodontics Classification System for Periodontal Disease

CHRONIC PERIODONTITIS

☞ Formerly called adult periodontitis

CASE TYPE I— GINGIVAL DISEASE (GINGIVITIS)	Inflammation of the gingiva characterized clinically by changes in color, form, position, surface appearance, and presence of bleeding and/or exudate ☞ No attachment loss is present and no bone loss seen radiographically
CASE TYPE II— EARLY PERIO-DONTITIS	• Progression of the gingival inflammation into the deeper periodontal structures and alveolar bone crest, with slight bone loss (may or may not be seen radiographically) • There is usually a slight loss of connective tissue attachment and alveolar bone ☞ Attachment loss of 1–2 mm is usually present
CASE TYPE III— MODERATE PERIODONTITIS	• A more advanced stage of periodontitis with increased destruction of the periodontal structures and noticeable loss of bone support (seen radiographically), possibly accompanied by an increase in tooth mobility • There may be furcation involvement in multirooted teeth; attachment loss of 3–4 mm is usually present
CASE TYPE IV— ADVANCED PERIODONTITIS	• Further progression of periodontitis with major loss of alveolar bone support (seen radiographically) usually accompanied by increased tooth mobility • Furcation involvement in multirooted teeth ☞ Attachment loss of > 4 mm is usually present
CASE TYPE V— REFRACTORY PERIODONTITIS	• Patients with multiple disease sites that continue to demonstrate attachment loss after appropriate therapy • These sites presumably continue to be infected by periodontal pathogens no matter how thorough or frequent the treatment provided • Patients with recurrent disease at single or multiple sites

AGGRESSIVE PERIODONTITIS

☞ Formerly called early-onset periodontitis

PREPUBERTAL	• Occurs between eruption of primary teeth and puberty • Can be localized or generalized
JUVENILE	May be generalized or localized and occurs during the circumpubertal period; familial distribution; relative paucity of microbial plaque; less acute signs of inflammation than expected due to the severity of disease
RAPIDLY PROGRESSIVE PERIODONTITIS	Age of onset 20s or later; most of the teeth are affected; clinical indications of inflammation may be less than expected

PERIODONTITIS AS A MANIFESTATION OF SYSTEMIC DISEASES

Several systemic diseases predispose the affected individuals to periodontitis, usually chronic periodontitis

NECROTIZING PERIODONTAL DISEASES

Acute inflammation with a distinctive erythema of the supporting structures
☞ Formerly known as "necrotizing ulcerative periodontitis"

PERIODONTAL ABSCESS

Associated with combinations of pain, swelling, color change, tooth mobility, extrusion of teeth, purulence, sinus tract formation, fever, lymphadenopathy, and radiolucency of the affected bone.
☞ Added category

GINGIVAL ABSCESS	Localized purulent infection that involves the marginal gingiva or interdental papilla
PERIODONTAL ABSCESS	Localized purulent infection within the tissues adjacent to the periodontal pocket that may lead to the destruction of periodontal ligament and alveolar bone

PERICORONAL ABSCESS	Localized purulent infection within the tissue surrounding the crown of a partially erupted tooth

PERIODONTIC-ENDODONTIC LESIONS

Infections of periodontal or endodontic origin may result in periodontitis and may be caused by plaque-associated periodontitis or endodontic infections that enter the periodontal ligament through the apical foramen or accessory canals
☛ Added category

DEVELOPMENTAL OR ACQUIRED DEFORMITIES AND CONDITIONS

These classifications are not separate diseases but increase susceptibility of periodontal diseases, or can influence treatment outcome
☛ Added category

MUCOGINGIVAL DEFORMITIES AND CONDITIONS AROUND THE TEETH	• Gingival/soft tissue recession • Lack of keratinized gingiva • Decreased vestibular depth • Aberrant frenum/muscle position • Gingival excess • Abnormal color ☛ Same for mucogingival deformities around dental implants
MUCOGINGIVAL DEFORMITIES AND CONDITIONS ON EDENTULOUS RIDGES	• Vertical and/or horizontal ridge deficiency • Lack of gingiva/keratinized tissue • Gingival/soft tissue enlargement • Aberrant frenum/muscle position • Decreased vestibular depth • Abnormal color

Assessment and Maintenance of Periodontal Disease

COMPONENTS OF COMPREHENSIVE PERIODONTAL ASSESSMENT

Examination of the periodontium should occur at each visit and comprehensive exams should be performed on all new patients and at least once a year for established patients; exam includes probing for bleeding, pocket depth, and loss of attachment, mobility, furcation involvement, recession, mucogingival problems, and radiographic bone loss

PHASES OF PATIENT CARE

CARE PLAN	Blueprint or guide that coordinates all treatment procedures and estimates the length of treatment to establish a healthy periodontal environment
PRELIMINARY PHASE	Treats emergency needs only; "getting the patient out of pain"
PHASE I	Focuses on controlling the etiologic influences responsible for dental disease; includes initial dental hygiene care, self-care education, diet control, removal of plaque-retentive factors, antimicrobial therapy, and dental caries management
PHASE II	Focuses on periodontal surgery, including placement of implants and endodontic therapy
PHASE III	Prosthetic therapy, including the final management of dental caries and exams to evaluate response to restorative procedures
PHASE IV	Maintenance including oral hygiene education, deposit removal, assessment, supportive therapy, and recall interval evaluation

STAGES OF INFLAMMATION IN THE PERIODONTAL LESION

Three stages of gingivitis (initial, early, and established) lesion and an advanced lesion of periodontitis

STAGE I (INITIAL LESION)	• Initial response of tissues to bacterial plaque; subclinical gingivitis • Vasodilation, margination, emigration, and migration of PMNs • Light alteration of the JE • Increase of gingival crevicular fluid • 2 to 4 days ☞ Clinical signs: none

STAGE II (EARLY LESION)	• Acute gingivitis • Continuation of initial lesion • Chronic inflammatory cells appear • JE invaginates with rete pegs • Ulceration in sulcular epithelium • Destruction of connective tissue fibers • 4 to 7 days • Clinical signs: redness, swelling, bleeding upon probing, loss of tissue tone
STAGE III (ESTABLISHED LESION)	• Chronic gingivitis • Plasma cells predominate • Chronic inflammation; blood vessels are congested and blood flow is impaired; increase in enzymes • Elongated rete pegs in JE extending deep into connective tissue; breakdown of connective fibers • 14+ days • Clinical signs: moderate to severe inflammation, underlying bluish hue, changes in consistency
STAGE IV (ADVANCED LESION)	• Transition from gingivitis to periodontitis • Continuation of changes in the established lesion • Inflammation extends into connective tissue attachment and alveolar bone • Repair manifests as fibrotic tissue • Bone resorption by osteoclasts and mononuclear cells • Time interval: dependent upon host response • Clinical signs: true periodontal pockets, attachment loss, and bone loss

GOALS OF PERIODONTAL THERAPY

Goals of periodontal therapy are to eliminate pain, inflammation, and bleeding; to reduce pathologic mobility and tooth loss; to restore function and tissue contour; and prevent disease recurrence

LOCAL THERAPY	Removal of plaque and all plaque retentive factors

SYSTEMIC THERAPY	Adjunct to control systemic complications that aggravate the disease

HEALING PROCESSES

REGENERATION	Growth and differentiation of new cells and intercellular substances to form new tissues or parts
REPAIR	Healing by scar; restores tissue at the same level on the root as the base of the preexisting pocket by a process of wound healing; may not restore original architecture or function
EPITHELIAL ADAPTATION	Close apposition of the gingival epithelium to the tooth without complete obliteration of the pocket
NEW ATTACHMENT	Embedding of new periodontal ligament fibers into new cementum and formation of a new gingival attachment

Stains

CLASSIFICATION OF STAINS

EXTRINSIC STAINS	External surface of the tooth ➻ May be removed
INTRINSIC STAINS	Occur within the tooth ➻ Cannot be removed
EXOGENOUS STAINS	Originate from sources outside the tooth ➻ May be extrinsic or intrinsic
ENDOGENOUS STAINS	Originate within the tooth ➻ Always intrinsic

EXTRINSIC STAINS

YELLOW STAIN	• Dull, yellowish discoloration of bacterial plaque • Associated with dental plaque • Usually from food pigments

GREEN STAIN	• Light or yellowish green to dark green • Embedded in dental plaque • Frequently superimposed by soft yellow or gray debris • Composed of chromogenic bacteria and fungi, decomposed hemoglobin, inorganic elements • Dark green: may become embedded in surface enamel as exogenous intrinsic stain • Demineralization is common under plaque
BLACK LINE STAIN	• Black calculus-like stain that forms near gingival margin • Continuous fine line that follows contour of gingival crest • Gingiva is firm • Teeth are usually clean and shiny • Composed of microorganisms, usually gram-positive rods embedded in intermicrobial substance • Mineralization is similar to the formation of calculus
TOBACCO STAIN	• Light brown to dark leathery brown or black • Incorporated in calculus deposits • Heavy deposits may become intrinsic • Composed of tar products
OTHER BROWN STAINS	• Brown pellicle: pellicle stains from various colors • Stannous fluoride: light brown, sometimes yellowish, after repeated use of stannous fluoride • Food sources: tea, coffee, soy sauce • Anti-plaque agents: chlorhexidine, alexidine used in mouthwashes • Betel leaf chewing
ORANGE AND RED STAINS	• Appear at the cervical third of tooth • Occurrence is rare • Composed of chromogenic bacteria

METALLIC STAINS FROM METAL-CONTAINING DUST OF INDUSTRY	• Copper or brass: green or bluish-brown • Iron: brown to greenish-brown • Nickel: green • Cadmium: yellow or golden brown • Industrial workers inhale dust
METALLIC STAINS FROM DRUGS	• Pigment of drug attaches to tooth substance • Black or brown stains

ENDOGENOUS INTRINSIC STAINS

PULPLESS TEETH	• Wide range of colors: light yellow-brown, gray, reddish-brown, bluish-black • Formulated from blood and other pulp tissue elements, root canal treatment, necrosis
TETRACYCLINES	• Absorbed by bones and teeth, and can be transferred through the placenta during the third trimester of pregnancy, and to a child in infancy and early childhood • Light green to dark yellow, or a gray-brown • Discoloration depends on dosage, and length of time drug was used
IMPERFECT TOOTH DEVELOPMENT	• Amelogenesis imperfecta: yellowish-brown, or gray-brown due to incomplete or missing enamel • Enamel hypoplasia: teeth erupt with white spots • Dental fluorosis: enamel hypomineralization from excessive ingestion of fluoride, teeth erupt with white spots that later become discolored and appear light or dark brown

EXOGENOUS INTRINSIC STAINS

RESTORATIVE MATERIALS	Silver amalgam: Gray or black discoloration around restoration

DRUGS	Stannous fluoride topical application: light to dark brown from tin oxide, frequently in occlusal pits and grooves

Plaque Deposits

BACTERIAL PLAQUE

Dense, nonmineralized mass of bacterial colonies in a gel-like intermicrobial matrix

LOCATION OF PLAQUE

SUPRAGINGIVAL PLAQUE	Above the gingival margin on the clinical crown of the tooth
SUBGINGIVAL PLAQUE	Below the gingival margin

FORMATION OF PLAQUE

STAGE I (PELLICLE FORMATION)	• Forms on the tooth and is an acellular (contains no bacteria or other cell forms) organic tenacious film that forms within minutes over exposed tooth surfaces • Composed of gylcoproteins from saliva • Microorganisms adhere to the pellicle ☛ Mode of attachment for calculus
STAGE II (BACTERIAL COLONIZATION)	• Microbial colony layers form from oral microflora that attaches to the pellicle and the bacteria grow and multiply • Intermicrobial substance is formed by saliva from polysaccharides that are sticky and aid in adhesion • Microcolonies form in layers; they meet and coalesce • Gram + microorganisms predominate • During this phase transition from an aerobic to an anaerobic environment occurs ☛ Polysaccharides are produced from dietary sucrose

STAGE III (MATURATION)	Increases in mass and thickness with continued bacterial multiplication, and adherence of bacteria to plaque surface

CHANGES IN PLAQUE MICROORGANISMS

DAYS 1 AND 2	Consists primarily of gram-positive cocci • Streptococci (dominant) • Streptococcus mutan • Streptococcus sanguis
DAYS 2 TO 4	Filamentous and slender rods grow and replace the cocci
DAYS 4 TO 7	Filamentous forms increase and mixed flora begin to appear with rods and fusobacteria
DAYS 7 TO 14	Gram-negative vibrios and spirochetes appear as well as anaerobic microorganisms
DAYS 14–21	Vibrios and spirochetes are prevalent • Gingivitis is clinically evident

SUBGINGIVAL PLAQUE

SOURCE	Subgingival plaque microorganisms proliferate apically
MICROORGANISMS	More anaerobic and motile organisms that are predominantly gram-negative
ATTACHED PLAQUE	• Plaque over the pellicle that is densely packed with microorganisms • Associated with calculus formation, root caries, and root resorption
UNATTACHED PLAQUE	Between layers of attached plaque, mostly gram-negative motile organisms
EPITHELIUM-ASSOCIATED PLAQUE	• Loosely attached to pocket epithelium • Gram-negative microorganisms and white blood cells • Microorganisms invade the connective tissue and are associated with periodontal disease

COMPOSITION OF PLAQUE	
INORGANIC COMPONENTS	Calcium, phosphorus, fluoride
ORGANIC COMPONENTS	Carbohydrates, proteins, lipids

Calculus Deposits

SUPRAGINGIVAL CALCULUS

Mineralized bacterial plaque on the clinical crown coronal to the gingival margin
☛ Frequent sites—lingual surfaces of mandibular anterior teeth and maxillary first and second molars adjacent to the ducts of salivary glands

SUBGINGIVAL CALCULUS

Mineralized bacterial plaque on tooth structure in the gingival sulcus and extends close to the bottom of the pocket
☛ Proximal surfaces are heaviest

CALCULUS FORMATION

MINERALIZATION	Filamentous microorganisms within the intermicrobial matrix provide the site for the deposition of minerals
SOURCES OF MINERALS	• Supragingival: Saliva • Subgingival: Gingival sulcus fluid, inflammatory exudate
CRYSTAL FORMATION	Hydroxyapatite, octocalcium, phosphate
MINERALIZATION	• Same for supra and subgingival calculus • Heavy calculus formers: higher salivary levels of calcium and phosphorus • Light calculus formers: higher levels of parotid pyrophosphate ☛ Pyrophosphate is a calcification inhibitor and used in anticalculus dentifrices
FORMATION TIME	10–20 days, with 12 days being the average

COMPOSITION OF CALCULUS

INORGANIC COMPONENTS	Calcium, phosphorus, carbonate, sodium, magnesium, potassium
FLUORIDE	Varies depending on concentration from drinking water, topical application, etc.
CRYSTALS	Two-thirds of inorganic matter is crystalline, mostly hydroxyapatite ☛ Same crystal present in enamel, dentin, cementum, and bone

MODES OF CALCULUS ATTACHMENT

ACQUIRED PELLICLE OR CUTICLE	• Superficial attachment • Pellicle is positioned between the calculus and the root surface • Easily removed
MECHANICAL LOCKING INTO MINUTE IRREGULARITIES	• Calculus is locked into tooth surface • Cemental irregularities include location of previous Sharpey's fibers, resorption lacunae, instrumentation grooves, cemental tears, to fragmentation; challenging to remove
DIRECT CONTACT BETWEEN CALCIFIED INTERCELLULAR MATRIX AND THE SURFACE	• Inorganic crystals of the tooth interlock with the mineralized plaque; hard to distinguish between the cementum and the calculus

➤ ORAL EVALUATION

LOCATION OF DENTAL CARIES

PIT AND FISSURE	In minute enamel faults ☛ Occlusal pits, buccal, lingual grooves
SMOOTH SURFACE	No pit, groove where bacterial plaque collects ☛ Proximal tooth surfaces, cervical thirds of teeth, and difficult to clean areas
ROOT SURFACE	On roots of teeth, most commonly found in elderly population due to gingival recession

FIGURE 7-15 Class I Carious Lesion

FIGURE 7-16
Class II Carious
Lesion

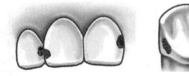

FIGURE 7-17 Class III Carious Lesion

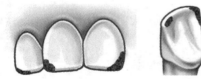

FIGURE 7-18 Class IV Carious Lesion

G.V. BLACK'S CLASSIFICATION OF CARIES

CLASS I	Cavities in pits or fissures 🗝 Examine: visual, exploration **Figure 7-15**
CLASS II	Cavities in proximal surfaces of premolars and molars 🗝 Examine: radiographs, color changes, loss of translucency, exploration of proximal surface **Figure 7-16**
CLASS III	Cavities in proximal surfaces of incisors and canines that do not involve the incisal angle 🗝 Examine: radiographs, transillumination; color changes, exploration **Figure 7-17**
CLASS IV	Cavities in proximal surfaces of incisors or canines that involve the incisal angle 🗝 Examine: visual, transillumination **Figure 7-18**
CLASS V	Cavities in the cervical one-third of facial or lingual surfaces (not pits or fissures) 🗝 Examine: direct visual, exploration **Figure 7-19**
CLASS VI	Cavities on incisal edges of anterior teeth and cusp tips of posterior teeth 🗝 Examine: direct visual **Figure 7-20**

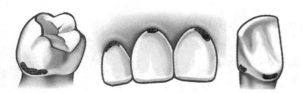

FIGURE 7-19 Class V Carious Lesion

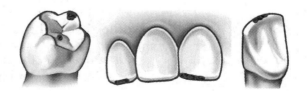

FIGURE 7-20 Class VI Carious Lesion

TYPES OF CARIES

RAMPANT CARIES	• Rapidly progressive decay requiring urgent intervention • Often associated with nursing bottle syndrome
ARRESTED CARIES	Demineralization–remineralization process
RECURRENT CARIES	New decay that occurs at margins of existing restorations

TOOTH ASSESSMENT

VENEER	Aesthetic tooth-colored material ☛ Used for malformed, discolored, or abraded facial surfaces of teeth
GOLD INLAY	Cast gold restoration placed within the tooth ☛ Does not cover the cusps
GOLD ONLAY	Cast gold restoration with cusp tips covered in gold ☛ Covers the cusps
GOLD FOIL	Noncasted gold restoration
FIXED BRIDGE	Replaces one or more missing teeth and consists of abutment and pontic teeth splinted together
DENTAL IMPLANTS	Osseointegrated anchor and abutment with a prosthetic tooth to replace one or more missing teeth
OVERHANG RESTORATION	Restorative material extends beyond natural tooth
DENTAL SEALANT	Plastic resin placed on occlusal surface to seal pits and fissures
ROOT CANAL	Removal of pulp tissue and replaced with endodontic material
DECALCIFICATION	Chalky white color usually softer than enamel ☛ Possibly an incipient carious lesion

ATTRITION	Mechanical wear due to forces of mastication
ABRASION	Mechanical wear due to improper tooth brushing or other oral habits
HYPOPLASIA	Enamel defects from systemic or traumatic influences
EROSION	Loss of tooth substance by chemical process ☞ Causes: chronic vomiting, lemons
FRACTURES OF TEETH	Horizontal, diagonal, vertical lines due to trauma to the face

➤ OCCLUSAL EVALUATION

Angle's Classification of Malocclusion

CLASS I (MESOGNATHIC) Figure 7-21	
MOLAR RELATIONSHIP	MB cusp of the maxillary first molar lines up approximately with the MB groove of the mandibular first molar
CANINE RELATIONSHIP	The maxillary canine is a half tooth posterior to the mandibular canine

CLASS II (RETROGNATHIC) Figure 7-22	
MOLAR RELATIONSHIP	MB cusp of the maxillary first molar falls approximately between the mandibular first molar and second premolar ☞ Overbite

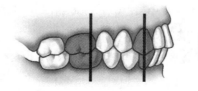

Class I

Mesognathic profile

FIGURE 7-21   Class I (Mesognathic) Occlusion

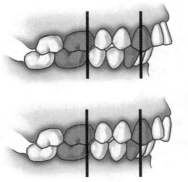
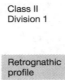
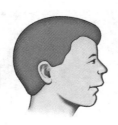

FIGURE 7-22 Class II (Retrognathic) Occlusion

CANINE RELATIONSHIP	The maxillary canine is a whole tooth anterior to the mandibular canine
CLASS II DIVISION 1	The mandible is retruded and all the maxillary incisors are protruded
CLASS II DIVISION 2	The mandibular anteriors are retruded and one or more of the maxillary incisors are retruded

CLASS III (PROGNATHIC)
Figure 7-23

MOLAR RELATIONSHIP	MB cusp of the maxillary first molar falls approximately between the mandibular first molar and the mandibular second molar ⚷ "Bulldog"
CANINE RELATIONSHIP	The maxillary canine falls posterior to the mandibular canine by a whole tooth width

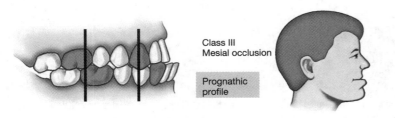

FIGURE 7-23 Class III (Prognathic) Occlusion

Malrelationships of Groups of Teeth

MALRELATIONSHIPS OF GROUPS OF TEETH	
CROSSBITE	Anterior: Maxillary incisors are lingual to the mandibular incisors Posterior: Maxillary or mandibular posterior teeth are either facial or lingual to their normal position; may be bilateral or unilateral **Figure 7-24**
EDGE-TO-EDGE	Incisal edges of anterior teeth occlude **Figure 7-25**
END-TO-END	Cusp tips of molars and premolars may be in occlusion **Figure 7-26**
OPEN BITE	Lack of occlusal or incisal contact; involves "vertical dimension" **Figure 7-27**
OVERJET	Refers to horizontal distance between lingual surfaces of maxillary anterior teeth and labial surfaces of mandibular anterior teeth **Figure 7-28**

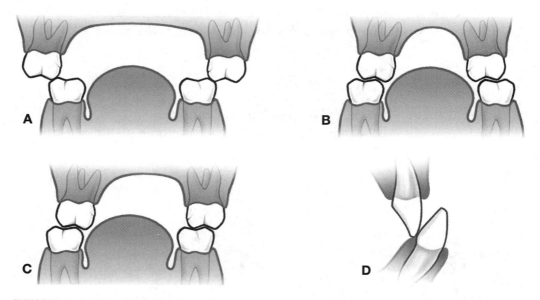

FIGURE 7-24 Crossbite: A) Mandibular Teeth Lingual to Normal Position; B) Mandibular Teeth Facial to Normal Position; C) Unilateral Crossbite—Right Side Normal, Left Side Mandibular Teeth Facial to Normal Position; D) Anterior Crossbite—Maxillary Teeth Lingual to Mandibular Teeth

OVERBITE	Vertical overlap: The vertical distance by which the maxillary incisors overlap the mandibular incisors
	Normal: Incisal edges of maxillary teeth within incisal third of mandibular teeth
	Moderate: Incisal edges of maxillary teeth are within middle third of mandibular teeth
	Deep (Severe): Incisal edges of maxillary teeth are within cervical third of mandibular teeth; when incisal edges of mandibular teeth are in contact with palatal tissue, overbite is classified as very deep or very severe
	Figure 7-29

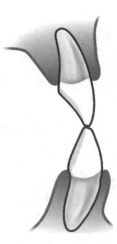

FIGURE 7-25 Edge-to-Edge Bite

➤ CLINICAL TESTING

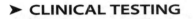

EXFOLIATIVE CYTOLOGY

Preliminary diagnosis

CLASSES OF DIAGNOSIS OF SMEARS	• Class I: normal
	• Class II: Minor atypia; no evidence of malignancy
	• Class III: Indeterminate; possible for cancer
	• Class IV: Suggestive of cancer; refer for biopsy
	• Class V: Positive for cancer; refer for biopsy

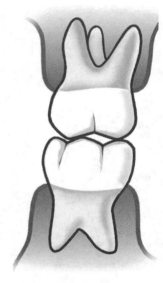

FIGURE 7-26 End-to-End Bite (Molar Are Cusp to Cusp)

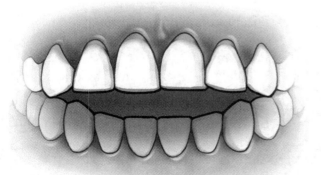

FIGURE 7-27 Open Bite

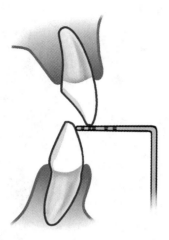

FIGURE 7-28 Overjet (Maxillary Incisors Are Facial to Mandibular; Measure Horzontal Distance)

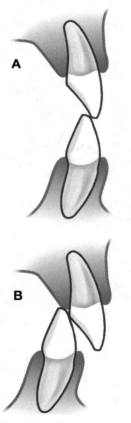

FIGURE 7-29 Overbite:
A) Normal Overbite;
B) Severe Anterior Overbite

BIOPSY

DEFINITION	Removal of tissue from the living organism for the purposes of microscopic examination and diagnosis
INDICATIONS FOR BIOPSY	• Any unusual lesion that cannot be identified • Lesions that do not heal within 2 weeks • Persistent, thick, white, hyperkeratotic lesion that does not break through the surface epithelium
TYPES OF BIOPSY	• Excisional biopsy—total excision of small lesion • Incisional biopsy—small section is removed for examination

TOLUDINE BLUE

INDICATIONS FOR USE	• Identify lesions that may be malignant • Follow-up for patients treated previously for oral cancer to aid in recognizing early tissue changes
PROCEDURE	Mouth rinse, or applied topically with cotton-tip applicator; post-rinse solution of 1% acetic acid
RESULTS	Lesions that retain the dye are considered suspicious and should be referred for a biopsy

PULP VITALITY TESTS

CLINICAL OBSERVATIONS	• Discoloration of tooth crown • Large carious lesion • Fracture • Fistula with opening into the oral cavity
RADIOGRAPHIC OBSERVATIONS	• Apical radiolucency • Bone loss with widened periodontal ligament space • Carious lesion close to pulp • Fractured tooth

INFLUENCING FACTORS TO PULP TESTING	• Degree of pulpal inflammation • Pain reaction threshold • Adjacent metal
MECHANICAL TESTS	Use explorer, end of mirror to tap on questionable tooth
HEAT THERMAL TESTS	Heated ball of gutta-percha
COLD THERMAL TESTS	Ice, cold air, or ethyl chloride
ELECTRICAL PULP TESTER	1. Explain procedure 2. Dry teeth 3. Apply a small amount of toothpaste to the tip 4. Apply tester tip and test at least one tooth other than the tooth in question 5. Place tester to middle or gingival third of tooth 6. Start rheostat at zero; advance slowly 7. Instruct the patient to signal when sensation is felt 8. Test each tooth at least twice and average the readings **Figure 7-30**
ELECTRICAL PULP TESTER READINGS	• Avoid contact with restorations • Avoid contact with soft tissues • Start at zero and slowly advance until sensation is felt • Test each tooth twice and average the readings

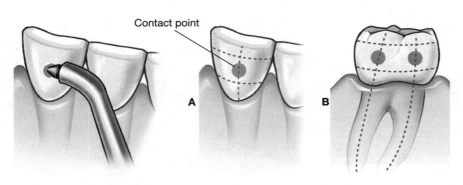

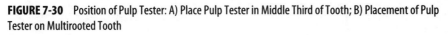

FIGURE 7-30 Position of Pulp Tester: A) Place Pulp Tester in Middle Third of Tooth; B) Placement of Pulp Tester on Multirooted Tooth

FALSE NEGATIVE RESPONSES	• Recently traumatized tooth • Pulp canal narrow and calcified • Premedication with analgesics • Newly erupted tooth

PERCUSSION

Tapping the tooth surface with fingers or an instrument to determine patient response

CHAPTER

8 Obtaining and Interpreting Radiographs

Demetra Daskalos Logothetis, RDH, MS

Tammy Teague RDH, BS

➤ PRINCIPLES OF RADIOPHYSICS

IONIZING RADIATION

Radiation that produces ions

PARTICULATE RADIATION

Tiny particles of matter that travel at high speeds in straight lines
Figure 8-1

ALPHA PARTICLES	Positively charged and contain two protons and two electrons
BETA PARTICLES	Negatively charged electrons that move at high speeds
PROTONS	Accelerated particles with a mass of 1 and a charge of +1
NEUTRONS	Accelerated particles with a mass of 1 and have no charge

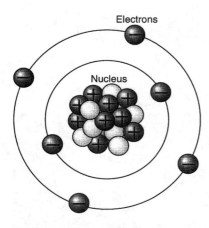

FIGURE 8-1 Diagram of an Atom

ELECTROMAGNETIC RADIATION
Figure 8-2

Movement of wavelike energy through space and matter
- Radio waves
- Visible light
- X- and gamma radiation
- Cosmic rays

ELECTROMAGNETIC SPECTRUM

Electromagnetic radiations that are organized according to their energies; all share the same properties:

- Travel at speed of light
- Have no electric charge
- Have no mass or weight
- Pass through space as particles and in a wavelike motion
- Give off an electrical field at right angles to their path of travel and a magnetic field at right angles to the electrical field
- Have high energies that are measurable and different

WAVELENGTH	<ul><li>The distance between two similar points on two successive waves</li><li>The shorter the distance between crests, the shorter the wavelength</li><li>The shorter the wavelength, the higher the energy and ability to penetrate matter</li><li>⚷ Determine the penetrating power of radiation</li></ul>

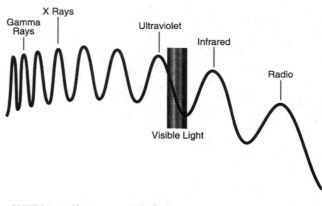

FIGURE 8-2 Electromagnetic Radiation

FREQUENCY	• Measure of the number of waves that pass a given point per unit of time • Inversely related to wavelength; example: frequency is high→wavelength is short, or vice versa • ☛ Measured in Hertz (Hz)
ENERGY	Measured in electron volts (eV) ☛ X-ray photons with high energy have high frequency and short wavelength

X-RADIATION PROPERTIES

- Invisible
- No mass or weight
- No charge
- Travel in straight lines
- Travel at speed of light
- Cause ionization
- Penetrate opaque tissues
- Produce image on photographic film

PRINCIPLES OF X-RAY PRODUCTION

The sudden slowing down or stopping of high-speed electrons produces X-ray photons; items needed to produce x-rays:

- Source of high-speed electrons
- Target for the high-speed electrons to interact or collide with, causing a release of large amounts of energy in the form of x-rays (1%) and heat (99%)
- Tungsten is used for x-ray targets due to its high melting point and good thermal conductivity

X-RAY TUBE

Critical to the production of x-rays

Figure 8-3

CATHODE	• Negative electrode consisting of tungsten wire filament • Supplies electrons to generate x-rays
ANODE	Positive electrode that converts electrons into x-ray photons

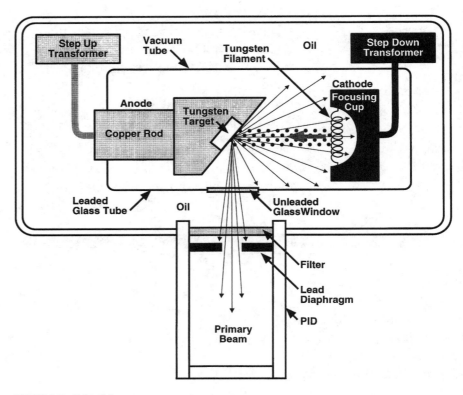

FIGURE 8-3 X-Ray Tube

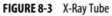

FOCUS CUP	Shapes cloud of electrons to strike the target or "focal spot"
POSITION-INDICATING DEVICE (PID)	Rectangular lead-lined area on the target of the anode that the focus cup directs the electron beam to the object and film ☞ The smaller the focal point, the sharper the radiographic image
TRANSFORMERS	Devices that alter electrical current (increase or decrease the voltage)
OIL	Insulates the x-ray tube and serves to dissipate heat

X-RAY TUBE OPERATION

AMPERAGE	Determines the available number of free electrons at the cathode filament ☞ Measured in milliamperes (mA)

VOLTAGE	Determines speed of travel (electrical pressure) that pushes electrons toward their target on the anode • Measured in kilovolts (kV) • Both milliamperes and kilovolts may be adjusted on the control panel
PRIMARY RADIATION	Penetrating x-ray beam produced at the target of the anode and exits the tubehead
SECONDARY RADIATION	Created when primary beam interacts with matter
SCATTER RADIATION	Secondary radiation resulting from x-ray that has deflected from the path by interacting with matter

WAVELENGTH

Determines energy and penetrating power
• Short wavelengths = higher penetrating power
• Long wavelengths = less penetrating power

QUALITY OF X-RAY BEAM (WAVELENGTH)

Describes penetrating ability of x-ray beam

Exposure Factors

DENSITY

- Darkness or blackness of film—changes occur from adjustment of kilovoltage peak
- Affected by kVp, mA, and exposure time, patient thickness, source-to-film distance
• Higher kV is used for dense or thick areas
• Increased density (darker) → kilovoltage peak is increased while milliamperage and exposure time stay the same
• Decreased density (lighter) → kilovoltage peak is decreased

CONTRAST

- Differentiation between sharp dark or light areas
- Affected by kVp, patient thickness and density, film contrast, and film processing

- Low kilovoltage (65–70 kVp) = high contrast representing more black and white areas with few shades of gray
- ☞ Useful for caries detection
- High kilovoltage (≥90 kVp) = low contrast representing more shades of gray with few black and white
- ☞ Useful for diagnosis of periodontal or periapical disease

KILOVOLTAGE

- Controls quality, quantity, and energy of x-ray beam
- Causes electrons to move from negative cathode to positive anode—determines the speed
- Affects contrast of densities on radiograph
- Kilovoltage peak (kVp): controlled on control panel; maximum voltage
- ☞ Voltage increased → speed of electrons increases→target is struck with greater force and energy → short wavelength → x-ray produced
- ☞ Voltage decreased → decreases the efficiency of x-ray production → reducing the penetrating qualities of the x-ray beam
- ☞ 1kV = 1000 volts, thus 90 kV = 90,000 volts
- ☞ Dental x-ray = 65–100 kV
  - ↓ 65 = inadequate penetration
  - ↑ 100 = over-penetration
  - 85–100 kV = more penetration of rays due to shorter wave lengths produced
  - 65–75 kV = less penetrating rays energy due to longer wave-lengths produced

EXPOSURE TIME

Measured in impulses and is the length of time in which x-rays are produced; adjustment in exposure time is required when kVp or mA are altered
- ☞ Most frequently altered exposure factor
- ☞ 60 impulses occur in 1 second

"KILOVOLTAGE PEAK RULE"
- When kilovoltage peak is increased by 15, exposure time should be decreased by one-half
- Conversely, when kilovoltage peak is decreased by 15, the exposure time should be doubled
- Example: 90 kVp at 0.5 seconds if decrease kVp to 75 exposure time must be increased to 1.0 seconds to create proper film density

MILLIAMPERAGE (mA)

- Ampere (A) = measures the number of electrons passing through cathode filament
- Controls quantity or number of x-rays produced
- ☞ 1 mA = 1/1000 A
- ☞ Dental radiographs require 7–15 mA
- Increase mA = increase temperature of cathode filament → increase number of electrons → increase in number of x-rays emitted from x-ray tube

MILLIAMPERE SECONDS (mAs)	mA × exposure time (seconds) = mAs ☞ Most significant density factor Example: 10 mA and 1.5 seconds results in 15 mAs (10 mA × 1.5 seconds = 15 mAs)
	If mA is increased to 15 mA, the time must be decreased to 1.0 seconds (15 mA × 1.0 seconds = 15 mAs)
	*Both will produce the same density of radiograph
	If you need less exposure time (difficult patient), increase mA to allow for decrease in exposure time ☞ Increase mA must decrease exposure time ☞ Decrease mA must increase exposure time
DENSITY RELATED TO mA	Increase in mA increases density → darker image Decrease mA decreases density → lighter image

BEAM INTENSITY

- Quantity and quality of x-rays
- Affected by the distance from the source of x-rays to the film
- Higher kVp = ↑ intensity of x-ray beam
- Higher mA = ↑ intensity of x-ray beam
- Increase in exposure time = ↑ intensity of x-ray beam
- Intensity of x-ray beam is reduced as distance is increased
- ☞ *Inverse square law:* The intensity of radiation is inversely proportional to the square of the distance from its source
- ☞ Filtration and collimation reduces intensity

➤ PRINCIPLES OF RADIOBIOLOGY

Effects of radiation on living tissue

IONIZATION

Occurs when x-rays strike patient's tissue

FREE RADICAL FORMATION

Occurs when x-ray photon ionizes water

DIRECT THEORY

Cell damage results when ionizing radiation directly hits critical areas

☛ Example: X-ray strikes DNA of cell, causing severe damage; occurs infrequently

INDIRECT THEORY

Absorption of x-ray photons within cell, causing production of toxins that damage cell

☛ Example: Free radical formation from absorbed x-ray photon in water creates toxins (e.g. H_2O_2) and causes cellular damage; occurs frequently due to high water content of cells

DOSE-RESPONSE CURVE

Illustrates the possible biologic responses to ionizing radiation

SOMATIC EFFECTS OF RADIATION

Somatic tissue includes all cells in the body with the exception of reproductive cells (sperm and ova); changes in these cells will not be passed to offspring

GENETIC EFFECTS OF RADIATION

Changes in genetic cells (mutations) are passed to succeeding generations; these effects cannot be detected in exposed patient

☛ Irreversible, permanent

LATENT PERIOD

Time between exposure to ionizing radiation and clinical symptoms (may be hours, weeks, months)
- ☛ Increase dose = decrease latent period

TISSUE SENSITIVITY

HIGH SENSITIVITY	• Lymphoid organs • Bone marrow • Testes • Intestines • Skin • Cornea
INTERMEDIATE SENSITIVITY	• Fine vasculature • Growing cartilage • Growing bone
LOW SENSITIVITY	• Salivary glands • Lungs • Kidneys • Liver • Optic lens • Muscle cells • Neurons

EFFECTS OF DENTAL X-RAY EXPOSURE

SKIN	Erythema can result with doses of 250 rad
EYES	Cataract formation can be induced with 200,000 mrem
THYROID	Malignant changes can occur with doses of 6 rad ☛ Thyroid is radiosensitive
BONE MARROW	Cancer risk, particularly leukemia ☛ Greatest somatic hazard from dental x-rays

➤ PRINCIPLES OF RADIOLOGIC HEALTH

Radiation Protection

PRESCRIBING RADIOGRAPHS

Number, type, and frequency are always based upon individual needs
☞ Medical history and clinical exams should be completed first to determine radiograph needs

FILTRATION

INHERENT FILTRATION	• 0.5 to 1.0 millimeter (mm) of aluminum • X-ray beam passes through unleaded glass window and oil ☞ Does not meet federal, state standards—more filtration is required
ADDED FILTRATION	• Placement of aluminum disks in path of x-ray beam; can be added in 0.5-mm increments • Reduce intensity of x-ray beam and are placed in path of beam in tubehead • Filter out long wavelengths, low-energy x-rays • Increased penetrating capability while reducing intensity ☞ Low-energy, long wavelengths are harmful and provide no diagnostic effect ☞ Filtration produces higher energy and a more penetrating beam
TOTAL FILTRATION	Sum of both inherent and added filtration (determined by federal regulations) • Machines operating at kilovoltages up to 70kVp 1.5 mm total filtration is required • Machines operating at 70 kVp or higher require 2.5 mm or total filtration

COLLIMATION

Lead plate with hole in middle to restrict size and shape of x-ray beam to reduce patient exposure
☞ Skin exposure to x-ray beam should not exceed 2.75 inches or 7 cm

POSITION-INDICATION DEVICE (PID)

Extension of tubehead used to direct beam

Types:

1. Conical (closed pointed plastic): produces scattered radiation (no longer manufactured, illegal and contraindicated in most states)
2. Rectangular and round: available in 8-inch and 16-inch cones

THYROID COLLAR

Lead collar that protects the thyroid

☛ Not recommended with extraoral films because it obscures information

LEAD APRON

Protects tissues from radiation

☛ Recommended for all patients during x-ray exposure

FILM SPEED

- Fast speed film is extremely effective in reducing x-ray exposure
- E speed film instead of D produces a 40% reduction in exposure
- F speed film instead of E speed film further reduces exposure by 20%

EXPOSURE FACTOR SELECTIONS

Limits x-ray exposure by adjusting kVp, mA, and exposure time

☛ Related to child vs. adult, missing teeth, tori, exostosis, cone length

INTENSIFYING SCREENS

- Used with extraoral film and screens fluorescence upon exposure to x-rays
- Decreases the exposure time by intensifying the effect of x-rays on the film
- Reduces patient radiation dose

OPERATOR PROTECTIONS

DISTANCE	Operator must stand at least 6 feet away from x-ray source at a 90–135° angle from primary beam if not behind a lead barrier **Figure 8-4**
MONITORING	Leakage monitoring through a film device from the State Health Department or manufacturer of x-ray equipment ☞ Records whole body radiation
FILM BADGE	Monitors x-radiation that reaches the body of the dental radiographer ☞ Should be worn when exposing radiographs

RADIATION EXPOSURE GUIDELINES

MAXIMUM PERMISSIBLE DOSE (MPD)	Whole body dose limit for occupational exposure = 5.0 rem/year (0.05 Sv/year) Whole body dose limit for pregnant radiation users and nonoccupationally exposed individuals = 0.5 rem/year (0.005 Sv/year)
MAXIMUM ACCUMULATED DOSE (MAD)	Accumulated lifetime dose determined by a formula based on worker's age: MAD = (N − 18) × 5 rem/year MAD = (N − 18) × 0.05 Sv/year

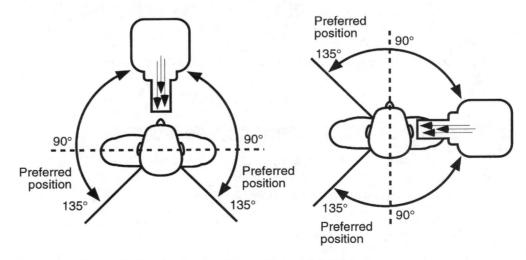

FIGURE 8-4   Operator Must Be 6 Feet Away From Primary Beam, at a 90°–135° Angle

	N = persons age 18 = minimum required age of radiographer 5 = rems per year ☛ Example MAD for 40-year-old radiation worker (40–18) × 5 = 110 rems
ALARA CONCEPT	• Patient radiation exposure must be kept to a minimum; "as low as reasonably achievable" • Determine if benefit of radiograph outweighs the risk of exposure

X-Ray Film

COMPOSITION

FILM BASE	Provides support to emulsion
ADHESIVE LAYER	On both sides of film base and serves as attachment of emulsion to base
EMULSION	Causes film to be sensitive to x-radiation; homogeneous mixture of gelatin and silver halide crystals
GELATIN	Suspends silver halide crystals over film base; absorbs processing solutions to interact with silver halide crystals
SILVER HALIDE CRYSTALS	Absorb radiation and store energy from the radiation ☛ Extremely sensitive to x-ray light
LATENT IMAGE FORMATION	During exposure the x-rays strike and ionize some silver halide crystals, forming a latent image; image becomes visible during processing procedures ☛ Latent means undeveloped but exposed ☛ Structures that permit passage of x-rays are radiolucent ☛ Structures that absorb x-rays are radiopaque and do not form a latent image

FILM EMULSION SPEED

Amount of radiation required to produce a radiograph
- Faster film speed, less radiation required
- Larger the silver halide crystals, the faster the film speed
- Larger crystals reduce the sharpness of the radiographic image; however, there is a reduction in patient exposure

EXTRAORAL FILMS

SCREEN FILM	Extraoral film used in a cassette between two intensifying screens; during exposure the screens convert the x-ray energy into blue or green light; film is sensitive to blue and green fluorescent light formed inside the cassette - Blue-sensitive film must be used with screens that produce blue light - Green-sensitive film must be used with screens that produce green light
NONSCREEN FILM	Exposed directly to x-rays, therefore not requiring screens Requires more exposure time, therefore not used often

INTENSIFYING SCREENS

- Transfer x-ray energy into visible light; the x-ray light, in turn, exposes the screen film
- Intensify the effect of x-rays on film
- Purpose is to reduce the radiation required to expose the film
- Smooth cardboard or plastic sheet coated with fluorescent crystals
- Use with panoramic, cephalometric film

➤ RADIOGRAPHIC TECHNIQUE

PARALLELING TECHNIQUE

Technique used to expose periapical films that are dimensionally accurate

CONCEPTS OF THE PARALLELING TECHNIQUE	- Film is placed parallel to the long axis of the tooth to be radiographed - Central ray of the x-ray beam is aimed perpendicular to the tooth (long axis) and film

Figure 8-5	• Film holders are utilized to stabilize the film and keep it parallel with the long axis of the tooth
GUIDELINES FOR THE PARALLELING TECHNIQUE	• Film is positioned to cover the teeth to be examined • Film is positioned parallel to the long axis; the film must be placed toward the middle of the oral cavity • Central ray is directed at a right angle to the film and long axis of the tooth • Central ray is directed through the contact areas • X-ray beam must be centered on the film to ensure that all of the film is exposed
ADVANTAGES OF THE PARALLELING TECHNIQUE	• Produces an image that is dimensionally accurate with maximum definition • Easy to learn and use • Can be accurately duplicated
DISADVANTAGES OF THE PARALLELING TECHNIQUE	• Placement of the film may be difficult because of the film-holding device; modifications may be necessary for children or adults with shallow palates or small mouths • Film-holding device used can be uncomfortable for the patient

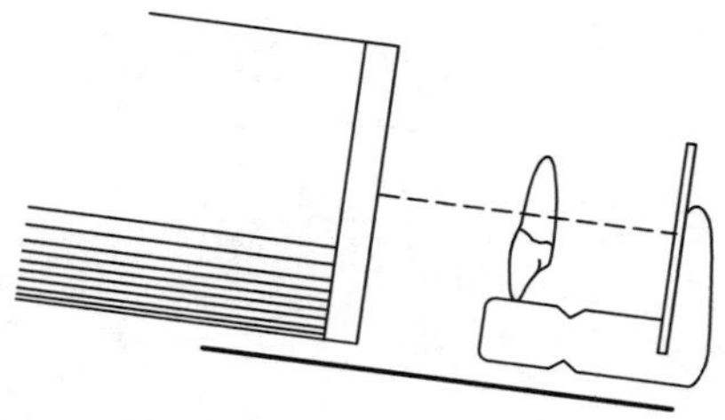

FIGURE 8-5

BISECTING TECHNIQUE

Used to expose periapical films; based on the geometric principle known as the rule of isometry

CONCEPTS OF THE BISECTING TECHNIQUE **Figure 8-6**	• The film is placed along the lingual surface of the tooth to be examined • An angle is formed where the film contacts the tooth and its long axis • An imaginary line that bisects the angle formed by the film and long axis of the tooth is visualized • The central ray of the x-ray beam is directed perpendicular to the imaginary bisector

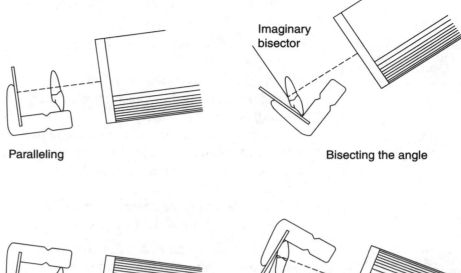

Paralleling

Bisecting the angle

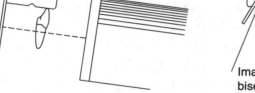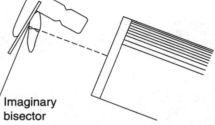

Paralleling

Bisecting the angle

FIGURE 8-6 Differences between Paralleling and Bisecting Techniques

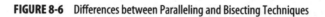

GUIDELINES FOR THE BISECTING TECHNIQUE	• The film is placed in a position that covers the teeth to be examined • The film is placed against the lingual surface of the teeth, with 1/8 of the film extending past the occlusal or incisal surface of the teeth and resting on the palate or alveolar tissues • The central ray of the x-ray beam is aimed perpendicular to the imaginary bisector that divides the angle formed by the long axis of the tooth and the film • The central ray of the x-ray beam is directed through the contact areas • The x-ray beam must be centered on the film to ensure coverage of the entire film
ADVANTAGES OF THE BISECTING TECHNIQUE	Can be used on patients with a shallow palate, children, or other patients that have difficulty with the film holder

DISADVANTAGES OF THE BISECTING TECHNIQUE	Image distortion occurs because of the use of a short PID and the difficulty in determining vertical angulation without a film holder

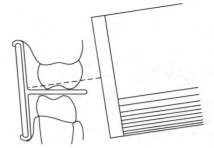

BITEWING TECHNIQUE

Best technique used to examine the interproximal surfaces of the teeth and crestal bone

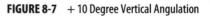

FIGURE 8-7   + 10 Degree Vertical Angulation

CONCEPTS OF THE BITEWING TECHNIQUE Figure 8-7	• Film placement is parallel to the crowns of the upper and lower teeth using a film holder or stick-on tab • A film holder or stick-on tab is used to stabilize the film • The central ray of the x-ray beam is directed through the contact areas of the teeth using a +10 degree vertical angulation
GUIDELINES FOR USING THE BITEWING TECHNIQUE	• The film is placed on the lingual surfaces of the teeth to be examined • The film is positioned parallel to the crowns of the upper and lower teeth and stabilized by a tab or holder • The central ray of the x-ray beam is directed at +10 degrees • The central ray of the x-ray beam is directed through the contact areas • The x-ray beam is centered on the film to ensure coverage of the entire film
VERTICAL BITEWINGS Figure 8-8	• Used to examine the level of alveolar bone when greater bone loss has occurred • The film is placed with the long portion of the tooth in a vertical direction as opposed to the horizontal direction normally used
DIFFICULTIES WITH BITEWING RADIOGRAPHS	Edentulous spaces and tori may cause problems with film placement; cotton rolls may be utilized to help stabilize film when edentulous areas are present and film holders may be needed for stabilization if large tori are present

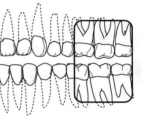

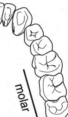

molar

FIGURE 8-8

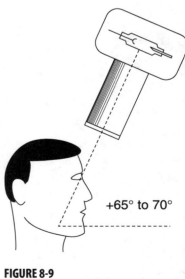

+65° to 70°

FIGURE 8-9

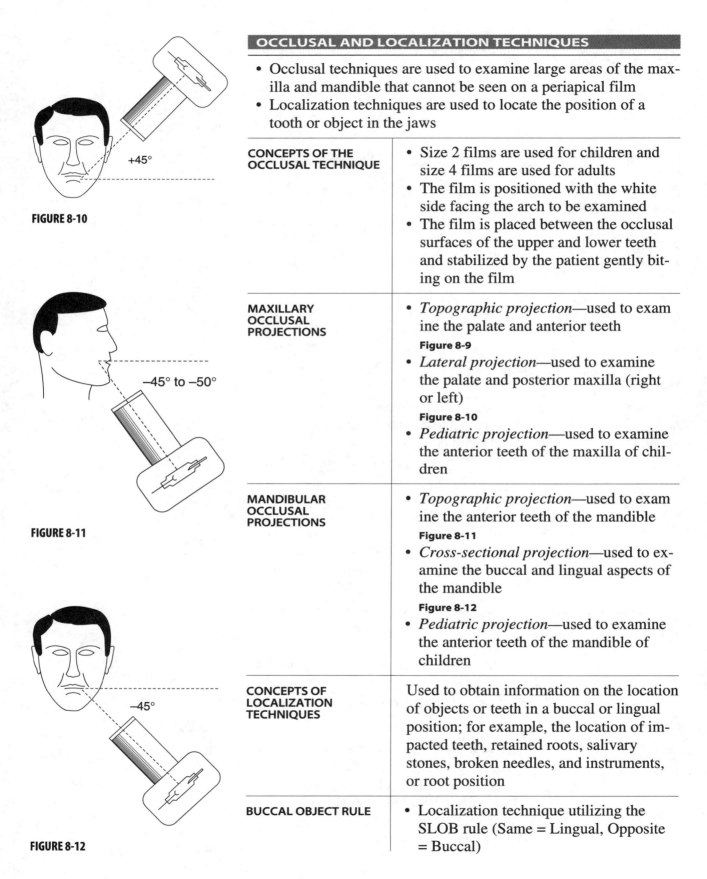

FIGURE 8-10

FIGURE 8-11

FIGURE 8-12

OCCLUSAL AND LOCALIZATION TECHNIQUES

- Occlusal techniques are used to examine large areas of the maxilla and mandible that cannot be seen on a periapical film
- Localization techniques are used to locate the position of a tooth or object in the jaws

CONCEPTS OF THE OCCLUSAL TECHNIQUE	• Size 2 films are used for children and size 4 films are used for adults • The film is positioned with the white side facing the arch to be examined • The film is placed between the occlusal surfaces of the upper and lower teeth and stabilized by the patient gently biting on the film
MAXILLARY OCCLUSAL PROJECTIONS	• *Topographic projection*—used to examine the palate and anterior teeth **Figure 8-9** • *Lateral projection*—used to examine the palate and posterior maxilla (right or left) **Figure 8-10** • *Pediatric projection*—used to examine the anterior teeth of the maxilla of children
MANDIBULAR OCCLUSAL PROJECTIONS	• *Topographic projection*—used to examine the anterior teeth of the mandible **Figure 8-11** • *Cross-sectional projection*—used to examine the buccal and lingual aspects of the mandible **Figure 8-12** • *Pediatric projection*—used to examine the anterior teeth of the mandible of children
CONCEPTS OF LOCALIZATION TECHNIQUES	Used to obtain information on the location of objects or teeth in a buccal or lingual position; for example, the location of impacted teeth, retained roots, salivary stones, broken needles, and instruments, or root position
BUCCAL OBJECT RULE	• Localization technique utilizing the SLOB rule (Same = Lingual, Opposite = Buccal)

- Two radiographs are exposed using different angulations (vertical when trying to locate vertically aligned objects and horizontally when locating horizontally aligned objects) and then the two x-rays are compared
- When the object being compared appears to have moved in the same direction as the shift of the PID, the object is positioned to the lingual; if the object moves in the opposite direction of the PID, the object is positioned on the buccal aspect

FIGURE 8-13 Clear Film

RIGHT-ANGLE TECHNIQUE	• Technique used primarily to locate objects in the mandible • A periapical film and occlusal film are compared to locate the object in three dimensions

Intraoral Exposure and Technique Errors

FILM EXPOSURE

Results in film that is either too dark or too light

FIGURE 8-14 Black Film

CLEAR FILM	Film was not exposed due to x-ray machine not being turned on, malfunctioning, or electrical failure **Figure 8-13**
BLACK FILM	The film was exposed to white light; only unwrap film with the use of a safelight **Figure 8-14**
DARK FILM	The film is overexposed because of excessive exposure time, kilovoltage, milliamperage, or a combination of these
LIGHT FILM	The film is underexposed due to inadequate exposure time, kilovoltage, milliamperage, or a combination of these **Figure 8-15**

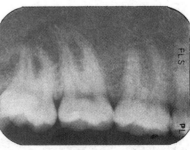

FIGURE 8-15 Light film

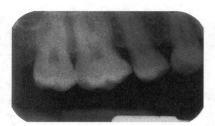

FIGURE 8-16 Apex of Tooth Missing

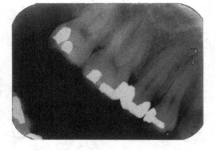

FIGURE 8-17 Tilted Occlusal Plane

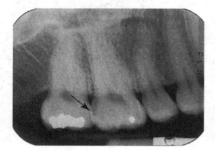

FIGURE 8-18 Overlapping Contacts of Molars

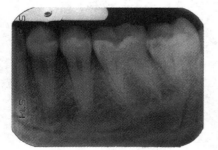

FIGURE 8-19 Blunted Roots

Radiographer Technique Errors

FILM PLACEMENT ERRORS WITH PERIAPICAL FILMS

Correctly placed films include the entire tooth, including the apex, and 2–3 mm of surrounding structures; the edge of the film should extend 1/8 inch beyond the incisal or occlusal surfaces and be parallel to them

APEX OF THE TOOTH DOES NOT APPEAR ON THE FILM	Film should be placed with only 1/8 inch of film beyond the incisal or occlusal surface **Figure 8-16**
OCCLUSAL PLANE APPEARS TILTED	The edge of the film must be parallel to the incisal or occlusal surfaces of the teeth **Figure 8-17**

ERRORS ASSOCIATED WITH ANGULATION IN PERIAPICAL FILMS

Horizontal angulation refers to the positioning of the PID in a side-to-side plane; vertical angulation refers to the positioning of the PID in an up-and-down plane.

OVERLAPPED CONTACTS APPEAR IN THE FILM	The central ray of the x-ray beam must be directed through the interproximal surfaces; horizontal angulation **Figure 8-18**
TEETH APPEAR SHORTENED WITH BLUNT ROOTS	Excessive vertical angulation of the PID was used **Figure 8-19**
TEETH APPEAR LONG AND DISTORTED ON THE FILM	Insufficient vertical angulation of the PID was used **Figure 8-20**
A CLEAR (UNEXPOSED) AREA APPEARS ON THE FILM (AKA CONE CUT)	The PID must be positioned so that the x-ray beam is centered over the film and the entire film is covered **Figure 8-21**

ERRORS ASSOCIATED WITH RADIOGRAPHER TECHNIQUE IN BITEWING FILMS

Film placement and angulation errors can occur when exposing bitewing radiographs

ERRORS IN FILM PLACEMENT OF BITEWING FILMS

Premolar bitewings must include the maxillary and mandibular premolars and distal contact areas of both canines
Figures 8-22 and 8-23
Molar bitewings must include the maxillary and mandibular molars and be centered over the mandibular second molar
Figures 8-24 and 8-25

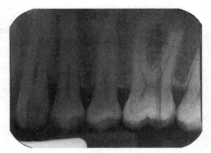

FIGURE 8-20 Elongated Roots

ERRORS WITH ANGULATION OF BITEWING FILMS

Error may be incorrect horizontal angulation or vertical angulation

OVERLAPPED CONTACTS	The central ray of the x-ray beam was not directed through the interproximal contacts **Figure 8-26**
DISTORTED IMAGES	Always use a +10 vertical angulation with bitewing films
CLEAR AREA (UNEXPOSED)	A cone cut occurs when the x-ray beam is not centered over the film and the entire film is not covered **Figure 8-27**

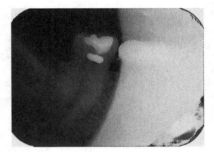

FIGURE 8-21 Cone Cut

OTHER TECHNIQUE ERRORS

STRETCHED AND DISTORTED IMAGES	The film may have been bent by the anatomy of the oral cavity or pressure; for example, a large palatal tori
APPEARANCE OF THIN RADIOLUCENT LINE	The film was creased and the emulsion of the film cracked, causing the line on the film **Figure 8-28**
DOUBLE IMAGES	The film was exposed twice **Figure 8-29**
BLURRED IMAGES	The patient moved during exposure of the film **Figure 8-30**
LIGHT FILM WITH A HERRINGBONE PATTERN	The film was placed in the mouth and exposed backward; the herringbone pattern is a result of x-ray passing through lead foil before striking film **Figure 8-31**

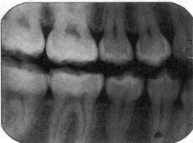

FIGURE 8-22 Correct Placement

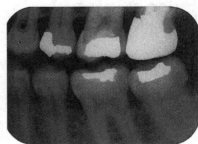

FIGURE 8-23 Incorrect Placement

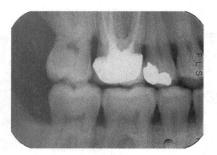

FIGURE 8-24 Correct Placement

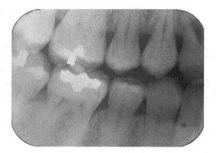

FIGURE 8-25 Incorrect Placement

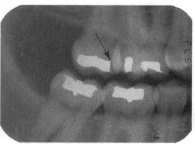

FIGURE 8-26 Overlapped Contacts

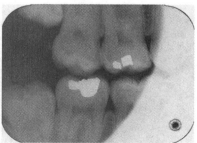

FIGURE 8-27 Cone Cut

Extraoral Radiography

PANORAMIC RADIOGRAPHY

Extraoral radiographic technique that is used to examine the upper and lower jaws on the same film

ADVANTAGES OF THE PANORAMIC X-RAY	• The entire maxilla and mandible are observed with more anatomic structure • Exposure is easy to learn and do • There is little discomfort to the patient
DISADVANTAGES TO THE PANORAMIC X-RAY FILM	• Images seen are not as sharp as periapical films • Images outside the focal trough are not seen • Distortion, magnification, and overlapping occur even with proper technique • Loss of detail

PANORAMIC PATIENT PREPARATION AND TECHNIQUE ERRORS

RADIOPAQUE ARTIFACT ON FILM	A ghost image is caused by the presence of metallic or radiodense objects that the patient has on or around their head or neck
RADIOPAQUE CONE-SHAPED ARTIFACT THAT OBSCURES THE MANDIBLE ON FILM	The presence of the thyroid collar will produce an undiagnostic film
RADIOLUCENT SHADOW THAT OBSCURES THE ANTERIOR TEETH ON FILM	The patient did not close his lips on the biteblock
RADIOLUCENT SHADOW THAT OBSCURES THE APICES OF THE MAXILLARY TEETH ON FILM	The patient did not lift his tongue to the roof of his mouth
SUPERIMPOSED HARD PALATE AND FLOOR OF THE NASAL CAVITY OVER THE ROOTS OF THE MAXILLARY TEETH	• There is a loss of detail in the maxillary incisor region or they appear blurred and magnified, or there is a reverse smile line on a film • The Frankfort plane is angled upward instead of being parallel to the floor (patient's chin is tilted up

BLURRED MANDIBULAR INCISORS	• There is less detail in the apices, the condyles are not visible, or there is an exaggerated smile line • The Frankfort plane was not parallel with the floor; the chin was too low or tipped downward
ANTERIOR TEETH APPEAR SKINNY AND OUT OF FOCUS ON THE FILM	The patient's teeth were not positioned in the groove on the biteblock; they were positioned too far forward; anterior to the focal trough
ANTERIOR TEETH APPEAR FAT AND OUT OF FOCUS ON THE FILM	The patient's teeth were not positioned in the groove on the biteblock; they were positioned too far back; posterior to the focal trough
RAMUS AND POSTERIOR TEETH APPEAR UNEQUALLY MAGNIFIED ON THE FILM	The patient's head is not centered; the mid-sagittal plane should be perpendicular to the floor and the midline is centered on the biteblock
RADIOPACITY APPEARS IN THE CENTER OF THE FILM	The patient's spine is visible on the film because the patient is not sitting or standing straight

EXTRAORAL PROJECTION TECHNIQUES

LATERAL JAW PROJECTION	• Body of the mandible film used to evaluate impacted teeth, fractures, and lesions located in the body of the mandible • Ramus of the mandible film used to evaluate impacted third molars, large lesions, and fractures that extend into the ramus of the mandible
LATERAL CEPHALOMETRIC PROJECTION	Film used to evaluate facial growth and development, trauma, and disease and developmental abnormalities
POSTEROANTERIOR PROJECTION	Film used to evaluate facial growth and development, trauma, and disease and developmental abnormalities, as well as the frontal and ethmoidal sinuses, orbits, and nasal cavity

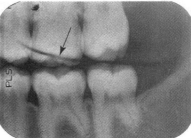

FIGURE 8-28 Creased Film Causes Radiolucent Line

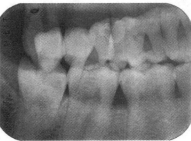

FIGURE 8-29 Double Image

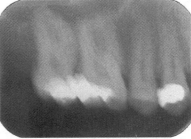

FIGURE 8-30 Blurred Image

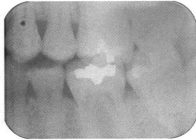

FIGURE 8-31 Herringbone Pattern

WATERS' PROJECTION	Film used to evaluate the maxillary sinuses, frontal and ethmoidal sinuses, orbits, and nasal cavity
SUBMENTOVERTEX PROJECTION	This film is used to evaluate the position of the condyle, base of the skull, and fractures of the zygomatic arch
REVERSE TOWNE PROJECTION	Film used to evaluate fractures of the condylar neck and ramus area
TRANSCRANIAL PROJECTION	Film used to evaluate the superior surface of the condyle and the articular eminence; used to evaluate the TMJ
TEMPOROMANDIBULAR JOINT TOMOGRAPHY	Film that evaluates the TMJ while blurring other areas

Digital Radiography

FUNDAMENTALS OF DIGITAL RADIOGRAPHY

A sensor is used to capture an image, break it into electronic pieces, and present and store the image on a computer; intraoral and extraoral images can be obtained

TYPES OF DIGITAL IMAGING	• Direct digital imaging • Indirect digital imaging • Storage phosphor imaging
ADVANTAGES OF DIGITAL RADIOGRAPHY	• Reduced x-ray exposure • Superior gray-scale resolution; greater contrast • Image is viewed much faster • Increased efficiency because the digital radiography does not interrupt patient care
DISADVANTAGES OF DIGITAL RADIOGRAPHY	• Sensors are thicker than intraoral film and may be uncomfortable for the patient • Sensors must be completely barrier-wrapped for infection control because they cannot be heat sterilized • Original digital image can be manipulated, so legal issues may arise • Software compatibility with offices

➤ RECOGNITION OF NORMALITIES AND ABNORMALITIES

RADIOGRAPHIC INTERPRETATION TERMINOLOGY

INTERPRET	To offer an explanation ☞ Performed by RDH and DDS
INTERPRETATION	An explanation of what is viewed on a radiograph
DIAGNOSIS	The identification of a disease or condition that is revealed through examination and analysis ☞ Performed by the dentist
RADIOPAQUE	Structure that resists the passage of the x-ray beam and limits the amount of x-rays that reach the film; light or white on film ☞ Remember P in paque stands for pale (white or light); example = alveolar bone and enamel
RADIOLUCENT	Structure that permits the passage of x-ray beam allows more x-rays to reach the film; appears dark or black ☞ Example = Caries, foramen, canals, pulp chambers

INTERPRETATION OF DENTAL CARIES ON RADIOGRAPHS

INTERPROXIMAL CARIES	Between two teeth; seen radiographically at or apical to the contact point; as caries spread through enamel to dentin it assumes a triangular configuration ☞ Bitewing radiographs are the radiograph of choice for viewing interproximal caries **Figure 8-32**
INCIPIENT INTER-PROXIMAL CARIES	Lesion seen on enamel only; caries extends less than halfway through the thickness of enamel; Class I lesion
MODERATE INTER-PROXIMAL CARIES	Lesion seen on enamel only, caries extends more than halfway through the thickness of enamel but does not involve the DEJ; Class II lesion

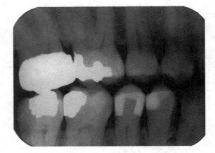

FIGURE 8-32 Incipient Caries

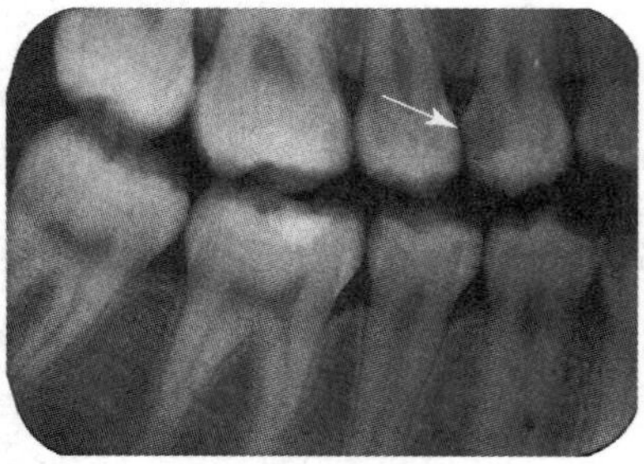

FIGURE 8-33 Severe Interproximal Caries

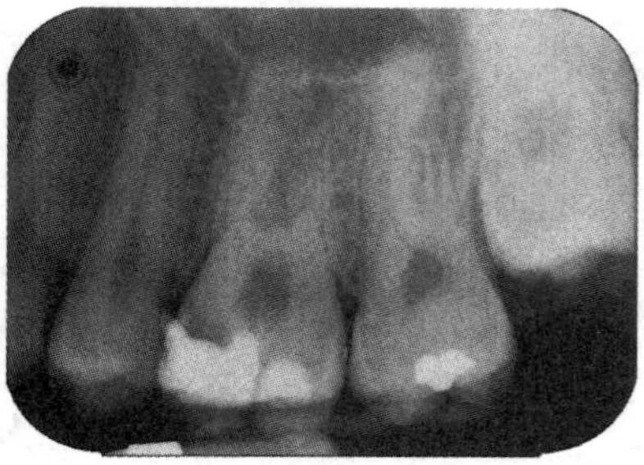

FIGURE 8-34 Root Surface Caries

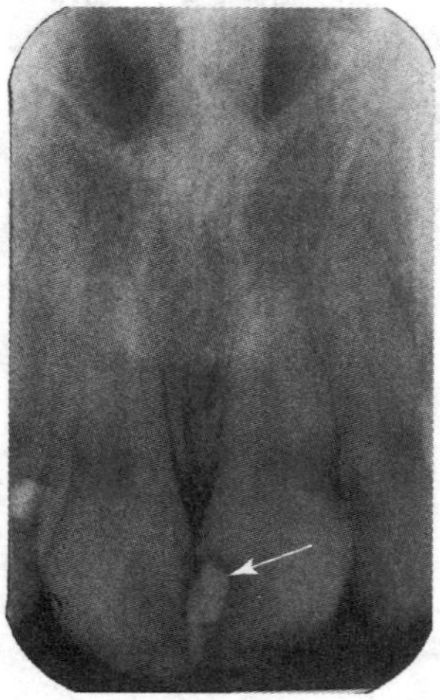

FIGURE 8-35 Recurrent Caries

ADVANCED INTER-PROXIMAL CARIES	Lesion that affects both enamel and dentin; caries extends through enamel into dentin but not more than half the distance to the pulp; Class III lesion
SEVERE INTER-PROXIMAL CARIES	Lesion involves enamel and dentin; caries extends through enamel, through dentin, and more than half the distance to the pulp; Class IV lesion ☛ Clinically appears as a cavitation or hole in the tooth **Figure 8-33**
INCIPIENT OCCLUSAL CARIES	Caries does not involve the DEJ and cannot be seen on the radiograph ☛ Must be detected with an explorer
MODERATE OCCLUSAL CARIES	Caries extends into dentin and appears as a thin radiolucent line under the enamel at the occlusal surface of the tooth
SEVERE OCCLUSAL CARIES	Caries extends into dentin and appears as a large radiolucency under the enamel of the occlusal surface of the tooth ☛ Clinically appears as a cavitation or hole in the tooth
BUCCAL AND LINGUAL CARIES	Caries that involve the buccal or lingual tooth surfaces; appears as a small, circular radiolucent area; however, they are difficult to detect on an x-ray because the superimposition of normal tooth structure ☛ Best detected by clinical exam with an explorer
ROOT SURFACE CARIES	Caries that involves only the cementum and dentin of root surfaces of the tooth; seen on an x-ray as a cupped-out or crater-shaped radiolucency just below the CEJ **Figure 8-34**
RECURRENT CARIES	Caries that occur adjacent to a preexisting restoration; appears as a radiolucency just beneath a restoration; occurs because of inadequate cavity preparation, defective margins, or incomplete removal of caries prior to the placement of the restoration **Figure 8-35**

| RAMPANT CARIES | Advanced and severe caries that affects numerous teeth
Figure 8-36 |

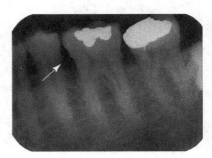

FIGURE 8-36 Rampant Caries

INTERPRETATION OF PERIODONTAL DISEASE ON RADIOGRAPHS

- Radiographs are used in conjunction with the clinical exam to evaluate the amount of bone present and determine the pattern, distribution, and severity of bone loss that has occurred as a result of periodontal disease; also used as a source of documentation
- A periapical radiograph taken with the paralleling technique is optimum for evaluating periodontal disease because the height of crestal bone is accurately recorded in relation to the root of the tooth

BONE LOSS	X-rays show the amount of bone remaining rather than the amount of bone loss; bone loss is estimated as the difference between the physiologic bone level and the height of the remaining bone; described in terms of pattern, distribution, and severity
PATTERN OF BONE LOSS: HORIZONTAL OR VERTICAL	Horizontal bone loss occurs in a plane parallel to the CEJ of adjacent teeth; vertical bone loss does not
DISTRIBUTION OF BONE LOSS: LOCALIZED OR GENERALIZED	Localized bone loss occurs in isolated areas and generalized bone loss occurs evenly over most areas
SEVERITY: MILD, MODERATE, OR SEVERE	• Mild bone loss—seen as crestal changes • Moderate bone loss—bone loss of 10–33% • Severe bone loss greater than 33%

CONTRIBUTING FACTORS OF PERIODONTAL DISEASE

| CALCULUS | Appears as a radiopaque pointed or irregular projection from the proximal root surface, radiopacity encircling the cervical portion of the tooth, or a nodular projection
Figure 8-37 |

FIGURE 8-37 Calculus

DEFECTIVE RESTORATION	X-rays help identify restorations with open or loose contacts, poor contour, uneven marginal ridges, and inadequate margins

INTERPRETATION OF TRAUMATIC LESIONS

FRACTURES	Breaking of a part; may affect the crowns or roots of teeth or bones of the maxilla or mandible, fractures appear as a radiolucent line at the site of the break ☛ Crown or root fracture are visible on a periapical; however a panoramic radiograph is used for jaw fractures
LUXATION	• Abnormal displacement of the teeth • Intrusion is the abnormal displacement of teeth into bone • Extrusion is the abnormal displacement of teeth out of bone
AVULSION	Complete displacement of a tooth from alveolar bone; x-ray will show a tooth socket without a tooth Figure 8-38
RESORPTION: PHYSIOLOGIC AND PATHOLOGIC	• Physiologic resorption is seen when the roots of primary teeth are resorbed as the permanent tooth moves in an occlusal direction • Pathologic resorption is a regressive alteration of tooth structure that is observed when a tooth is subjected to abnormal stimuli; may be internal or external
EXTERNAL RESORPTION	• Seen along the periphery of the root and most often affects the apices of teeth, the apical region appears blunted and the root appears shorter than normal • Often associated with reimplanted teeth, abnormal mechanical forces, trauma, or tumors and cysts Figure 8-39
INTERNAL RESORPTION	• Occurs due to infection within the crown or root of a tooth and involves the pulp chamber, pulp canals, and dentin

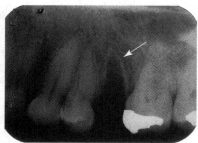

FIGURE 8-38 Avulsion

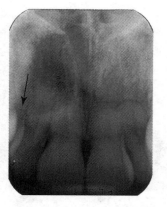

FIGURE 8-39 External Resorption

- Appears on an x-ray as round to ovoid radiolucency in the midcrown or mid-root portion of the tooth
- Etiology unknown
  Figure 8-40

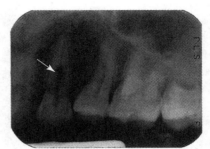

FIGURE 8-40 Internal Resorption

INTERPRETATION OF PULPAL LESIONS

Involves evaluation of the pulp cavity, chambers, and canals

PULPAL SCLEROSIS	Diffuse calcification of the pulp chamber and pulp canals of teeth that results in a pulp cavity of decreased size
PULPAL OBLITERATION	• Irritants such as attrition, caries, etc., may cause the production of secondary dentin, which results in the obliteration of the pulpal cavity; on an x-ray the affected tooth does not appear to have a pulp chamber or canals • Teeth are nonvital and do not require treatment
PULP STONES	• Calcifications that appear as round, cylindrical, or ovoid radiopacities in the pulp chamber or canal • Do not cause symptoms and do not require treatment **Figure 8-41**

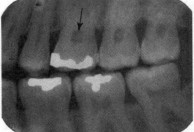

FIGURE 8-41 Pulp Stone

INTERPRETATION OF PERIAPICAL LESIONS

Lesions located around the apex of the tooth that may appear radiolucent or radiopaque

RADIOLUCENT PERIAPICAL LESIONS	Lesions that appear dark on an x-ray and cannot be diagnosed by x-rays alone
PERIAPICAL GRANULOMA	Localized mass of chronically inflamed granulation tissue at the apex of a nonvital tooth; seen on the x-ray initially as a widened periodontal ligament space at the apex of the root, in time it will widen and appear as a round or ovoid radiolucency; the lamina dura is not visible

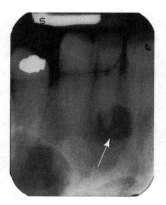

FIGURE 8-42 Periapical Cyst

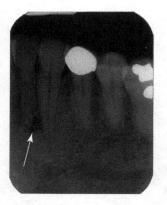

FIGURE 8-43 Periapical Abcess

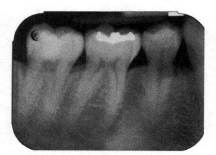

FIGURE 8-44 Sclerotic Bone

PERIAPICAL CYST	• Most common cyst in the oral cavity; develops over a prolonged period of time when cystic degeneration takes place within a periapical granuloma as a result of pulpal death and necrosis • Appears on an x-ray as a round or ovoid radiolucency **Figure 8-42**
PERIAPICAL ABCESS	• A localized collection of pus in the periapical region of a tooth that results from pulpal death may be acute or chronic • X-ray may show no changes or an increased widening of the periodontal ligament space; chronic abscesses appear as a round or ovoid apical radiolucency with poorly defined margins near or at site **Figure 8-43**

RADIOPAQUE PERIAPICAL LESIONS

Lesions that can be diagnosed by their radiographic appearance, clinical information, and patient history

CONDENSING OSTEOITIS	AKA chronic focal sclerosing osteomyelitis; a well-defined radiopacity that is seen below the apex of a nonvital tooth with a history of long-standing pulpitis; requires no treatment ☛ Most common radiopacity observed in adults, most commonly affects the mandibular first molar
SCLEROTIC BONE	AKA osteosclerosis or idiopathic periapical osteosclerosis; is a well-defined radiopacity that is seen below the apices of vital, noncarious teeth; asymptomatic and requires no treatment **Figure 8-44**
HYPERCEMENTOSIS	Excess deposition of cementum on root surfaces; visible on an x-ray as excess amount of cementum along all or part of a root surface; asymptomatic and does not require treatment

Normal Anatomic Landmarks Visual on Radiographs

BONY LANDMARKS OF THE MAXILLA

Present on maxillary periapical radiographs

INCISIVE FORAMEN	Appears as a small ovoid or round radiolucent area located between the roots of the maxillary incisors **Figure 8-45**
SUPERIOR FORAMINA OF THE INCISIVE CANAL	Appears as two small radiolucent areas located superior to the apices of the maxillary central incisors **Figure 8-46**
MEDIAN PALATINE SUTURE	Appears as a thin radiolucent line located between the two maxillary central incisors **Figure 8-47**
LATERAL FOSSA	Appears as a radiolucent area between the maxillary canine and lateral incisors; may be distinct or not present at all **Figure 8-48**
NASAL CAVITY	Appears as a large radiolucent area above the maxillary incisors
NASAL SEPTUM	Appears as a vertical radiopaque partition that divides the nasal cavity; may be superimposed over the median palatine suture
FLOOR OF THE NASAL CAVITY	Appears as a dense radiopaque band located above the maxillary incisors **Figure 8-49**
ANTERIOR NASAL SPINE	Appears as a V-shaped radiopacity at the midline of the floor of the nasal cavity **Figure 8-50**
INFERIOR NASAL CONCHAE	Appears as a diffuse mass within the nasal cavity
MAXILLARY SINUS	Appears as a radiolucent area located above the apices of the maxillary premolars and molars **Figure 8-51**
SEPTA WITHIN THE MAXILLARY SINUS	Appear as radiopaque lines located within the sinus **Figure 8-52**

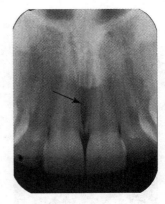

FIGURE 8-45 Incisive Foramen

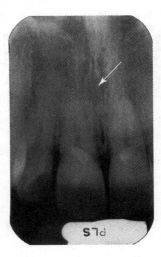

FIGURE 8-46 Superior Foramina of Incisive Canal

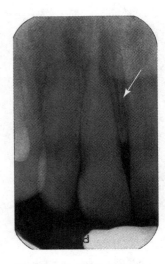

FIGURE 8-47 Median Palatine Suture

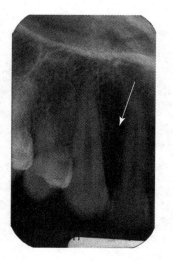

FIGURE 8-48   Lateral Fossa

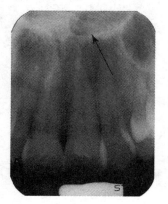

FIGURE 8-49   Floor of Nasal Cavity

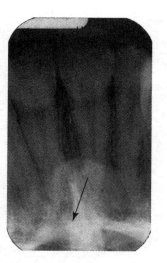

FIGURE 8-50   Anterior Nasal Spine

NUTRIENT CANALS WITHIN THE MAXILLARY SINUS	Appear as narrow radiolucent lines between two thin radiopaque lines
INVERTED Y	Appears as a radiopaque upside-down Y formed by the intersection of the maxillary sinus and nasal cavity; located above the maxillary canine **Figure 8-53**
MAXILLARY TUBEROSITY	Appears as a radiopaque bulge distal to the maxillary third molar **Figure 8-54**
HAMULUS	Appears as a radiopaque hook-like projection posterior to the maxillary tuberosity
ZYGOMATIC PROCESS OF THE MAXILLA	Appears as a radiopaque U- or J-shaped area located superior to the maxillary first molar **Figure 8-55**
ZYGOMA	Appears as a diffuse, radiopaque band that extends distally from the zygomatic process of the maxilla **Figure 8-56**

BONY LANDMARKS OF THE MANDIBLE

Includes the three main parts of the mandible: the ramus, body, and alveolar process

GENIAL TUBERCLES	Appears as a ring-shaped radiopacity located below the apices of the mandibular incisors **Figure 8-57**
LINGUAL FORAMEN	Appears as a small radiolucent area located below the apices of the mandibular incisors **Figure 8-58**
MENTAL RIDGE	Appears as a thick radiopaque band that extends from the incisors to the premolar region; may be superimposed over mandibular teeth **Figure 8-59**

MENTAL FOSSA	Appears as a radiolucent area above the mental ridge Figure 8-60
MENTAL FORAMEN	Appears as a small ovoid or round radiolucent area located between the apices of the mandibular premolars Figure 8-61
MYLOHYOID RIDGE	Appears as a dense radiopaque band that extends downward and forward from the molar area Figure 8-62
MANDIBULAR CANAL	Appears as a radiolucent band outlined by two thin radiopaque lines that is located in the mandibular molar apices area Figure 8-63
INTERNAL OBLIQUE RIDGE	Appears as a radiopaque band that extends downward and forward from the ramus Figure 8-62
EXTERNAL OBLIQUE RIDGE	• Appears as a radiopaque band that extends downward and forward from the anterior border of the ramus, usually ends in the mandibular third molar region • The internal and external oblique may be superimposed; if they are shown separately, the superior band is the external oblique and the inferior band is the internal oblique Figure 8-64
SUBMANDIBULAR FOSSA	Appears as a radiolucent area in the molar region below the myohyoid ridge Figure 8-65
CORONOID PROCESS	Appears on the maxillary molar film as a long triangular radiopacity superimposed over or below the maxillary tuberosity Figure 8-66

NORMAL TOOTH ANATOMY

ENAMEL	Appears as the outermost radiopaque layer of the crown of the tooth Figure 8-67

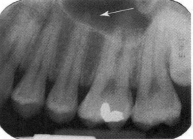

FIGURE 8-51 Maxillary Sinus

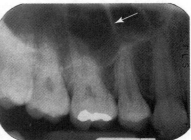

FIGURE 8-52 Septa

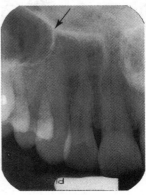

FIGURE 8-53 Inverted Y

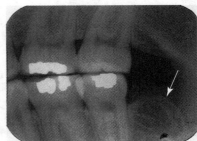

FIGURE 8-54 Maxillary Tuberosity

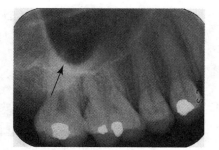

FIGURE 8-55 Zygomatic Process of the Maxilla

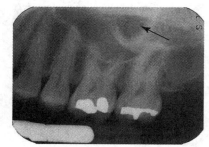

FIGURE 8-56 Zygoma

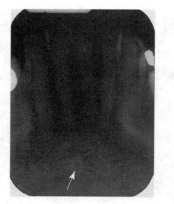

FIGURE 8-57 Genial Tuberacles

DENTIN	Appears as the less radiopaque layer beneath enamel **Figure 8-68**
PULP CAVITY	Appears as the radiolucent area inside the tooth; size and shape vary **Figure 8-69**

ALVEOLAR BONE	
LAMINA DURA	Appears as a dense radiopaque line that surrounds the root of the tooth **Figure 8-70**
PERIODONTAL LIGAMENT SPACE	Appears as a thin radiolucent line around the root of the tooth **Figure 8-71**

Normal Anatomic Landmarks on a Panoramic Radiograph
Figure 8-72

BONY LANDMARKS OF THE MAXILLA	
MASTOID PROCESS	Appears as a rounded radiopacity located posterior and inferior to the TMJ area
STYLOID PROCESS Figure 8–72b	Appears as a long radiopaque spine that extends from the temporal bone anterior to the mastoid process
EXTERNAL AUDITORY MEATUS Figure 8–72i	Appears as a round or ovoid radiolucency anterior and superior to the mastoid process
GLENOID FOSSA	Appears as a concave radiopacity superior to the mandibular condyle
ARTICULAR EMINENCE Figure 8–72k	Appears as a rounded radiopaque projection of the bone located anterior to the glenoid fossa
LATERAL PTERYGOID PLATE	Appears as radiopaque projection of bone distal to the maxillary tuberosity region
PTERYGOMAXILLARY FISSURE	Appears as radiolucent area between the lateral pterygoid plate and the maxilla

MAXILLARY TUBEROSITY Figure 8–72o	Appears as a radiopaque bulge distal to the third molar region
INFRAORBITAL FORAMEN Figure 8–72s	Appears as a round or ovoid radiolucency inferior to the orbit
ORBIT Figure 8–72w	Appears as a round radiolucent area with the radiopaque borders located above the maxillary sinus
INCISIVE CANAL	Appears as a tube-like radiolucent area with radiopaque borders located between the maxillary central incisors
INCISIVE FORAMEN Figure 8–72z	Appears as a small ovoid or round radiolucency located between the roots of the maxillary central incisors
NASAL CAVITY	Appears as a large radiolucent area above the maxillary incisors
NASAL SEPTUM Figure 8–72y	Appears as a vertical radiopaque partition that divides the nasal cavity
HARD PALATE Figure 8–72u	Appears as a horizontal radiopaque band superior to the apices of the maxillary teeth
MAXILLARY SINUS AND FLOOR Figure 8–72q	Appears as paired radiolucent ovals located above the apices of the maxillary premolars and molars; the floor appears as a radiopaque line
ZYGOMATIC PROCESS OF THE MAXILLA Figure 8–72p	Appears as a U- or J-shaped radiopacity located superior to the maxillary first molar region
ZYGOMA	Appears as a radiopaque band that extends posteriorly from the zygomatic process of the maxilla
HAMULUS	Appears as a radiopaque hook-like projection of bone that is located posterior to the maxillary tuberosity

BONY LANDMARKS OF THE MANDIBLE

MANDIBULAR CONDYLE Figure 8–72j	Appears as a rounded radiopaque projection extending from the posterior border of the ramus

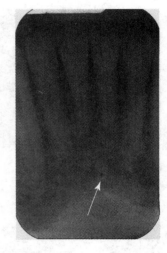
FIGURE 8-58 Lingual Foramen

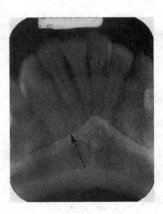
FIGURE 8-59 Mental Ridge

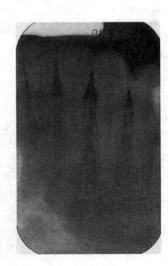
FIGURE 8-60 Mental Fossa

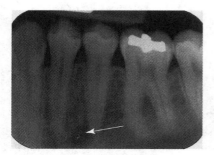

FIGURE 8-61 Mental Foramen

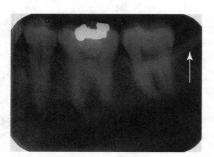

FIGURE 8-62 Mylohyoid Ridge and Internal Oblique Ridge

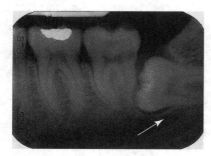

FIGURE 8-63 Mandibular Canal

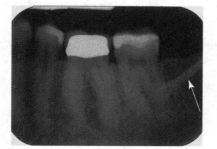

FIGURE 8-64 External Oblique Ridge

CORONOID NOTCH	Appears as a radiopaque concavity located distal to the coronoid process
CORONOID PROCESS Figure 8–72n	Appears as a triangular radiopacity posterior to the maxillary tuberosity region
MANDIBULAR FORAMEN Figure 8–72f	Appears as a round or ovoid radiolucency centered within the ramus of the mandible
LINGULA	Appears as an indistinct radiopacity anterior to the mandibular foramen
MANDIBULAR CANAL	Appears as a radiolucent band outlined by two radiopaque lines inferior to the apicies of the mandibular molars and premolars
MENTAL FORAMEN Figure 8–72ee	Appears as a smoll ovoid or round radiolucency located in the apical region of the mandibular premolars
MENTAL RIDGE	Appears as a thick radiopaque band that extends from the mandibular premolars to the incisors
MENTAL FOSSA	Appears as a radiolucent area above the mental ridge
LINGUAL FORAMEN Figure 8–72cc	Appears as a small radiolucent dot located below the apices of the mandibular incisors
GENIAL TUBERCLES Figure 8–72cc	Appear as a ring-shaped radiopacity surrounding the lingual foramen
INFERIOR BORDER OF THE MANDIBLE Figure 8–72dd	Appears as a dense radiopaque band that outlines the lower border of the mandible
MYLOHYOID RIDGE	Appears as a dense radiopaque band that extends downward and forward from the molar region
INTERNAL OBLIQUE RIDGE	Appears as a dense radiopaque band that extends downward and forward from the ramus
EXTERNAL OBLIQUE RIDGE Figure 8–72aa	Appears as a dense radiopaque band that extends downward and forward from the anterior border of the ramus of the mandible

OBTAINING AND INTERPRETING RADIOGRAPHS ■ 429

ANGLE OF THE MANDIBLE Figure 8–72d	Appears as the radiopaque bony structure that joins the mandible and the ramus

AIR SPACE IMAGES ON A PANORAMIC FILM

PALATOGLOSSAL AIR SPACE	Appears as a horizontal radiolucent band located above the apices of the maxillary teeth
NASOPHARYNGEAL AIR SPACE Figure 8–72h	Appears as a diagonal radiolucency located above the soft palate and uvula

SOFT TISSUE IMAGES ON A PANORAMIC RADIOGRAPH

TONGUE	Appears as a radiopaque area superimposed over the maxillary posterior teeth
SOFT PALATE AND UVULA Figure 8–72g	Appear as diagonal radiopacity extending posteriorly and inferiorly from the maxillary tuberosity area
EAR Figure 8–72c	Appears as a radiopaque shadow that extends anteriorly and inferiorly from the mastoid process

Processing Errors

UNDERDEVELOPED FILM

LIGHT FILM	Prevent by checking temperature of developer, and increase developing time if needed

OVERDEVELOPED FILM

DARK FILM	Prevent by checking temperature of developer, and decrease developing time if needed

RETICULATION OF EMULSION

CRACKED LOOK ON FILM	Results from sudden temperature changes Prevent by checking temperatures of processing solutions and water bath

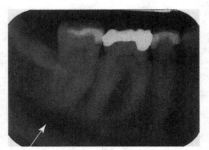

FIGURE 8-65   Submandibular Fossa

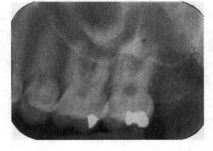

FIGURE 8-66   Coronoid Process

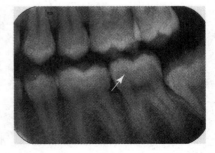

FIGURE 8-67   Enamel

FIGURE 8-68   Dentin

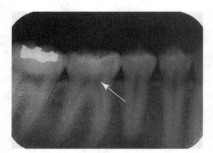

FIGURE 8-69   Pulp

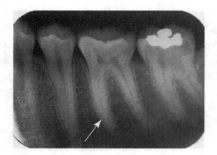

FIGURE 8-70   Lamina Dura

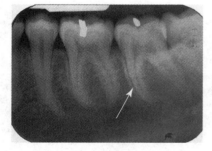

FIGURE 8-71   Periodontal Ligament Space

CHEMICAL CONTAMINATION

DEVELOPER SPOTS	Dark spots on film occurs when developer comes in contact with film before processing
FIXER SPOTS	White spots on film occurs when fixer comes in contact with film before processing
YELLOW-BROWN STAINS	Results from old developer or fixer, insufficient fixation time, or insufficient rinsing

FILM HANDLING

DEVELOPER CUT-OFF	Straight radiopaque border on film resulting from low level of developer solution
FIXER CUT-OFF	Black line on film resulting from a low level of fixer solution
OVERLAPPED FILMS	White or dark areas on film occurs when films come in contact during processing
STATIC ELECTRICITY	Black blanching lines on the film resulting from opening the film packet rapidly
FOGGED FILM	Overall gray appearance; film lacks image due to improper safelighting, improper film storage, or expired film
SCRATCHED FILM	Radiolucent lines from fingernail, film rack; emulsion is removed from film by mechanical means

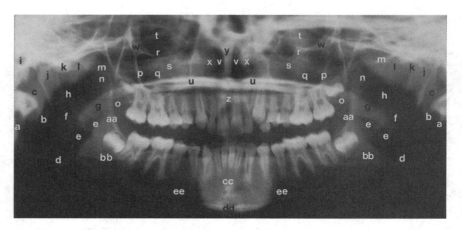

FIGURE 8-72   Anatomic Landmarks on a Panoramic Radiograph

9 Planning and Managing Dental Hygiene Care

Demetra Daskalos Logothetis, RDH, MS

Carla Loiacono, RDH, MS

➤ INFECTION CONTROL

Infectious Diseases

ROUTES FOR TRANSMISSION OF MICROBIAL AGENTS IN DENTISTRY	
DIRECT CONTACT	Infectious lesions, blood, or saliva
INDIRECT TRANSMISSION	Transfer of microorganism from a contaminated intermediate object
SPLATTER	Blood, saliva, or nasopharyngeal secretions directly splattered onto skin or mucosal
AEROSOLS	Airborne transfer of microorganisms

HEPATITIS A	

Caused by hepatitis A virus and is more common in children and young adults

TRANSMISSION	Person to person, fecal-oral route, generally through fecal contamination ☛ Unsanitary conditions
INCUBATION	15 to 50 days
SIGNS AND SYMPTOMS	• Preicteric phase—flu-like symptoms • Icteric phase—jaundice

IMMUNITY	Presence of anti-HAV in serum
PREVENTION	• Sanitation and personal hygiene • Instrument sterilization, disposable barriers • Handwashing, public health control of water contamination

HEPATITIS B

Major cause of acute and chronic hepatitis, cirrhosis; DNA virus

TRANSMISSION	Blood and other body fluids
MODE OF TRANSMISSION	• Percutaneous—IV, IM, subcutaneous • Needle stick exposure • Perinatal • Exchanging contaminated needles • Sexual exposure
INCUBATION	2–6 months
SIGNS AND SYMPTOMS	• Jaundice—usually lasts 6 weeks • Flu-like symptoms • Carrier state—individual with the HbsAg marker in blood serum for more than 6 months
IMMUNITY	Presence of anti-HbsAg in serum

HEPATITIS C

Originally called non-A, non-B hepatitis

TRANSMISSION	Percutaneous exposure to contaminated blood, contaminated needles, needle stick exposure
INCUBATION	2 weeks to 6 months
SIGNS AND SYMPTOMS	Can be insidious, with no clinical symptoms

HEPATITIS D

Delta hepatitis virus (hepatitis D) cannot cause infection except in the presence of HBV infection

| TRANSMISSION | • Superimposed on HbsAg carriers, occurs mostly in persons who have multiple exposures to HBV
• Transmission similar to HBV |

HEPATITIS E

Clinical course and distribution is similar to hepatitis A

| TRANSMISSION | Contaminated water, person to person, fecal-oral route |
| PREVENTION | Sanitary disposal of wastes, handwashing |

TUBERCULOSIS

Etiologic agent—*Mycobacterium tuberculosis*

TRANSMISSION	• Inhalation of fresh droplets containing tubercle bacilli • Aerosols created by ultrasonics, handpieces, and air water spray
PREDISPOSING FACTORS	• Immunosuppressive conditions • Systemic conditions that lower resistance to infection ☞ HIV, diabetes, congenital heart disease, chronic lung disease, alcoholism
INCUBATION PERIOD	As long as 12 weeks
SYMPTOMS	• Early—low-grade fever, loss of appetite, weight loss, slight cough • Late—persistent cough, fever (usually late afternoon) night sweats, weakness ☞ Diagnosis is by tuberculin test and chest radiograph
TREATMENT	Multiple antituberculosis drugs for 6 months ☞ Isoniazid, pyrazinamide, ritampin
MANAGEMENT	Defer treatment until patient is no longer infectious

VARICELLA-ZOSTER VIRUS (VZV)

CHICKENPOX	• Highly contagious disease transmitted by direct contact • Rash that becomes vesicular and then scabs
SHINGLES	• Reactivation of VZV in adulthood • Localized unilateral eruptions associated with nerve endings

CYTOMEGALOVIRUS (HCMV)

TRANSMISSION	• Virus is excreted in saliva, cervical secretion, semen, and urine • Mother's infection may infect the infant in utero, in the birth canal, or through breast milk; contact with body fluids; inhalation of respiratory droplets
DISEASE PROCESS	• Infants—most severe form of infection • May cause mental retardation, microcephaly, motor disabilities, anemia, and chronic liver disease • Adults—symptomatic infection is rare

HERPES SIMPLEX VIRUS

HERPES LABIALIS (COLD SORE)	• HSV-1 and HSV-2 cause genital and oral-facial infection that cannot be distinguished • Triggered by stress, sunlight, illness, or trauma • Healing may take up to 10 days • Autoinfection is possible
HERPETIC WHITLOW	• Herpes simplex infection of the fingers • Autoinfection is possible to lips from fingernail biting
OCULAR HERPES	Herpes lesion to the eye from splashing saliva or fluid from infected person
CLINICAL MANAGEMENT OF HERPES	Postpone dental treatment on patient with active lesion ☛ Possible transmission to others, auto-inoculation possible

HIV INFECTION

Infection with the human immunodeficiency virus (HIV-1)

TRANSMISSION	• Sexual contact • Blood and blood products—contaminated needles, transfusion, needle stick exposure • Perinatal

Exposure Control

UNIVERSAL PRECAUTIONS

Protective barriers should be used if contacting blood, saliva, and mucous membranes

UNIFORM	• Long sleeves and fitted cuffs, closed front and at neck • Never wear uniform outside clinic practice setting • Must be washed separately at water temperature of 60–70°C and dried at 110°C • ☞ Synthetic material is more effective
FACE MASK	• Change facemask between patients or if mask gets wet • Place and adjust mask before handwashing • Wear mask during and after procedures that produced aerosols
PROTECTIVE EYEWEAR	• Goggles with shields on both sides • Side shield can be used for patients with prescription lens • Face shields ensure maximum coverage • ☞ Face mask must be worn under shield • ☞ Clean and disinfect between patients
HANDWASHING	• Wash hands before and after patient care with antimicrobial liquid soap • Short handwashing method—three latherings and three rinses in 30 seconds • Surgical hand scrub—soft brush lather and scrub hands for 10 minutes

GLOVES	• Nonsterile single-use—examination, treatment (latex, nonlatex) • Sterile single-use—surgical procedures • Hands must be washed before gloving • Should extend over cuffs of long-sleeved clinic attire • Changed between patients or during long procedures (can get breakage after 50 minutes) • Double gloving not recommended by CDC, OSHA
LATEX HYPER-SENSITIVITY	• Exposure from inhalation of powder in gloves, mucosal contact, donning gloves • Urticaria, dermatitis, respiratory reactions, anaphylaxis • Individuals at risk—occupational exposure, many documented allergies, multiple surgical procedures • Management—no latex in treatment room • Have latex-sensitive patient box stocked with latex-free products
PATIENT PRERINSING	• Utilize chlorhexidine as a patient pre-rinse prior to use of aerosol-producing instruments • Ultrasonics, prophy jet

Chemical Disinfectants

CHEMICAL DISINFECTANT LEVELS

HIGH LEVEL	Inactivates spores and all forms of bacteria, fungi, and viruses • 2.0–3.2% glutaraldehyde preparations
INTERMEDIATE LEVEL	• Inactivates all forms of microorganisms but does not destroy spores • Kills *Mycobacterium tuberculosis* • Formaldehyde, chlorine compounds, iodophor, alcohols, complex phenols

LOW LEVEL	Inactivates vegetative bacteria, certain viruses; does not destroy spores, tubercle bacilli, nonlipid viruses, or fungi ☛ Quaternary ammonium compounds, simple phenols and detergents

IDEAL CHARACTERISTICS

- Broad spectrum
- Fast acting
- Nontoxic
- Surface compatibility—should not cause corrosion or disintegration of materials
- Residual effect
- Easy to use
- Odorless
- Economical

GLUTARALDEHYDES

ACTION	Kill microorganisms by damaging their proteins and nucleic acids ☛ Example—Cidex
DISADVANTAGES	- Caustic to skin - Corrosive to some instruments, and must be rinsed with sterile water after removal from bath - Not used as a surface disinfectant because of fumes

IODOPHORS

ACTION	- Broad spectrum antimicrobial with powerful germicidal action, where iodine is released slowly - Tuberculocidal - Bacteriocidal - Virucidal ☛ 1 part iodophor to 213 parts of distilled water; inactivated by hard water ☛ Example—Biocide

DISADVANTAGES	• Must be prepared daily • May discolor some surfaces

CHLORINE COMPOUNDS

ACTION	• Act primarily by oxidation; broad spectrum • Tuberculocidal • Bacteriocidal • Virucidal • ☞ Sodium hypochlorite
DISADVANTAGES	• Must be prepared daily • Unpleasant odor • Corrodes metals

COMPLEX PHEONOLS

ACTION	• Cytoplasmic poisons by penetrating cell walls and denature intracellular proteins • Broad spectrum with residual activity • Tuberculocidal • ☞ Example—Chlorhexidine
DISADVANTAGES	• Not sporicidal • Must be prepared daily

Classification of Instruments and Equipment

CRITICAL ITEMS

Penetrate soft tissue or bone and have the greatest potential for transmitting infection

STERILIZATION AND DISINFECTION	All critical items must be sterile or disposed
EXAMPLES	Needles, curets, explorers, probes, ultrasonic tips

SEMICRITICAL ITEMS

Touch intact mucous membranes or oral fluids; have a lower potential for transmitting infection
☞ Do not penetrate soft tissue or bone

STERILIZATION AND DISINFECTION	Sterile or have high level of disinfection
EXAMPLES	Mirror, radiographic biteblock, ultrasonic and slow speed handpieces

NONCRITICAL ITEMS

Do not touch mucous membrane

STERILIZATION AND DISINFECTION	Intermediate level of disinfection, which kill *Mycobacterium tuberculosis,* hepatitis B virus, and HIV ☛ Should be covered with barriers
EXAMPLES	Light handles, safety glasses, x-ray equipment

Instrument Processing

ULTRASONIC PROCESSING

Prior to sterilization to prevent manual cleaning of instruments
☛ Manual cleaning is dangerous and difficult

ADVANTAGES	• Reduce danger to clinician • Decrease in aerosol production from hand scrubbing • Cleaner instruments prior to sterilization • Decrease chance of penetrating tissue during hand scrubbing
PROCEDURE	• Avoid overloading • Use manufacturer's guidelines for length of time • Drain, rinse, and dry instruments before sterilization

MANUAL CLEANING

PROCEDURE	• Wear utility gloves and mask • Use long-handled brush with detergent under running water • Rinse and dry before packaging

STERILIZATION

TESTS FOR STERILIZATION	Ampule, vial, or strip with microorganism is placed in package to be sterilized, and incubated following sterilization • Steam autoclave—*Bacillus stearother-mophilus* • Dry heat oven—*Bacillus subtilis* • Chemical vapor—*Bacillus stearother-mophilus* • Ethylene oxide—*Bacillus subtilis* • Records should show dates and outcomes
MOIST HEAT: STEAM UNDER PRESSURE	• Sterilization from heat and moisture • Space between objects is critical to allow heat and steam to penetrate • Presterilized instruments (i.e., after placing in ultrasonic) must be cleaned and dried • Standard procedure—121°C (250°F) at 15 pounds pressure for 15 minutes; 30 minutes for heavy loads • Destroys all microorganisms, spores, and viruses • May corrode instruments
DRY HEAT	• Used for instruments that cannot be steam sterilized • Sterilization by heat conducted from exterior surface to the interior surface • Standard procedure—160°C (320°F) for 2 hours or 170°C (340°F) for 1 hour; timing must start after temperature has been reached
CHEMICAL VAPOR STERILIZER	• Sterilization by alcohols, formaldehyde, ketone, acetone, and water heated under pressure to produce a gas • Tightly wrapped instruments will not permit penetration of vapors • Cannot be used on plastics, liquids, and heat-sensitive handpieces • Standard procedure—127° to 132°C (260°F to 270°F); 20–40 pounds pressure for 20 minutes minimum

ETHYLENE OXIDE	• Sterilization by gas using ethylene oxide • Almost all material can be sterilized with no damage to material • Standard procedure—10–16 hours, aeration after completion for at least 24 hours • ☛ Not commonly found in dental offices • ☛ Common in hospitals or clinics

UNIT WATER LINES

- Biofilm of microorganisms forms on inside of water lines overnight
- Flush all water lines at least 3–5 minutes at the beginning and at the end of each day
- Run water through water syringes for 30 seconds before and after each patient
- Use disinfecting agent followed by rinse at the end of each day

OCCUPATIONAL EXPOSURE MANAGEMENT

PROCEDURE FOLLOWING EXPOSURE	• Immediately wash wound with antibacterial soap and rinse well • Blood testing for HbsAg and anti-HIV for patient and clinician on same day of exposure

➤ RECOGNITION OF AND PROVISION FOR EMERGENCY SITUATIONS

Emergency Situations

SYNCOPY

Decreased circulation to the brain

SYMPTOMS	• *Early:* Pallor, sweating nausea, rapid heard rate (pulse), tachpnea (rapid breathing) • *Late:* Papillary dilation, yawning, decreased blood pressure, bradycardia (slow pulse), convulsive movements, unconsciousness

PATIENT PLACEMENT	Trendelenburg (feet up, head down)
TREATMENT	• Establish airway • Loosen tight clothing • Spirits of ammonia • Oxygen at 6 liter flow • Cold compress to face • Monitor and record vitals • Reassure and comfort patient when they awaken
UNRESPONSIVE TO SYNCOPY TREATMENT	• Patient does not awaken after 1 minute • Vital signs unstable → consider hypoglycemia, seizure, cerebrovascular accident, cardiac arrest, transient ischemic attack (TIA) → call EMS

POSTURAL HYPOTENSION (ORTHOSTATIC HYPOTENSION)

Drop in blood pressure when quickly moving from supine to upright position

SYMPTOMS	Same as syncopy but related to supine positioning
PATIENT PLACEMENT	Return to Trendelenburg position
TREATMENT	• Establish airway • Assess ABCs • Oxygen at 6 liter flow • Monitor vitals
UNRESPONSIVE TO TREATMENT	Same as syncopy
DENTAL CONSIDERATION	Raise chair slowly

RESPIRATORY FAILURE

Difficulty breathing or cessation of breathing

SYMPTOMS	• Loss of consciousness • Labored breathing or cessation of breathing • Cyanosis • Dilated pupils

TREATMENT	• Check for foreign objects in mouth • Establish airway • Begin CPR if needed • Monitor vital signs

OBSTRUCTED AIRWAY

Foreign body in larynx and pharynx

SYMPTOMS	Ineffective cough, choking, gasping with effort, labored breathing, unable to speak, panicky
PATIENT PLACEMENT	Supine if unconscious, otherwise upright
TREATMENT	• Conscious patient: perform Heimlich maneuver • Unconscious patient: activate EMS, tilt head backward and attempt to open airway → Perform abdominal thrusts

HYPERVENTILATION

Respiratory alkalosis caused by excessive exhalation of carbon dioxide

SYMPTOMS	Light-headedness, rapid breathing, confusion, feeling of suffocation
PATIENT PLACEMENT	Upright
TREATMENT	• Calm and reassure the patient • Ask patient to breath deeply into a paper bag to enrich carbon dioxide or into cupped hands if no paper bag is available ☛ Carbon dioxide is indicated, NOT oxygen

ASTHMATIC ATTACK

Spasm and constriction of the bronchi

SYMPTOMS	Difficulty breathing, wheezing, anxiety
PATIENT PLACEMENT	Upright

TREATMENT	• Administer bronchodilator (albuterol) • Administer oxygen 6 liters • Activate EMS if condition worsens

ANGINA PECTORIS

Insufficient blood supply to cardiac muscle; may be precipitated by stress, anxiety, or exercise

SYMPTOMS	Pain in chest, vital signs satisfactory, pallor, faintness, difficulty breathing
PATIENT PLACEMENT	Upright
TREATMENT	• Administer nitroglycerin 0.2–0.6 mg sublingually • Administer oxygen • Reassure patient • ☛ Without prompt relief from second dose of nitroglycerin, treat as myocardial infarction

MYOCARDIAL INFARCTION

Occlusion of coronary vessels

SYMPTOMS	• Severe pain in chest, which may radiate to shoulder, neck, arms • Pallor, cold, clammy skin • Cyanosis • Weakness and anxiety
PATIENT PLACEMENT	Upright
TREATMENT	• Symptoms are not relieved with nitroglycerin • Monitor vital signs • Basic life support • Administer oxygen • Alleviate anxiety • Activate EMS

URTICARIA OR PURUITUS

- Caused by allergy
- Delayed reaction

SYMPTOMS	• Urticaria—red eruption on face, neck, hands, or arms • Pruritus—itching of these areas
PATIENT PLACEMENT	Upright
TREATMENT	• Administer Benadryl (diphenhy-dramine), 25–50 mg • Follow-up, prescribe oral antihistamines

ANAPHYLACTIC SHOCK

Severe allergic reaction (⊶ Immediate reaction)

SYMPTOMS	• Progressive respiratory and circulatory failure, wheezing, erythema, urticaria, angioedema (localized swelling of mucous membranes) • Profound drop in blood pressure
PATIENT PLACEMENT	Supine
TREATMENT	• Rapid treatment with epinephrine 3–5 mL 1:1000 solution • Basic life support

STROKE

Obstruction of blood vessels of brain

SYMPTOMS	Muscle weakness, loss of consciousness, confusion, headache, dizziness, nausea, paralysis, convulsions

TREATMENT	Transient ischemic attack (TIA): • Upright positioning • Monitor vital signs • Refer for immediate medical examination CVA (conscious patient): • Semi-reclining position • Monitor vital signs • Seek medical assistance • Administer oxygen CVA (unconscious patient): • Supine position • Record vital signs • Provide basic life support • Administer oxygen • Activate EMS

SEIZURE

SYMPTOMS	Excitement, tremors, muscular contractions, trance-like state
PATIENT PLACEMENT	Leave patient in dental chair
TREATMENT	Open airway, administer oxygen, allow patient to sleep after during post-convulsive stage ☛ Do not force anything between patient's teeth

HYPOGLYCEMIA

SYMPTOMS	Sudden onset; confusion; skin is moist, cold, pale
PATIENT PLACEMENT	Semi-reclining, supine if patient is unconscious
TREATMENT	Conscious patient: • Administer sugar cubes, apple juice, frosting • Observe patient Unconscious patient: • Basic life support • Administer oxygen • Monitor vital signs

- Activate EMS—administer intravenous glucose

Emergency Kit Medications

ADRENALIN

ACTION AND USES	Anti-allergic drug—to combat undue reactions to drugs such as penicillin or to combat severe asthmatic attack
DOSAGE	1:1000 IM or IV

BENEDRYL

ACTION AND USES	Same as adrenalin
USUAL DOSAGE ADMINISTRATION	25–50 mg

AMINOPHYLLIN

ACTION AND USES	Same as adrenalin
USUAL DOSAGE	250 mg

NITROGLYCERINE/AMYL-NITRATE

ACTION AND USES	Coronary vessel dilator in angina pectoris
USUAL DOSAGE	0.2–0.6 tablets sublingual

AMMONIA

ACTION AND USES	Irritant—increases respiratory rate
USUAL DOSAGE	1 inhalant, break under nose

WYAMINE SULFATE

ACTION AND USES	Vasopressor—to combat falling blood pressure
USUAL DOSAGE	30 mg/cc IV

VALIUM

ACTION AND USES	Depressant—to combat convulsions
USUAL DOSAGE	10 mg IV preferred

TALWIN

ACTION AND USES	To combat severe pain
USUAL DOSAGE	30 mg IM, subcutaneous, or IV

ATROPINE

ACTION AND USES	Parasympathetic depressant—to prevent vagal syncopes
USUAL DOSAGE	0.4 mg adults .01 mg/kg/dose children Subcutaneous, IM, or IV

TIGAN

ACTION AND USES	To combat nausea
USUAL DOSAGE	2 mL tid or qid IM

➤ INDIVIDUALIZED PATIENT EDUCATION

PLANNING INDIVIDUALIZED PROGRAM

PERSONAL BACKGROUND	Collect and apply information about the patient: • Education • Attitude regarding oral health care • Personal homecare and frequency • Dexterity • Age and physical, mental abilities • Patient motivation
FIRST LESSON	Increase patient awareness to bacterial plaque: • Discuss the formation and relationship to periodontal disease and caries formation • Develop plaque control program

	• Use illustrations and demonstrations in patient's own mouth to identify inflamed areas • Use disclosing solution to identify masses of plaque, record a plaque score • Keep instruction simple: first flossing, then brushing techniques
SECOND LESSON	Evaluate patient's homecare: • Evaluate gingiva with patient • Apply disclosing solution, compare present with past plaque scores • Review and extend knowledge

➤ INSTRUCTION FOR PREVENTION AND MANAGEMENT OF ORAL DISEASE

Diet and Caries

CARIES

HOST FACTORS	The major factors involved in the formation of dental caries are: 1. Food 2. Bacterial plaque 3. Saliva 4. Tooth factors ☞ Caries microorganisms—Streptococcus mutans, Streptococcus sobrinus, Lactobacilli
BACTERIA	• Streptococcus mutans—Gram + nonmotile bacteria with a spherical or coccoid morphology • Streptococcus sobrinus • Lactobacilli—Gram + nonmotile rods that do not form spores, grows optimally under anaerobic conditions; metabolically both oxidative and fermentive

CRITICAL pH

- A pH of less than 5.5
- The pH of dental plaque that results in demineralization of tooth structure and caries formation

TIME

- The length of time the pH of bacterial plaque is less than 5.5
- After sugar and/or starch is eaten, plaque is below the critical pH for approximately 20–30 minutes

CARIOGENIC FOODS

- Have the potential to cause caries
- Foods that can be fermented by oral bacteria to produce acids, which lower the pH of dental plaque
- ⚷ Also called fermentable carbohydrates

SUGARS	Sugars (mono- and disaccharides), which include glucose, fructose, maltose, sucrose, and lactose
EXAMPLES OF FOODS THAT CONTAIN SOME FORM OF SUGAR	Table sugar, brown sugar, fruit, juices and fruit cocktails, dried fruits such as raisins and apples, white or chocolate milk, ice cream, frozen and fruit-flavored yogurt, honey, baked beans, molasses, syrup, cookies, granola and granola bars, plain and sweetened cereals, potato and corn chips, jams and jellies, pancakes, muffins, cake, icing, biscuits, candies, gum, sodas, ketchup, and many brands of peanut butter ⚷ Taste sweet ⚷ Fresh fruit is the least cariogenic ⚷ Can also include cough drops, cough syrup, antacids
COOKED STARCHES	Complex carbohydrates such as flour, pasta, potatoes, cereals, and rice that have been cooked by baking, boiling, or frying
EXAMPLES OF FOODS THAT CONTAIN COOKED STARCH	White and whole wheat bread, pastries, doughnuts, whole grain cereals, rice, pasta, potato dishes, crackers, pretzels, popcorn, corn and flour tortillas, pizza dough, and rolls ⚷ Often these foods do not taste sweet
COMBINED FOODS	• Foods that contain cooked starch and one or more types of sugars have a potential to cause dental caries equal to or greater than sucrose

- Many of the foods listed under simple sugars fall into this category such as sweetened cereals, pastries, granola, pancakes, muffins

OTHER FACTORS RELATED TO FOOD AND CARIES

QUANTITY	• Amount of sugar and/or starch eaten • The greater the amount eaten at each meal or snack, the greater the potential for caries formation
FREQUENCY	• Number of times sugar and/or starch are eaten during the day • The greater the frequency of eating meals and snacks that contain sugar and/or starch, the greater the potential for caries formation • The number of times when the pH of plaque is below 5.5
PHYSICAL FORM	• The form in which sugar and starch are eaten • Sugars and starches eaten in the form of a solid, along with the stickiness of the food, increases the potential for caries formation • Sugar consumed in a liquid form has a lower caries potential • The stickiness of a food is related to its ability to be retained on tooth structure • Starchy foods such as chips, crackers, and bread are retentive as much or more than foods with just sugar
TIME OF DAY	• At what times sugar and/or starch are eaten during the day • There is more potential for caries formation if sugars and starch are eaten as a snack without fat or protein • When sugar and/or starch are eaten during meals containing fat and protein, caries potential is decreased

DIETARY RECOMMENDATIONS TO REDUCE THE POTENTIAL FOR CARIES FORMATION

- Eat foods with low amounts of sugars and/or cooked starches
- Limit snacking on foods with sugar and/or starch
- Eat sugar with a meal
- Limit the number of meals and snacks
- Use moderate amounts of sugar substitutes
- Refer to food labels for the total amount of carbohydrate and sugars in foods
- Use spices such as allspice, cinnamon, ginger, and nutmeg to enhance the flavor of foods that contain low amounts of sugar
- Clear mouth with water or unsweetened beverages after eating foods containing sugar and/or starch

PRINCIPLES OF DIETARY COUNSELING

FORM A TREATMENT PLAN FOR DIETARY ASSESSMENT AND COUNSELING	Assess patient willingness and motivation
OBTAIN A RECORD OF FOOD INTAKE	• Ask patient to keep a record of all food and beverage intake for a specified length of time, usually 3–5 days • Have client include the use of cough drops, cough syrup, gum, candy, etc
REVIEW THE DIET RECORD WITH THE PATIENT	• Ask if anything else was consumed at each meal or snack time • Ask about beverage intake and condiment use (ketchup, mustard, mayonnaise, soy sauce, honey, etc.)
CODE FOOD ITEMS	• Code each food item according to the food groups of the food guide pyramid • Estimate the number of servings of each food according to food group • Code foods that contain sugar and/or cooked starches • Code foods according to physical form
ASSESS FOOD INTAKE	• Tally the number of servings from each food group • Note food groups and/or number of servings that were deficient or excessive • Tally the number and physical form of sugars/starches eaten

COUNSEL PATIENT	• Discuss with patient the findings of the dietary assessment • Have patient suggest foods they like that could be added or substituted to make their diet more healthful and to reduce caries potential • Help patient set realistic and measurable dietary goals • Stress making small changes that can be maintained
REASSESS DIET	• Determine time interval for reassessment • Evaluate behavior and dietary changes • Help patient set new goals if needed

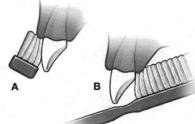

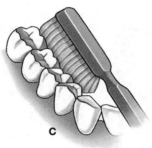

FIGURE 9-1 Sulcular Brushing—Filament Tips at 45-Degree Angle to Long Axis of Tooth

Plaque Control

BRUSHING TECHNIQUES

BASS METHOD: SULCULAR BRUSHING	• For all patients • Bristle positioning—45° to apex; in sulcus • Motion—vibratory, short horizontal strokes; jiggle, sweep occlusally **Figure 9-1**
COLLIS METHOD: SIMULTANEOUS SULCULAR	• Collis curved brush • Indicated for patients with limited range of motion; caregivers • Bristle positioning—curved filaments apically (filaments enter sulcus at 45° automatically) • Motion—back-and-forth strokes **Figure 9-2**
ROLLING STROKE METHOD	• Children • Bristle positioning—apically against attached gingiva • Motion—sweep in arch occlusally
MODIFIED STILLMAN	• Bristle positioning—45° to apex; part on gingival margin, part on cervix of tooth • Motion—rolling stroke (sweep occlusally) after vibratory pulsing **Figure 9-3**

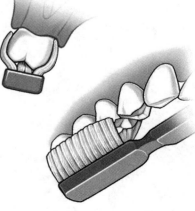

FIGURE 9-2 Collis Simultaneous Sulcular— Curved Filaments Placed Over the Crown

CHARTERS METHOD	• Excellent for cleaning orthodontic appliances, plaque from abutment teeth under gingival border of fixed bridge • Bristle positioning—45° to occlusal or incisal plane • Motion—circular vibratory • Disadvantages—bristles do not clean subgingivally, and requires high degree of dexterity **Figure 9-4**
FONES: CIRCULAR METHOD	• Used commonly to teach school children • Bristle positioning—90° to tooth • Motion—circular vibratory • Disadvantages—may be detrimental if brushing is too vigorous **Figure 9-5**
LEONARD: VERTICAL METHOD	• Bristle positioning—right angles to the long axes of the teeth • Motion—vertical, vigorous, up-and-down stroke
HORIZONTAL	• Bristle positioning—90° to tooth • Motion—horizontal stroke • Considered detrimental, may produce abrasion

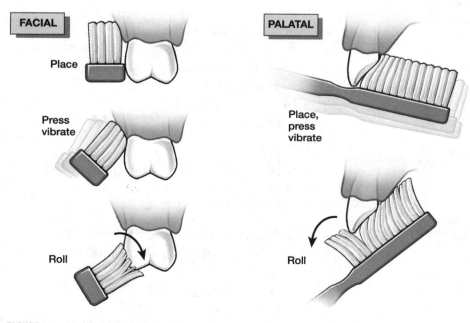

FIGURE 9-3   Modified Stillman Method

SMITH'S METHOD: PHYSIOLOGIC	• Bristle position—at occlusal surface • Motion—sweep gingivally

INTERPROXIMAL CLEANING

⚷ Col area is not keratinized and is vulnerable to bacterial invasion
Figure 9-6

FLOSS	• Removes plaque and debris • Polishes surfaces • Massages interdental papilla • Aids in identifying subgingival calculus, overhanging restorations, caries
FLOSS HOLDER	Recommended for: • Patients with disabilities • Manual dexterity problems • Caretakers • Patients with strong gag reflexes
FLOSS THREADER	Carries floss: • Through embrasure areas • Gingiva of abutment teeth • Under pontics • Around orthodontic appliances
KNITTING YARN	Recommended for: • Wide proximal spaces • Mesial and distal abutments • Isolated teeth **Figure 9-7**

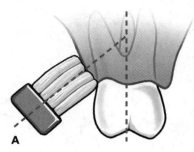

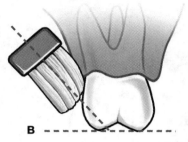

FIGURE 9-4 A) Stillman Method; B) Charter's Methods

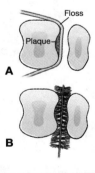

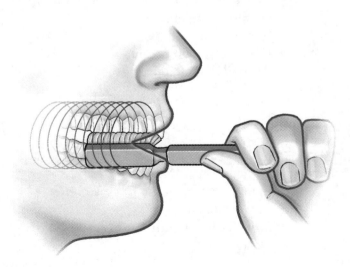

FIGURE 9-5 Fones Method—Circular Motion Extending from Maxillary to Mandibular Gingiva

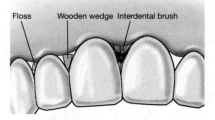

FIGURE 9-6 Interproximal Cleaning: An Interdental Brush (B) is More Effective than Floss (A) in Interproximal Spaces

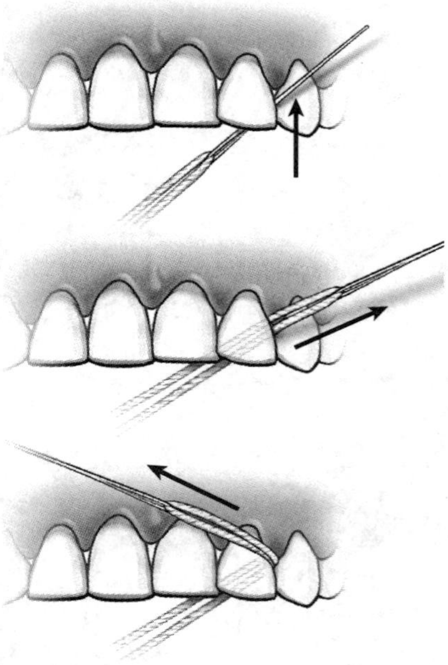

FIGURE 9-7   Knitting Yarn

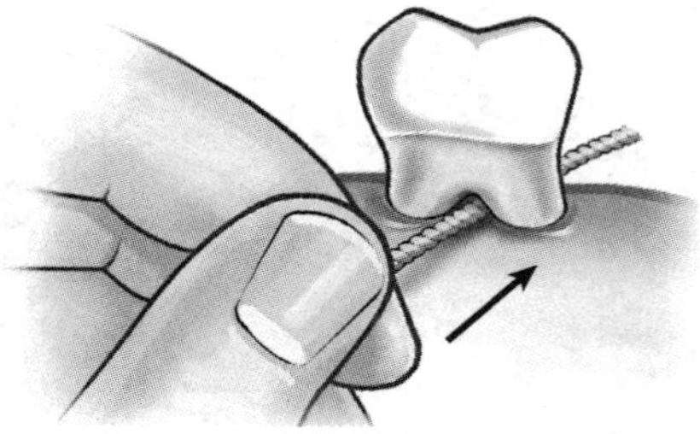

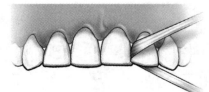

FIGURE 9-8   Pipe Cleaner—Used to Clean Exposed Furcation

FIGURE 9-9   Gauze Strip—Used Adjacent to Endentulous Area, in Interproximal Spaces, or Distal to Posterior Teeth

PIPE CLEANER	Recommended for • Exposed proximal surfaces • Open furcation areas • Separated teeth **Figure 9-8**
GAUZE STRIP	Recommended for • Widely spaced teeth • Teeth adjacent to edentulous areas • Abutment teeth **Figure 9-9**
INTERDENTAL TIP STIMULATOR	Recommended for: • Plaque removal in interdental area where embrasures are open • Reshaping and recontouring gingiva after periodontal surgery • Massaging interdental tissue
PERIO AIDS (TOOTHPICK HOLDERS)	Recommended for: • Plaque removal along gingival margin and within sulcus • Cleaning of concave proximal surfaces • Exposed furcations • Around orthodontic surfaces **Figure 9-10**
WOODEN WEDGE	Indicated for proximal tooth surfaces where gingival tissue is missing **Figure 9-11**
INTERPROXIMAL BRUSH	Recommended for: • Mesial and distal surfaces adjacent to edentulous spaces • Exposed furcations • Wide-open embrasures • Around dental appliances

Oral Conditions

ORAL CANCER

COMMON SITES	• Lateral border of the tongue • Lower lip • Floor of the mouth • Oropharynx

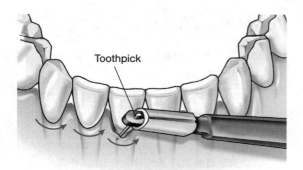

FIGURE 9-10 Perio Aid (Toothpick Holder)

COMMON SIGNS OF ORAL CANCER	• Ulceration—loss of skin surface • Erythema—red lesion • Induration—hard • Fixation—nonmobile lesion • Chronicity—failure to heal • Lymphadenopathy—hardening and enlarged lymph nodes • Adnenopathy—disease of glands • Leukoplakia—white patch
SELF-EXAMINATION	Instruct patient to: • Identify sores, swellings, lumps on face, neck, mouth that do not heal within 2 weeks • Report persistent hoarseness • Check facial symmetry • Check for changes in skin color, size of moles • Check cheeks, lips by retracting with fingers and view for color variations, ulcerations, swellings, lumps • Check under tongue by lifting to roof of mouth; use gauze to grasp tongue and evaluate the sides of tongue
RISK FACTORS FOR ORAL CANCER	• Tobacco abuse—smoking and smokeless tobacco • Alcohol use

FIGURE 9-11 Wooden Wedge

TOBACCO CESSATION

FOUR STEPS OF INTERVENTION	1. Ask patient about tobacco use in nonjudgmental manner 2. Advise patient to stop using tobacco products by clearly stating the consequences 3. Assist patient in taking the necessary steps to stop by setting a quit date; remove all tobacco products; avoid people who use tobacco 4. Arrange patient follow-up services ☞ 4 As—Ask, Advise, Assist, Arrange

ORAL HABITS

BRUXISM	• Oral manifestations—decrease in canine height and flattening of incisal and occlusal surfaces • Suggested patient interventions—night guard, stress management protocols
THUMBSUCKING	• Oral manifestations—open-bite, tongue thrusting, protruding teeth, anterior overjet, deep narrow palate • Suggested patient interventions—make child aware of habit, restrict movement of hand to mouth, incentive program, orthodontic evaluation

IMPLANTS

ENDOSSEOUS	• Implant placed "in bone" • Two-stage system—first surgery consists of installing the implant and covering with mucosal for several months to allow osseointegration; second stage consists of attaching abutment to cylinder; prosthesis follows ☞ Cylindrical (root form), flat (blade) **Figure 9-12**

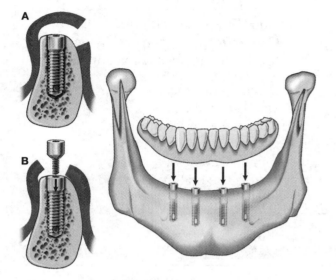

FIGURE 9-12 Endosseous Implant

SUBPERIOSTEAL	• "Under the periosteum" or "on bone" • Surgical flap exposes bone for impression to be taken; metallic unit is placed in second surgical step, four posts protrude to hold denture • Used on severely resorbed ridge **Figure 9-13**
TRANSOSTEAL	• "Through the bone" • 5–7 pins fitted to the inferior border of mandible and connected by a crossbar

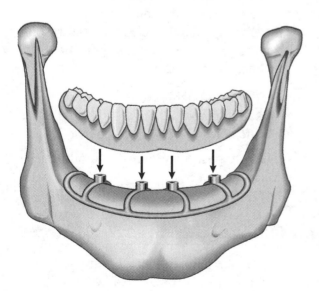

FIGURE 9-13 Subperiosteal Implant

PATIENT CHARACTERISTICS INDICATIONS	• Good physical condition • Commitment to good oral hygiene • Sufficient quality and quantity of bone
PATIENT CHARACTERISTICS CONTRAINDICATIONS	• Bleeding disorders • Uncontrolled diabetes • Connective tissue disorders • Chronic steroid therapy • Immunosuppressive therapy • Inadequate oral hygiene and patient motivation

DENTAL APPLIANCES

ORTHODONTIC APPLIANCES	• Daily home fluoride application to prevent demineralization • Oral irrigation techniques • Power assisted brushing
CARE OF FIXED PARTIAL DENTURES	• Brushing—Charters method is helpful • Knitting yarn • Pipe cleaner • Interdental brush ☛ Cantilever—supported by one or more teeth at one end only
CARE OF REMOVABLE PARTIAL DENTURES	• Rinsing—after each meal • Immersion—rinse and brush first
CARE OF COMPLETE DENTURES	• Rinsing—after each meal • Immersion—rinse and brush first • Mechanical denture cleaners—ultrasonics, magnetic, and agitating mechanisms; used with immersion agent
DENTURE IMMERSION AGENTS	• Alkaline hypochlorite • Alkaline peroxide • Dilute acids
ABRASIVE CLEANSERS FOR BRUSHING	• Denture pastes and powers, toothpastes • Baking soda

POST-OPERATIVE INSTRUCTION FOR EXTRACTIONS

EXODONTIA— REMOVAL OF TEETH	• Apply ice pack to face: 20 minutes on, 20 minutes off for first 24 hours

- Apply heat after 24 hours
- Common to have blood in saliva for 12 hours after surgery
- Nausea may develop from pain medication
- Maintain good nutrition—cold liquid diet the first day
- Do not drink any beverage through a straw, rinse mouth vigorously; drink carbonated beverages for first 24 hours
- ☛ May cause dry socket by sloughing away blood clot

➤ ANXIETY AND PAIN CONTROL

Reduction of Stress

APPOINTMENT SCHEDULING	
NEW PATIENT	First appointment should be consultation and assessment to build rapport and evaluate level of anxiety
TIME OF APPOINTMENT	• Plan according to patient health requirements • Usually morning appointment when patient is well rested
WAITING TIME	• Minimize waiting time • Morning appointments will reduce chance of long waits
EATING REQUIREMENTS	Help prevent hypoglycemia, and hunger
LENGTH OF APPOINTMENT	Limit to patient's durability

MEDICATION	
PREMEDICATION	When indicated by physician and dentist
PAIN CONTROL	Topical anesthetics or local anesthetics to reduce pain during treatment
PATIENT'S PERSONAL MEDICATIONS	Instruct patient to bring medications needed in case of an emergencies ☛ Asthma, angina pectoris

POST-TREATMENT CARE	
POST-CARE INSTRUCTIONS	For prevention and relief of discomfort
FOLLOW-UP	Telephone call for anxious patient

Pain Control

DEFINITIONS	
LOCAL ANESTHESIA	The loss of sensation in a circumscribed area of the body as a result of the depression of excitation in nerve endings or the inhibition of the conduction process in peripheral nerves
PAIN	A protective mechanism manifested by an environmental change in an excitable tissue
PAIN THRESHOLD	A level of excitability that once reached elicits an impulse, which is an electrical message from one part of the body to another
PAIN PERCEPTION THRESHOLD	The physioanatomical process by which an impulse is generated following application of an adequate stimulus ☞ Differs little among healthy individuals
PAIN REACTION THRESHOLD	The psychophysiological process representing the individual's overt manifestation of the unpleasant perceptual process that occurred ☞ May differ significantly among individuals
STIMULUS	An environmental change in an excitable tissue • Chemical—citric acid • Thermal—hot/cold sensations • Mechanical—toothbrush/instrument • Electrical—electrical toothbrushes
IMPULSE	A wave of excitation initiated by a stimulus; electrical message from one part of body to another (it has to be a minimal threshold stimulus)

MINIMAL THRESHOLD LEVEL (MTL)	Stimulus of sufficient magnitude to stimulate nerve impulse; different nerve fibers (depending on size of fiber) have different MTL
ALL-OR-NONE PRINCIPLE	• Once nerve is excited impulse will travel full length of fiber without additional stimulus • Impulse travels same speed from any stimulus, which exceeds minimum threshold level

Physiology of the Peripheral Nerves

IONS IN NERVE TRANSMISSION

- Na+ (Sodium)—predominately in extracellular fluid
- K+ (Potassium)—predominately in intracellular fluid
- Cl- (Chloride)—predominately in extracellular fluid, and does not diffuse through the nerve sheath, regardless of the stage of nerve transmission

☞ Because of a sodium pump located within the cell membrane, the positively charged sodium molecules are forced outside the nerve cell; as the sodium leaves the intracellular fluid, a state of negativity is created inside the nerve cell; once the sodium ion is transported out of the cell, it is not able to diffuse back into the intracellular fluids because of the relative impermeability of the nerve membrane to this ion

NERVE CONDUCTION Figure 9-14

RESTING POTENTIAL	Balance exists between positive sodium ions on the outside of the nerve membrane and negative potassium ions on the inside of the membrane
DEPOLARIZATION	• A stimulus, which may be chemical, thermal, mechanical, or electrical in nature (such as pain), produces excitation of the nerve fiber, which leads to increase in permeability of the cell membrane to sodium ions • The rapid influx of sodium ions to the interior of the nerve cell causes a depolarization of the nerve membrane from the resting level to its firing threshold

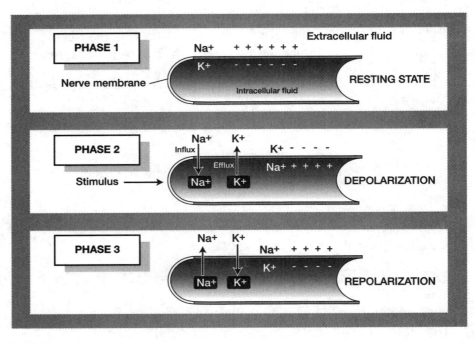

FIGURE 9-14 Nerve Conduction

REPOLARIZATION	• The sodium pump actively transports the sodium ions out of the nerve cell while potassium ions diffuse to the inside of the nerve cell • The nerve's resting potential are reestablished
ABSOLUTE REFRACTORY PERIOD	Period where nerve will not fire no matter what intensity of stimulus applied
RELATIVE REFRACTORY PERIOD	Nerve will fire only if greater than usual stimulus is applied

Pharmacology of Local Anesthetics

LOCAL ANESTHETICS

Refer to drugs used to provide temporary anesthesia (loss of sensation) or pain relief or pain control to a specific or localized area of the body

IDEAL LOCAL ANESTHETICS

- Potent local anesthesia
- Reversible local anesthesia
- Absence of local reactions
- Absence of systemic reactions
- Rapid onset
- Satisfactory duration
- Adequate tissue penetration
- Low cost
- Stability in solution (long shelf-life)
- Ease of metabolism and excretion

CHEMICAL PROPERTIES Figure 9-15

AROMATIC LIPOPHILIC GROUP	Composed of the aromatic ring structure, ensures that the anesthetic agent is able to penetrate the lipid-rich nerve membrane where impulse conduction is blocked
INTERMEDIATE CHAIN	This linkage determines whether the local anesthetic agent is classified as an ester or an amide
HYDROPHILIC AMINO GROUP	When combined with hydrochloric acid, allows the anesthetic to diffuse through the interstitial fluid in the tissues to reach the nerve

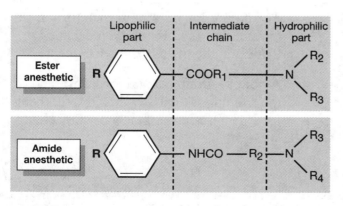

FIGURE 9-15 Chemical Structure of Ester Anesthetic and Amide Anesthetic

ACTIONS

INTERRUPT NERVE CONDUCTION	Block ability of membrane to undergo changes, which occur when nerves fire
VASODIALATION	• Increase in rate of absorption of the local anesthetic • Increase in blood levels and therefore increase risk of anesthetic toxicity • Decrease duration of action • Increased bleeding at the site of injection

PROPERTIES AND IONIZATION FACTORS

BASE FORM	Lipophilic (fat soluble) and un-ionized (not charged) ⚷ Penetrates the nerve
SALT FORM	Hydrophilic (water soluble) and ionized (charged) ⚷ Form in the cartridge
EQUILIBRIUM	The salts of local anesthetics exist as both uncharged molecules called the free base (RN) and positively charged molecules called the cation (RNH) ⚷ Ionization equilibrium depends on pH and pKa
EQUILIBRIUM QUATION	$RNH+ \Leftrightarrow RN + H+$ ⚷ Local anesthetics are weak bases and occur as an equilibrium between their two forms, lipophilic and hydrophilic
pKa	The proportion of drug in each form is determined by the pKa of the local anesthetic and the pH of the environment
INFECTION	Acidic environment and lower pH, and the amount of freebase are reduced, therefore, dental anesthesia is more difficult to attain

PHARMACOKINETICS

The body's handling of local anesthetics

ABSORPTION	First to the site of administration, then to the circulation, which carries it to the body ☞ Determined by degree of ionization ☞ Dependant on the vascularity of the tissue
DISTRIBUTION	Once absorbed, the drug is distributed throughout the body into the systemic circulation
METABOLISM (BIO-TRANSFORMATION) OF ESTERS	Hydrolyzed in the blood by plasma pseudocholinesterase (an enzyme)
METABOLISM OF AMIDES	Metabolized by the liver ☞ Prilocaine is metabolized by lungs as well as the liver
EXCRETION	Kidney is the primary excretory organ for both esters and amides
INFLUENCES OF ADVERSE REACTIONS AND TOXICITIES	• Nature of the drug • Concentration of the drug and dose • Route of administration • Rate of administration • Vascularity • Age • Weight of patient • Health of patient • Route and rate of metabolism and excretion

COMPOSITION

VASOCONSTRICTOR	Added to local anesthetic solution to delay absorption, reduce toxicity, and prolong duration
ANTIOXIDANT	Included to retard oxidation of epinephrine ☞ Sodium bisulfite or metabisulfite
SODIUM HYDROXIDE	Alkalinizes the pH of the solution to between 6 and 7
SODIUM CHLORIDE	Makes solution isotonic

SHORT-ACTING AMIDE LOCAL ANESTHETICS

☞ Pulpal anesthesia about 30 minutes

LIDOCAINE 2% **(XYLOCAINE)**	36 mg/carpule 4.4 mg/kg 300 mg maximum recommended dose (MRD)
MEPIVACAINE 3% **(CARBOCAINE)**	54 mg/carpule 4.4 mg/kg 300 mg MRD
PRILOCAINE 4%	72 mg/carpule 6 mg/kg 400 mg MRD

INTERMEDIATE-ACTING LOCAL AMIDE ANESTHETICS

☞ Pulpal anesthesia about 60 minutes

LIDOCAINE 2% **1:100,000 AND** **1:50,000 EPINEPHRINE**	36 mg/carpule 4 mg/kg 300 mg MRD
MEPIVACAINE 2% **1:200,000 AND** **1:20,000** **LEVONORDEFRIN**	54 mg/carpule 4 mg/kg 300mg MRD
PRILOCAINE 4% **1:200,000** **EPINEPHRINE**	72 mg/carpule 6 mg/kg 400 mg MRD
ARTICAINE 4% **1:100,000 AND** **1:200,000 EPINEPHRINE**	72 mg/carpule 7 mg/kg 500 mg MRD

LONG-ACTING AMIDE LOCAL ANESTHETICS

☞ Pulpal anesthesia 90+ minutes

BUPIVACAINE 0.5% **1:200,000 EPINEPHRINE**	9 mg/carpule 1.3 mg/kg 90 mg MRD
ETIDOCAINE 1.5% **1:200,000 EPINEPHRINE**	27 mg/carpule 8 mg/kg 400 mg MRD

DOSAGES (MRD)

DETERMINE MG PER CARPULE CALCULATED BY CONCENTRATION OF SOLUTION	Example: 2% solution $$2\% = \frac{2\text{ g}}{100\text{ mL}} \times \frac{2000\text{ mg}}{100\text{ mL}}$$ $$= \frac{20\text{ mg}}{1\text{ mL}} = 20\text{ mg / mL}$$ amount in 1 carpule = $$\frac{20\text{ mg}}{1\text{ mL}} \times \frac{1.8\text{ mL}}{\text{carpule}} = 36\text{ mg / carpule}$$ ☛ Carpule of anesthetic contains 1.8 mL of solution 1 g = 1000 mg
DETERMINE MRD BASED ON PATIENT'S WEIGHT IN KG	Example: Using Lidocaine 2%, on 125-pound patient 125 ÷ 2.2 = 57 kg 57 kg × 4.4 mg/kg = 251 mg MRD ☛ lbs ÷ 2.2 = kg ☛ Each local anesthetic has set mg/kg determined by manufacturer
DETERMINE MAXIMUM NUMBER OF CARPULES THAT CAN BE ADMINISTERED	Example: Using Lidocaine 2%, on 125-pound patient Determine MRD, which is 251 mg 251 mg ÷ 36 mg = 6.9 carpules ☛ Divide mg per carpule by MRD

Topical Local Anesthetics

INDICATIONS

- To provide regional (topical) analgesia at the site of application for patient comfort
- Avoid using ester topical anesthetics on patients with a history of allergic reactions to many sources

☛ Patients allergic to ester anesthetics should be given an amide topical anesthetic

AGENTS

BENZOCAINE	Ester of PABA Hurricaine gel used in dentistry (20%)

LIDOCAINE 2–5%	Amide
TETRACAINE 2%	Ester of PABA

Pharmacology of Vasoconstrictors

ROLE OF VASOCONSTRICTOR

- Increased safety by decreasing reuptake of local anesthetic by blood vessels
- Increased duration
- Decreased dose required
- Increased hemostasis—less blood because of shutdown of vessels
- Counteracts vasodilatation action of local anesthetic

MECHANISM OF ACTION OF VASOCONSTRICTOR

Exert their action directly on the adrenergic receptors

☞ Alpha (α) effects of vasoconstrictors cause constriction of blood vessels, decreasing the amount of blood flow to the site of injection, thereby decreasing systemic absorption of the local anesthetic

SYSTEMIC EFFECTS OF VASOCONSTRICTORS

- Cardiac excitability
- Increased heart rate
- Increased force of contraction
- Increased stroke volume and cardiac output
- Increase in diastolic and systolic pressures
- Increase in myocardial oxygen consumption

ADVERSE REACTIONS TO VASOCONSTRICTORS

- Anxiety
- Apprehension
- Nervousness
- Increased blood pressure
- Increased heart rate

INACTIVATION OF VASOCONSTRICTORS

Major—termination of drug action takes place primarily due to re-uptake of the drug by adrenergic nerves
- Monoamine oxidase (MAO)
- Catechol-o-methyltranserase (COMT)

AGENTS

EPINEPHRINE (ADRENALIN)	Concentrations: • 1:20,000 • 1:30,000 • 1:50,000 • 1:100,000 • 1:200,000 ☞ Oxidizes easily so bisulfite is added ☞ Most commonly used in dentistry
LEVONORDEFRIN (NEO-COBEFRIN)	Concentration—1:20,000

DOSAGES OF VASOCONSTRICTORS

DETERMINE MG PER CARPULE CALCULATED BY CONCENTRATION OF SOLUTION	Example: Using 1:100,000 concentration $1:100,000 = \dfrac{1000 \text{ mg}}{100,000 \text{ mL}} = \dfrac{1 \text{ mg}}{100 \text{ mL}}$ $= \dfrac{0.1 \text{ mg}}{1 \text{ mL}}$ $0.1 \times 1.8 \text{ mL/carpule}$ $= .018 \text{ mg/carpule}$ ☞ Carpule contains 1.8 mL of solution
MRD OF VASO-CONSTRICTORS	• Healthy patient, .2 mg • Compromised patient, .04 mg for epinephrine and .2 mg for Levonordephrin

DETERMINE MAXIMUM NUMBER OF CARPULES	Example: Epinephrine 1:100,000 Determine mg per carpule = .018 (as determined above) Healthy patient .2 ÷ .018 mg = 11.1 carpules Compromised patient .04 ÷ .018 = 2.2 carpules ⚷ Local anesthetic and vasoconstrictor must be calculated separately and lower of the two maximum doses is MRD, called the limiting factor

Medical History Review for Local Anesthetics

ABSOLUTE CONTRAINDICATION

- Requires that the offending drug not be administered to the individual under any circumstances
- The administration of such a drug is contraindicated in all situations because it substantially increases the possibility of a life-threatening risk for the patient

RELATIVE CONTRAINDICATION

Signifies that it is preferable to avoid administration of the suspected drug because there is the increased possibility that an adverse reaction may occur; however, if an acceptable substitute is not available, the drug may be used judiciously

⚷ Administer the minimal dose that still produces sufficient pain control

VASOCONSTRICTOR/DRUG INTERACTIONS

⚷ Epinephrine and other vasoconstrictors should be used with great caution or eliminated entirely when patients are taking the following drugs

MONOAMINE OXIDASE INHIBITORS (MAOIs)	• Monoamine oxidase is one of the two enzymes responsible for the inactivation of epinephrine and norepinephrine • If the activity of MAO is inhibited by the action of certain drugs, then the systemic effects of epinephrine result

	• MAO inhibitors are occasionally pre-scribed for patients with hypertension or psychological depression ☞ Phenylzine (Nardil), tranylpromine (Parnate), isocarboxazid (Marplan)
TRICYCLIC ANTI-DEPRESSANTS	• Prescribed for the treatment of neurotic or psychotic depression; when epineph-rine is given to patients taking these drugs, the pressor (blood pressure rais-ing) activity of the epinephrine is poten-tiated two to four times • If the patient also has arrhythmias, the situation is of even greater concern ☞ Amitriptyline (Elavil), doxepin (Sinequan, Adapin), nortriptyline (Pamelor), imipramine (Tofranil), desipramine (Norpramin, Pertofrane), protriptyline (Vivactil), trimipramine (Surmontil), amoxapine (Asendin)
ANTIHYPERTENSIVES (BETA BLOCKERS)	Like the tricyclic antidepressants, the anti-hypertensives potentiate the action of epi-nephrine and other adrenergic amines by increasing the pressor potency two to six times ☞ Propranolol (Inderal), metoprolol (Lo-pressor), atenolol (Tenormin), timolol (Blocadren), nadolol (Corgard), pindolol (Visken)
CARDIAC DRUGS	Digitalis glycosides are used for the treat-ment of congestive heart failure; the com-bination of digitalis glycosides and epinephrine increases the potential for cardiac arrythmias
ANTIDIABETIC AGENTS	• Oral hypoglycemic agents—epinephrine and other sympathomemic amines in-hibit the peripheral glucose uptake by the tissues and increase glucose release by the liver • Hyperglycemia can result • Epinephrine is, therefore, an antagonist to antidiabetic agents ☞ Insulin, chlorpropamide (Diabinese), glyburide (Diabeta), glypizide (Glucotrol)

COCAINE	A patient who you suspect may be taking cocaine will present with an increased risk for arrythmias

ESTER-DERIVATIVE LOCAL ANESTHETIC DRUG/DRUG INTERACTIONS

CHOLINESTERASE INHIBITORS	• Frequently prescribed for the treatment of myasthenia gravis and glaucoma • Patients taking cholinesterase inhibitors should not be given ester derivative local anesthetics • Ester derivatives are metabolized primarily in the bloodstream by plasma cholinesterase • If cholinesterase is inhibited, then the ester derivatives are more slowly broken down and systemic toxicity may result
SULFONAMIDES	• Procaine and other ester-type local anesthetics undergo hydrolysis to para-aminobenzoc acid (PABA), a major metabolic by-product; sulfonamides competitively inhibit PABA in microorganisms • PABA derivatives, therefore, may antagonize the antibacterial activity of sulfonamines, rendering them ineffective
ATYPICAL PLASMA-CHOLINESTERASE	• Relative to esters • Slow to metabolize esters • ☛ Use amide local anesthetics

AMIDE-DERIVATIVE LOCAL ANESTHETIC DRUG/DRUG INTERACTIONS

CIMETIDINE (TAGAMET)	Inhibits hepatic metabolism of amides by decreasing hepatic blood flow, therefore, increasing risk of toxic overdose
BETA BLOCKERS	• One type of antihypertensive—inhibits metabolism of amides by decreasing hepatic blood flow, therefore, increasing risk of toxic overdose • Not all antihypertensives behave in this manner, see PDR for specific interactions

CARDIOVASCULAR DISEASE	No vasoconstrictors—absolute contraindication if: • Blood pressure greater than normal 200/115 • Not after a heart attack or stroke • Unstable angina (uncontrolled) • Cardiac arrhythmia—refractory arrhythmia • Heart failure—(relative) may not tolerate lying down for treatment, increase risk for toxicity
LIVER DISEASE	• Relative contraindication to amides • Possible risk of toxicity ☞ Prilocaine can be used because is metabolized primarily in the lungs
KIDNEY DISEASE	No contraindications; use judiciously
UNCONTROLLED HYPERTHYROIDISM	Absolute contraindication ☞ Could cause thyroid crisis, thyroid storm (loss of speech, bulging eyes)

PREGNANCY/ PLACENTAL BARRIER/ FETAL IMPLICATIONS	• Relative contraindication
	• Use as little as possible, try not to use in 1st trimester
	• FDA Categories
	  • Category B: lidocaine, prilocaine
	  • Category C: mepivacaine, bupivacaine, procaine

MALIGNANT HYPERTHERMIA	• Relative contraindication to amides • Complications associated with the administration of general anesthesia • Recategorized as relative because research has shown that amide local anesthetics are not likely to trigger episode • Unusual hereditary condition • Will cause patient to have high fever during surgery (Dantrolene treats symptom)
METHEMOGLOBINEMIA	Prilocaine and articaine when administered in large doses, and topical anesthetic benzocaine can cause the inability to carry oxygen ☞ Clinical cyanosis occurs

AGE	More susceptible to maximum permissible dose ☞ Reduce dose in children and elderly patients
BLEEDING DISORDERS	• Hemophiliac patients: need to use caution not to puncture artery; infiltrate instead of block injection • Hematoma could be a life-threatening situation • Should bleeding occur, use pressure and ice
UNCONTROLLED DIABETES	• Absolute contraindication to vasoconstrictors; risk of hyperglycemia • Refer to physician
PHEOCHROMO-CYTOMA	• Absolute contraindication • Tumor in adrenal gland • Produces adrenal insufficiency • Rule of two's: 20 mg cortisone for 2 weeks or longer within past two years
UNCONTROLLED HYPERTHYROIDISM	• Absolute contraindication to vasoconstrictors • May precipitate an exaggerated response to the vasopressor, resulting in cardiac stimulation

Local Anesthesia Armamentarium

SYRINGES

BREECH-LOADING, METALLIC, ASPIRATING, CARTRIDGE TYPE	Most commonly used syringe for the administration of an intraoral local anesthetic **Figure 9-16**

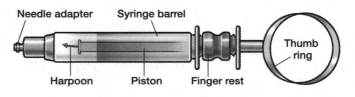

Needle adapter · Syringe barrel · Thumb ring · Harpoon · Piston · Finger rest

FIGURE 9-16 Breech-loading Aspirating Syringe

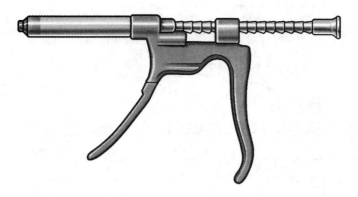

FIGURE 9-17 Pressure-type Syringe

PRESSURE-TYPE SYRINGE	Used when administering a periodontal ligament (PDL) injection, which provides pulpal anesthesia to one tooth **Figure 9-17**
JET INJECTOR	Delivers .05 to .2 mL of anesthetic agent to the mucous membranes at a high pressure via small openings called jets **Figure 9-18**

NEEDLES

Virtually all needles used in oral healthcare today are made of stainless steel, are presterilized by the manufacturer, and are disposable

BEVEL	The angled surface of the needlepoint that is directed into the tissues **Figure 9-19**
SHANK	Length of the needle from the point to the hub

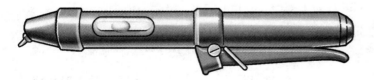

FIGURE 9-18 Jet Injector

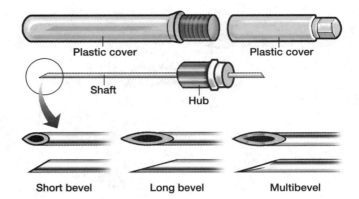

Plastic cover   Plastic cover

Shaft   Hub

Short bevel   Long bevel   Multibevel

FIGURE 9-19 Parts of Needle and Types of Bevels

HUB	Plastic or metal piece that attaches the needle onto the syringe • Plastic syringe adapter is not threaded so must be pushed onto syringe while being screwed on • Metal syringe adapter is prethreaded
SYRINGE PENETRATING END	Punctures the rubber diaphragm of cartridge and tip rests within the cartridge
COLORED SHIELD	Protects the part of the needle that is inserted into the tissues
GAUGE	Diameter of the lumen of the needle • Higher the gauge number, the smaller the diameter of the lumen • Most commonly used needles are 25, 27 • Recommended to use 25-gauge needle for those injections that pose a high risk of aspiration or when a significant depth of soft tissue must be penetrated • 27-gauge may be used for all other injections • 30-gauge is not recommended ☞ Advantages of larger gauge needles • Less deflection • Greater accuracy • Needle breakage less likely to occur • Aspiration of blood is more reliable through larger lumen
LENGTH	• Long: 1 5/8 in. or 40 mm measured from hub to the needle tip

	• Preferred for those injections that require penetration of significant soft tissue (inferior alveolar and infraorbital nerve blocks) • Short: 1 in. or 25 mm • Recommended when not penetrating significant tissue **Figure 9-20**
INSERTION	• Needles should not be inserted to the hub • Retrieval is very hard if the needle is embedded in the tissue • The face of the bevel is directed parallel to bone
DISPOSAL	Comply with OSHA guidelines, which is to recap the needle utilizing "scoop" method and place in a "sharps" disposal container
PAIN ON INSERTION	• Due to dull needle • Prevention: change needle after 3 to 4 injections
PAIN ON WITHDRAWAL	• Due to barbs on needle tip • Prevention: run tip backward over sterile gauze square, barbs will snag gauze

CARTRIDGE

🔑 Holds 1.8 mL of local anesthetic solutions

INGREDIENTS	• Local anesthetic drug • Vasoconstrictor drug • Preservative for vasoconstrictor (usually sodium bisulfite) • Sodium chloride • Distilled water

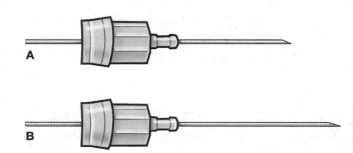

FIGURE 9-20 Needle Lengths: A) Short; B) Long

BUBBLES	• Small bubbles (1–2mm in diameter) may at times be seen in a cartridge; this is nitrogen gas that was bubbled into the anesthetic solution during the manufacturing process to preclude oxygen, which destroys the vasoconstrictor; these bubbles are harmless and can be ignored **Figure 9-21** • Large bubbles (larger than 2mm) are an indication that the solution has been frozen; because sterility of the solution is no longer guaranteed, the cartridge should not be used **Figure 9-22**
EXTRUDED STOPPER	• Accompanied by a large bubble in the cartridge; is an indication the solution has been frozen and should be discarded • No bubble indicates that the cartridge has probably been stored too long in chemical disinfecting solution ☛ Will produce burning sensation upon injection **Figure 9-23**
STICKY STOPPER	Does not advance smoothly through the glass cylinder when pressure is applied to the thumb ring
CORRODED CAP	May be observed if it has been immersed in quaternary compounds
RUST ON THE ALUMINUM CAP	Signifies that a cartridge has broken or leaked in the metal container
LEAKAGE DURING INJECTION	Off-center perforation of the needle into the diaphragm of the cartridge
BURNING ON INJECTION	• Normal response to pH of drug • Cartridge containing sterilizing solution • Overheated cartridge • Vasoconstrictor pH outdated solutions

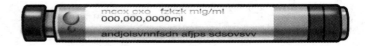

FIGURE 9-21   Small Bubbles in Cartridge

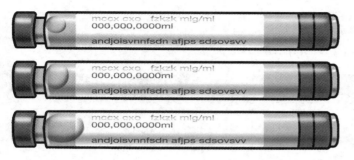

FIGURE 9-22

SUPPLEMENTARY ARMAMENTARIUM	
TOPICAL ANTISEPTICS	• Reduce the risk of introducing surface microorganisms into the tissue, which could result in infection • Contain iodine ⚷ Caution against patients allergic to iodine
TOPICAL ANESTHETIC	• Applied to the mucous membrane prior to the initial needle penetration to anesthetize the terminal nerve endings • Concentration is high to facilitate diffusion of the drug through the mucous membranes • Small amounts should be applied to avoid toxicity • Apply to injection site for 1–2 minutes ⚷ Most contain ester local anesthetics such as benzocaine; possible allergic reaction to these agents is greater than amide topical anesthetics
HEMOSTAT, FORCEPS, COTTON PLIERS	Used to remove a needle from the soft tissues in case the needle breaks off within tissue

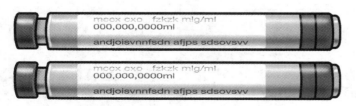

FIGURE 9-23 A) Frozen Carpule—Large Bubble and Extruded Stopper; B) Stored in Disinfecting Solution—Extruded Stopper

➤ ADMINISTERING LOCAL ANESTHETICS

Classification of Injections

CLASSIFICATION OF ADMINISTRATION TECHNIQUES Figure 9-24	
NERVE BLOCK ANESTHESIA	Injection of local anesthetic solution close to a nerve trunk • Has the advantage of blocking sensations from a large portion of the anatomy with a single injection ☞ Disadvantage: major blood vessels frequently accompany nerve trunks, and the possibility of accidentally piercing an artery or vein is significantly enhanced
FIELD BLOCK ANESTHESIA	A form of regional anesthesia commonly employed in the maxillary arch; injection of local anesthetic solution close to large terminal nerve branches
INFILTRATION ANESTHESIA	• Provides pain relief solely in the area bathed by the drug solution • Only terminal nerve endings are affected by infiltration • Usually employed for soft tissue anesthesia
TOPICAL ANESTHESIA	Surface application of a local anesthetic to block free nerve endings supplying the mucosal surfaces

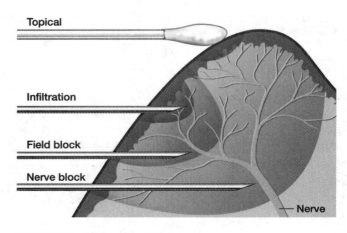

Topical

Infiltration

Field block

Nerve block

Nerve

FIGURE 9-24 Administration Techniques

Maxillary Injections

Refer to Head and Neck Anatomy section in Chapter 1 to review trigeminal nerve

INFRAORBITAL INJECTION (IO) Figure 9-25

TEETH	Pulpal anesthesia of the maxillary central incisor, lateral incisor, and canine; 60% maxillary premolars, mesiobuccal root of the first molar
GINGIVA/BONE/ ADJACENT TISSUES	Lower eyelid, lateral aspect of the nose, upper lip, buccal and labial periodontal tissues, and bone overlying these same teeth
PENETRATION SITE	Height of mucobuccal fold above the first premolar
LANDMARKS	Mucobuccal fold, infraorbital notch, infraorbital ridge, infraorbital depression, infraorbital foramen
DEPOSIT LOCATION	Upper rim of the infraorbital foramen, the needle should gently contact bone when reaching the deposition site
DEPTH OF PENETRATION	Long needle, 25-gauge 1/2 the needle length
TECHNIQUE	• Locate infraorbital foramen • Maintain pressure with your finger over the foramen during injection, massage • Bevel toward bone • Insert needle at height of mucobuccal fold above first premolar until bone is gently contacted • Aspirate and deposit

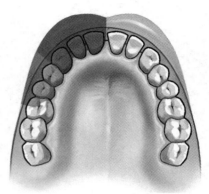

FIGURE 9-25 Darkened Area Shows Anesthesia Provided from IO Injection

MIDDLE SUPERIOR ALVEOLAR (MSA) INJECTION Figure 9-26

TEETH	Pulpal anesthesia of 1st and 2nd maxillary premolars and mesiobuccal root of maxillary 1st molar

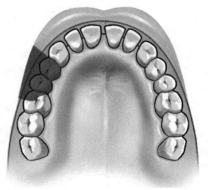

FIGURE 9-26 Darkened Area Shows Anesthesia Provided by MSA Injection

GINGIVA/BONE/ ADJACENT TISSUES	Buccal periodontal tissue and bone over same teeth
PENETRATION SITE	Height of mucobuccal fold above apex of maxillary second premolar
LANDMARKS	Mucobuccal fold, second premolar
DEPOSIT LOCATION	Above (3–5mm) the apical region of the second premolar
DEPTH OF PENETRATION	Short, 25- or 27-gauge 1/4 of the needle length
TECHNIQUE	Parallel to long axis of the 2nd maxillary premolar above the apex Aspirate and deposit
ADVERSE EFFECTS	Pain from injecting too close to periosteum or too rapid deposition

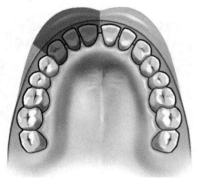

FIGURE 9-27 Darkened Area Shows Anesthesia Provided by ASA Injection

ANTERIOR SUPERIOR ALVEOLAR (ASA) INJECTION
Figure 9-27

TEETH	Pulpal anesthesia of maxillary central, lateral, and cuspid
GINGIVA/BONE/ ADJACENT TISSUES	Facial periodontium and bone overlying these teeth
PENETRATION SITE	Height of mucobuccal fold slightly mesial to the canine eminence
LANDMARKS	• Mucobuccal fold • Canine eminence • Depression located just anterior to the canine eminence
DEPOSIT LOCATION	Apical region of canine
DEPTH OF PENETRATION	Short needle, 25- or 27-gauge 1/4 of needle
TECHNIQUE	• Angle needle from lateral toward the bone above the apex of the cuspid • Aspirate and deposit
ADVERSE EFFECTS	Scrape periosteum from injecting too close to periosteum or too rapidly

POSTERIOR SUPERIOR ALVEOLAR (PSA) INJECTION
Figure 9-28

TEETH	Pulpal anesthesia of the 3rd, 2nd, and 1st maxillary molars entirely in 60%; mesiobuccal root anesthetized in 40%
GINGIVA/BONE/ ADJACENT TISSUES	Buccal periodontium and bone overlying these teeth
PENETRATION SITE	Height of mucobuccal fold opposite the distal portion of the second molar
LANDMARKS	• Mucobuccal fold • Second molar • Maxillary tuberosity • Maxillary occlusal plane • Midsaggital plane
DEPOSIT LOCATION	Posterior and superior to the posterior border of the maxilla at the PSA nerve foramina
DEPTH OF PENETRATION	Short needle, 25- or 27-gauge 3/4 of needle length
TECHNIQUE	• Upward 45 degrees to occlusal plane; inward and backward 45 degrees to midsaggital plane • Aspirate and deposit
ADVERSE EFFECTS	• Needle inserted too far posterior and superior may tear maxillary artery or pterygoid plexus of veins, resulting in hematoma • Mandibular anesthesia

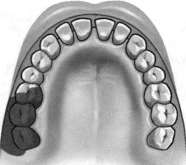

FIGURE 9-28 Darkened Area Shows Anesthesia Provided by PSA Injection

NASOPALATINE (NP) INJECTION Figure 9-29

TEETH	None
GINGIVA/BONE/ ADJACENT TISSUES	Hard palate and overlying soft tissue of the maxillary anterior teeth bilaterally
PENETRATION SITE	Lateral to the incisive papilla
LANDMARKS	• Maxillary central incisors • Incisive papilla

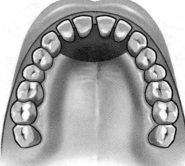

FIGURE 9-29 Darkened Area Shows Anesthesia Provided by NP Injection

DEPOSIT LOCATION	Incisive foramen beneath the incisive papilla
DEPTH OF PENETRATION	No more than 4–6 mm or until bone is lightly contacted 27-gauge short needle
TECHNIQUE	• 45–90 degrees to tissue at the edge of incisive papilla, watch for blanching of the tissue • Use pressure anesthesia • Aspirate and deposit
ADVERSE EFFECTS	Because of the density of the tissues, the anesthetic solution may appear around the needle penetration site during administration

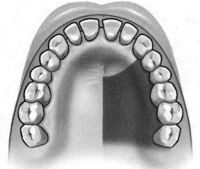

FIGURE 9-30 Darkened Area Shows Anesthesia Provided by GP Injection

GREATER PALATINE (GP) INJECTION Figure 9-30

TEETH	None
GINGIVA/BONE/ADJACENT TISSUES	Hard palate and overlying soft tissue maxillary third molar—the first premolar on side injected
PENETRATION SITE	Slightly anterior to the greater palatine foramen
LANDMARKS	Greater palatine foramen located at the junction of the maxillary alveolar process and palatine bone distal to the maxillary second molar
DEPOSIT LOCATION	Greater palatine nerve located between soft tissue and bone of the hard palate
DEPTH OF PENETRATION	No more than 5–7 mm or until palate is lightly contacted 25- or 27-gauge short needle
TECHNIQUE	• Advance syringe from opposite side of mouth at right angle to target area • Use pressure anesthesia, topical and swab • Aspirate and deposit

Mandibular Injections

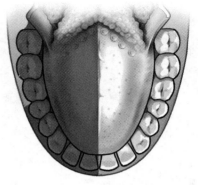

FIGURE 9-31 Darkened Area Shows Anesthesia Provided by a Combination of IA and L Injections

INFERIOR ALVEOLAR (IA) INJECTION Figure 9-31	
TEETH	Mandibular teeth to midline
GINGIVA/BONE/ ADJACENT TISSUES	• Body of mandible • Inferior portion of the ramus • Facial tissue from the second premolar to midline • Lower lip on side of injection
PENETRATION SITE	Middle of pterygomandibular triangle at the height of the coronoid notch (6–10 mm above the occlusal plane of the mandibular molars)
LANDMARKS	• Anterior border of ramus • External oblique ridge • Coronoid notch • Internal oblique ridge • Pterygomandibular raphe • Pterygomandibular triangle • Mandibular occlusal plane
DEPTH OF PENETRATION	• Until bone is lightly contacted, 2/3 to 3/4 of the needle length inserted, withdrawal needle 1mm • Long needle, 25-gauge
DEPOSIT LOCATION	Superior to the mandibular foramen at the inferior alveolar nerve before it enters the foramen
TECHNIQUE	• Locate pterygomandibular triangle • Place thumb on the greatest depression (coronoid notch) • Roll your finger medially to locate the internal oblique ridge • The point of penetration is between the internal oblique ridge and the pterygomandibular raphe • Syringe barrel rests on premolars of opposite side
ADVERSE EFFECTS	• Transient facial paralysis from deposition in parotid gland • Hematoma • Avoid by always contacting bone prior to deposting anesthesia

LINGUAL (L) INJECTION

TEETH	None
GINGIVA/BONE/ ADJACENT TISSUES	Lingual gingival tissue to the midline, anterior 2/3 of the tongue and floor of the oral cavity
PENETRATION SITE	Same as IA
LANDMARKS	Same as IA
DEPTH OF PENETRATION	After depositing solution for IA, withdraw needle until 1/2 its length remains in tissues
TECHNIQUE	Same as IA
ADVERSE EFFECTS	"Shocking" pain if lingual nerve is touched

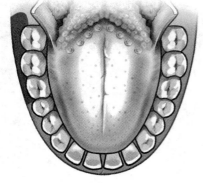

FIGURE 9-32 Darkened Area Shows Anesthesia Provided by B Injection

BUCCAL (B) INJECTION Figure 9-32

TEETH	None
GINGIVA/BONE/ ADJACENT TISSUES	Buccal soft tissues to the mandibular molars
PENETRATION SITE	In vestibule, distal and buccal to the most distal molar in the quadrant
LANDMARKS	Mandibular molars, vestibule, mucobuccal fold
DEPTH OF PENETRATION	1–4 mm, until bone is lightly contacted
DEPOSIT LOCATION	Buccal nerve as it passes over the anterior border of the ramus
TECHNIQUE	• Administer after IA • Penetrate mucous membrane until bone is contacted • Aspirate and deposit
ADVERSE EFFECTS	Trismus of tendonous attachment of temporalis, ballooning of tissue

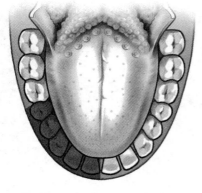

FIGURE 9-33 Darkened Area Shows Anesthesia Provided by Incisive and Mental Injections

INCISIVE AND MENTAL INJECTIONS Figure 9-33

TEETH	2nd premolar to central

GINGIVA/BONE/ ADJACENT TISSUES	Facial soft tissues from the mental foramen anterior to midline, lower lip, skin of chin
PENETRATION SITE	Mucobuccal fold directly over the mental foramen
LANDMARKS	Mucobuccal fold, mandibular premolars, mental foramen
DEPTH OF PENETRATION	1/4 length of short 25- or 27-gauge needle
DEPOSIT LOCATION	Directly over mental foramen, usually between the apices of the first and second premolars
TECHNIQUE	• Locate mental foramen • Pull tissue laterally, advance needle to level of foramen • Aspirate and deposit; massage area to achieve incisive injection ☛ If soft tissue anesthesia only, do not massage

Complications

NEEDLE BREAKAGE

CAUSES	• Sudden, unexpected movement • Poor technique
PREVENTION	• Inform the client about the procedure • Use long, large-gauge needle when penetrating a significant amount of tissue • Never bend the needle • Advance the needle slowly • Never force a needle against firm resistance such as bone • Do no change direction while needle is embedded in tissue • Never insert needle to hub
MANAGEMENT	• Remain calm • Instruct the client not to move; keep your hand in patient's mouth • Attempt to remove needle fragment if needle is protruding • If you cannot remove refer to oral surgeon • Document incident

PAIN DURING INJECTION	
CAUSES	• Careless injection technique • Dull needle from multiple injections • A barbed needle from hitting bone • Rapid deposit of solution
PREVENTION	• Adhere to proper techniques for injections • Use sharp disposable needles • Apply topical anesthetic prior to injection • Use sterile anesthetic agents • Inject slowly • Store anesthetic solutions at room temperature

BURNING DURING INJECTION	
CAUSES	• Local anesthetic with a vasoconstrictor that is more acidic than the tissue • Contamination of anesthetic in disinfecting solution • Heated cartridge • Expired solution • Solution deposited too rapidly
PREVENTION	• Store cartridge in a dark place at room temperature, do not store in chemical disinfectants • Check expiration date • Inject slowly

HEMATOMA	

Swelling and discoloration of the tissue resulting from effusion of blood into extravascular spaces

CAUSES	Inadvertent puncture of blood vessel, particularly an artery ☞ Most common after PSA or IA injection
PREVENTION	• Be attentive to anatomical detail • Modify injection technique depending on patient's mouth • Use a short needle for the PSA

	• Minimize the number of needle insertions • Maintain appropriate technique
MANAGEMENT	• If swelling appears, apply direct pressure to the site of bleeding for at least 2 minutes • Apply ice to the region—warm the next day • Inform patient of possibility of soreness and limited movement • Advise patient that swelling and discoloration will disappear after 7 to 14 days • Dismiss patient when bleeding has stopped

FACIAL PARALYSIS

Loss of motor function of the facial expression muscles

CAUSES	• Parotid gland located on the posterior border of the ramus—local anesthetic solution deposited into the parotid gland during IA injection where the facial nerves pass • To avoid—always contact bone before depositing solution during IA injection
PREVENTION	• Adhere to techniques recommended for IA • Needle should always contact bone to avoid depositing solution in parotid gland
MANAGEMENT	• Reassure the patient; paralysis lasts only a few hours • Instruct patient to remove contact lenses • Ask the patient to close their eyelid manually to keep cornea lubricated • Document

PARESTHESIA

Prolonged anesthesia for many hours or days following injection

CAUSES	• Irritation to nerve following injection of agent contaminated in disinfecting solution • Edema places pressure on nerve • Trauma of nerve sheath from needle contacting nerve during injection • Hemorrhage into or around neural sheath
PREVENTION	• Store dental cartridges properly • Avoid placing cartridges in disinfectant • Follow proper technique
MANAGEMENT	• Reassure patient • Arrange exam with dentist • Consultation with oral surgeon • Record incident

TRISMUS

Spasm of the muscles of mastication that results in soreness and difficulty opening the mouth

CAUSES	• Trauma to the muscles in the infratemporal space following injection • Multiple needle insertions • Contaminated solution with disinfectant • Depositing large amounts of solution in restricted areas, causing distension of tissues • Hemorrhage that leads to muscle dysfunction • Low-grade infection
PREVENTION	• Store anesthetic properly • Use sharp, sterile, disposable needles • Follow appropriate injection control protocol • Use minimal effective amount of solution and deposit slowly
MANAGEMENT	• Arrange for exam from dentist • Heat therapy • Direct patient to open and close mouth and move mandible from side to side for 5 minutes every 3–4 hours

- Infection—antibiotic treatment
- If severe pain, refer to oral surgeon
- Record incident

INFECTION

PREVENTION	<ul><li>Use sterile, disposable needle</li><li>The needle should be sheathed prior to injection and immediately after</li><li>Use appropriate infection control guidelines when handling the anesthetic cartridges</li><li>Store anesthetic in original container, and wipe off diaphragm with disinfectant if necessary</li><li>Use topical antiseptic</li></ul>

EDEMA

Swelling of the tissues

CAUSES	<ul><li>Trauma during injection</li><li>Administration of contaminated solution</li><li>Hemorrhage</li><li>Infection</li><li>Allergic response</li></ul>
PREVENTION	<ul><li>Follow appropriate infection control protocol when storing and handling components of local anesthetic armamentarium</li><li>Observe guidelines for administering atraumatic injections</li><li>Conduct an adequate preanesthetic patient assessment</li></ul>

TISSUE SLOUGHING

Surface layers of epithelium may be lost

CAUSES	<ul><li>Sterile abscess may develop after prolonged ischemia, usually on palate (vasoconstrictor)</li><li>Tissue irritation caused by topical anesthetic</li></ul>

PREVENTION	• Use topical anesthetics appropriately—limit to 1–2 minutes • Avoid high concentrations of vasoconstrictors

SOFT TISSUE TRAUMA

CAUSES	Lip, tongue, or cheek trauma results when patient inadvertently chews or bites tissues while numb
PREVENTION	• Select anesthetic agent with duration appropriate for length of appointment • Warn patient not to eat, drink, or test anesthesia area by biting • Place cotton roll between teeth and soft tissue • Use warning stickers on child to remind parent that child is numb

➤ LOCAL ANESTHETIC EMERGENCIES

Local Anesthetic Overdose

Overly high blood levels of a drug in various organs and tissues

CAUSES OF OVERDOSE

- Biotransformation of the anesthetic is unusually slow
- Elimination of the anesthetic from the body through the kidneys is unusually slow
- The total dose administered is too large
- Absorption of the anesthetic from the site of injection is unusually rapid
- The anesthetic is administered intravascularly

PREVENTION OF OVERDOSE

- Medical history review is very important
- Ester LA biotransformed in the blood by enzyme pseudocholinesterase, which causes the drug to undergo hydrolysis to para-aminobenzoic acid
- Patients with familial history of atypical pseudocholinesterase may be unable to detoxify the drug

- Calculation of maximum permissible dose is very important
- Age of patient and physical status (need to adjust dose accordingly)
- Addition of a vasoconstricting drug in the local anesthetic solution reduces the systemic toxicity of the anesthetic agent by slowing absorption into cardiovascular system
- Limit area of use of topical anesthetics—topicals are administered in high concentrations
- Know your anatomy
- Always aspirate
- Use 25- or 27-gauge needle
- Aspirate in two planes
- Administer drug slowly
- History of liver disease may indicate some hepatic dysfunction, and inability to biotransform amide drugs

CLINICAL MANIFESTATIONS OF LOCAL ANESTHETIC OVERDOSE REACTION

EARLY SIGNS AND SYMPTOMS	• Talkative, restless, apprehensve, excited • Tremors or convulsions—if too large dose or IV injection • Increased blood pressure and/or pulse rate
LATE SIGNS AND SYMPTOMS	• Convulsions, followed by depression • Drop in blood pressure • Weak, rapid pulse or bradycardia • Apnea • Unconsciousness • Death

TREATMENT OF OVERDOSE

- Protect patient during the convulsive period (consider 10 mg Valium IV—if convulsive period is prolonged longer than 15 minutes)
- Call paramedics
- Record vitals
- Supportive therapy (oxygen at 6 liter flow, maintain blood pressure)
- Treat bradycardia (0.4 mg Atropine IV)
- Gently restrict limbs, move all instrument trays away and keep hands and materials out of patient's mouth

Epinephrine Overdose

CAUSES OF OVERDOSE

- More likely to develop if concentrations of epinephrine greater than 1:100,000 are administered
- ⚷ Greater potential for epinephrine overdose in patients with cardiovascular disease

PREVENTION OF OVERDOSE

- Use the lowest effective concentration of epinephrine needed to produce the desired effect and carefully observe dosage guidelines
- Reduce total dose of vasoconstrictor to avoid systemic complications in patients with cardiovascular disease
- IV injection may produce an epinephrine overdose
- Know drug interactions and decrease dose accordingly
- ⚷ For patients with cardiovascular disease and patients taking drugs that interact with epinephrine, decrease dose to .04 mg

CLINICAL MANIFESTATIONS

SIGNS AND SYMPTOMS	
	- Fear, anxiety
	- Tenseness
	- Restlessness
	- Throbbing headache
	- Tremor
	- Perspiration
	- Weakness
	- Dizziness
	- Pallor
	- Respiratory difficulty
	- Palpitations
	- Sharp elevation in blood pressure
	- Elevated heart rate
	- Cardiac dysrhythmias

TREATMENT

- Terminate procedure
- Position patient upright

- Reassure patient
- Basic life support, as indicated
- Monitor vital signs
- Activate EMS, if needed
- Administer oxygen, if needed
- Allow patient to recover and discharge

Allergic Reactions

CAUSES OF ALLERGIC REACTIONS

- Most often in response to ester local anesthetics
- Amide allergic reactions are extremely rare
- Reports of allergy to sodium bisulfite are numerous
- ☞ Sodium bisulfite—preservative in vasoconstrictors

PREVENTION OF ALLERGIC REACTIONS

- Preanesthetic assessment is the primary measure for prevention
- A patient with multiple allergies has an increased potential for allergic reactions to medications (avoid esther topical anesthetics)
- Dialogue history is very important to determine true allergic reaction

MILD ALLERGIC REACTION

CLINICAL MANIFESTATIONS OF MILD ALLERGIC REACTION	• Mild pruritis (itching) • Mild urticaria (rash) • Angioedema (localized swelling of extremities, lips, tongue, pharynx, larynx)
TREATMENT OF MILD ALLERGIC REACTION	• Diphenhydramine (Benedryl) 25–50 mg IV or IM • Repeat up to 50 mg every 6 hours p.o. for 2 days

SEVERE ALLERGIC REACTIONS

CLINICAL MANI-FESTATIONS OF SEVERE ALLERGIC REACTIONS	Skin reaction: • Severe pruritus • Severe urticaria Mucous membrane rhinitis Angioedema—swelling of lips, eyelids, cheeks, pharynx, and larynx May progress to anaphylactic shock • Cardiovascular—fall in blood pressure • Respiratory—wheezing, choking, cyanosis, hoarseness • Dypsnea • Central nervous system—loss of consciousness, dilation of pupils
TREATMENT OF SEVERE ALLERGIC REACTION	• Epinephrine 1:1000 0.3–0.5 cc IV, IM or SC (contraindication: severe hypertension) • Theophylline ethylenediamine (Aminophylline), 250–500 mg IV over 10 minutes (contraindication: hypotension) • Steroids—Hydrocortisone sodium succinate (Solucortef), 100 mg IV • Record vitals • Cardiopulmonary resuscitation (if indicated) ☞ Caution: Since aminophylline may cause hypotension, it should be given with extreme caution to asthmatic patients who are also hypotensive

➤ RECOGNITION AND MANAGEMENT OF COMPROMISED PATIENTS

Patient with Diabetes Mellitus

Group of metabolic disorders resulting in hyperglycemia (abnormal increase in blood glucose)

TYPES OF DIABETES

TYPE I DIABETES	• Insulin-dependent diabetes mellitus • Commonly in young children, but may occur at any age • Hereditary, but not as common as Type II

	• Symptoms—polyuria, polyphagia, thirst, mimic flu
TYPE II DIABETES	• Non insulin-dependent diabetes mellitus • Occurs in adults usually after 40 years of age, but may occur younger • Risk factors—obesity and poor nutrition • Symptoms—can have same symptoms as Type I, delayed healing, fatigue

EFFECTS OF DIABETES RELATED TO DENTAL CARE

- Impaired healing
- Increases susceptibility to infections
- Inflammation may increase patient's insulin requirements
- Insulin reactions
- Long-term problems—nephropathy, vascular disease, blindness

DENTAL HYGIENE TREATMENT CONSIDERATIONS

- Appointment time should be in morning or alternate, after lunch
- Well-controlled patient—no alterations in treatment
- Uncontrolled diabetes—postpone treatment until diabetes is controlled
- Be aware of systemic complications related to diabetes and treat appropriately (hypertension, congestive heart failure, angina, renal failure)

ORAL COMPLICATIONS

- Accelerated periodontal disease
- Xerostomia
- Delayed healing
- Increased susceptibility to infection
- Candidiasis

Patients with Cardiovascular Disease

RHEUMATIC HEART DISEASE

Heart valve damage following rheumatic fever
⚷ Caused by beta-hemolytic group A streptococcal pharyngeal infection

DENTAL MANAGEMENT	• Patient is susceptible to infective endocarditis • Antibiotic premedication • Explain importance of high level of oral hygiene to prevent increased amount of bacteria in oral cavity

MITRAL VALVE PROLAPSE

Leaflets of mitral valve are damaged and tight closure of valve is compromised causing regurgitation (oxygenated blood backs up) of blood

DENTAL MANAGEMENT	Pretreatment antibiotic is indicated

INFECTIVE ENDOCARDITIS

Disease caused by microbial infection of the heart valves
☛ Infection must be promptly controlled or patient may develop heart failure leading to death

DENTAL MANAGEMENT	• Complete medical history with specific questions regarding history of rheumatic fever, congenital heart defects, prosthetic valves, or past occurrences of infective endocarditis • Pretreatment antibiotics

ISCHEMIC HEART DISEASE

Results from oxygen deprivation to the myocardium as a result of coronary atherosclerosis

MANIFESTATIONS OF ISCHEMIC HEART DISEASE	• Angina pectoris
DENTAL MANAGEMENT	• Stress reduction • Myocardial infarction may occur during dental procedure • Premedication with valium 5–10 mg

- Terminate procedure if patient becomes fatigued
- Nitroglycerin tablet, should angina occur

CONGESTIVE HEART FAILURE

- Complex symptoms that can occur from many different specific disease processes
- Heart failure develops when the heart can no longer function as a pump and causes a collection of fluids in various organs

DENTAL MANAGEMENT	<ul><li>No dental care until patient is under good medical management</li><li>Upright position during treatment</li><li>Bleeding and prothrombin times prior to surgery</li><li>Terminate procedure if patient becomes fatigued</li><li>If patient is taking digitalis, may be more prone to nausea</li><li>Anticoagulants should be reduced (takes 3–4 days)</li><li>Antihypertensive agents—reduce vasoconstrictor to .04 mg when administering local anesthetics</li></ul>

MYOCARDIAL INFARCTION

Most serious manifestation of ischemic heart disease
☛ "Heart attack"; left coronary artery is most often affected

DENTAL MANAGEMENT	<ul><li>No routine dental care until at least 6 months following infarction</li><li>Morning appointments</li><li>Bleeding tendency if patient is on anticoagulants</li><li>Terminate procedure if patient becomes fatigued</li></ul>

CONGENITAL HEART DISEASE

Anomalies of the structure of the heart following irregularities in development during the first 9 weeks in utero

VENTRICULAR SEPTAL DEFECTS	• Left to right shunt • Oxygenated blood from the lung is normally pumped by the left ventricle to the aorta, passes through defect back to right ventricle • Small defects—heart murmur • Large defects—heart enlarges to compensate for overload • 80% are located in the membranous septum just below the aortic valve
PATENT DUCTUS ARTERIOSUS	• Left to right shunt • Ductus that connects the pulmonary artery to the aorta usually closes within a few hours of birth; if it does not, there is flow from the aorta into the pulmonary artery, causing blood from the aorta to pass back into the lungs • Heart compensates to provide the body with oxygenated blood and becomes overburdened • Surgery is recommended before 2 years of age
TETROLOGY OF FALLOT	• Right to left shunt • Lesion consists of ventricular septal defect, and pulmonary stenosis that causes reduced venous return from the lungs • "Blue baby"
PULMONARY STENOSIS	Malformation that obstructs blood flow that leads to right ventricular dilation and hypertrophy
COARCTATION OF THE AORTA	Localized constriction at or distal to the left subclavian artery from the aorta, resulting in narrowed pulse pressure distal to the obstruction • Absent or weak pulses in lower limbs
DENTAL MANAGEMENT OF CONGENITAL HEART DEFECTS	Prevention of infective endocarditis

Patients with Bleeding Disorders

CLASSIFICATION OF BLEEDING DISORDERS

NONTHROMBO-CYTOPENIC PURPURAS	• Infections, chemical, or certain allergies may alter the structure and function of vascular wall resulting in bleeding problem • Platelets may be defective and unable to perform their proper functions, caused by genetic defects, drugs (aspirin, NSAIDs, penicillin, cephalothins) ⚷ Normal numbers of platelets
THROMBOCYTOPENIC PURPURAS	• Caused by radiation, various systemic diseases (leukemia) and have a direct effect on bone marrow ⚷ Total platelet count is reduced
DISORDERS OF COAGULATION	• Inherited—hemophilia • Acquired—liver disease (liver produces all the coagulation factors) • Acquired—vitamin deficiency; if vitamin K is not produced will result in decreased plasma level of prothrombin • Anticoagulation drugs—heparin, Coumadin

PHASES OF BLEEDING CONTROL

• Vascular phase—immediately following injury → vasoconstriction
• Platelet phase—platelets become sticky and produce plugs to seal off openings
• Coagulation phase—initiated by two separate mechanisms: extrinsic (outside blood vessel) and intrinsic (within blood vessel)

DENTAL MANAGEMENT

• Screen patient for bleeding times
• Oral complications—spontaneous bleeding, prolonged bleeding, petechiae, hematomas
⚷ Avoid PSA and IA injections

LABORATORY TESTS

- Prothrombin time—normal = 11–15 seconds
- Activated partial thromboplastin time—normal = 25–35 seconds
- Thrombin time—normal = 9–13 seconds
- Bleeding time—normal = 1 to 6 minutes
- Platelet count—normal = 140,000 to 400,000/mm^3

BLOOD DYSCRASIAS

See Pathology (Chapter 5)

Patients with Liver Disease

STAGES OF ALCOHOLIC LIVER DISEASE

FATTY INFILTRATE	• Enlargement of the liver • Completely reversible
ALCOHOLIC HEPATITIS	• Diffuse inflammatory condition of the liver • Characterized by destructive cellular changes, some of which may be irreversible, which lead to necrosis
CIRRHOSIS	• Most serious • Irreversible condition characterized by abnormal regeneration • Progressive deterioration of the metabolic and excretory functions of the liver

DENTAL MANAGEMENT OF LIVER DISEASE

- Bleeding tendencies
- Inability to metabolize and detoxify certain drugs
- ☞ Limit dose of amide local anesthetics

COMMON DENTAL DRUGS METABOLIZED BY THE LIVER

LOCAL ANESTHETICS	• Amides • Lidocaine • Mepivacaine • Prilocaine

ANALGESICS	• Aspirin • Tylenol • Codine • Demerol
SEDATIVES	• Valium • Barbiturates
ANTIBIOTICS	• Ampicillin • Tetracycline

HEPATITIS

See Infection Control section

Patients with Neurologic Disorders

EPILEPSY

TYPES OF SEIZURES	Partial (focal, local) • Simple partial seizure—without loss of consciousness • Complex partial seizure—simple partial seizure with loss of consciousness • Partial seizures evolving to general tonic-clonic convulsions
	Generalized • Convulsive seizures—absence seizures, atypical absence seizures, myclonic seizures, atonic seizures • Nonconvulsive seizures—tonic-clonic seizures, tonic seizures, clonic seizures
SIGNS AND SYMPTOMS OF SEIZURE	Tonic-clonic convulsions (grand-mal seizure) • Sudden cry • Muscle rigidity, uncoordinated beating movements of the limbs
ORAL COMPLICATIONS	• Phenytoin-induced gingival hyperplasia • Fractured teeth following grand-mal seizure • Injury to lips and tongue due to biting during seizure

DENTAL MANAGEMENT	• Prevent occurrence of generalized tonic-clonic seizure by decreasing psychotic stress and apprehension, fatigue, flashing lights and noises • Maintain optimal oral hygiene because plaque and gingivitis are complicating factors to phenytoin-induced gingival overgrowth • Surgical reduction of gingival hyperplasia, if indicated
ANTICONVULSANT MEDICATIONS	• Phenytoin dilantin • Carbemazepine (Tegretol)—drug interation with propoxphene and erythromycin • Phenobarbital (Luminal) • Valproic acid—drug interaction with aspirin and NSAIDs

STROKE

Result of focal necrosis of brain caused by chronic cerebrovascular disease

PREDISPOSING FACTORS	• Atherosclerosis • Hypertension • Smoking • Cardiovascular disease • Diabetes mellitus
SIGNS AND SYMPTOMS	• Transient ischemic attack (TIA)—small strokes that last only a few minutes with no damage as a result of the attack • Sudden and temporary weakness or numbness on one side of the body • Temporary loss of speech • Temporary loss of vision, usually in one eye • Dizziness, unsteadiness, sudden falls
DENTAL MANAGEMENT	• Short appointment • Bleeding tendencies due to anticoagulant medications

Patients with Adrenal Insufficiency

Hypofunction of the adrenal cortex

ADRENAL CORTEX

Produces three adrenal steroids:

GLUCOCORTICOIDS	• Cortisol—responsible for regulation of carbohydrates, fat and protein metabolism, vascular reactivity, inhibition of inflammation, maintenance of homeostatis during physical and emotional stress • Responses to stress→hypothalamus releases corticotropin-releasing hormone (CRH)→stimulates pituitary production and secretion of adrenocorticotropic hormone (ACTH)→stimulates adrenal cortex to produce and secrete cortisol
MINERALOCORTICOIDS	Aldosterone secreted by adrenal cortex to balance extracellular and intercellular sodium and potassium
ANDROGENS	Dehydroepiandrosterone secreted by adrenal cortex; effects are the same as testicular androgens but of relatively low importance

PRIMARY ADRENOCORTICAL INSUFFICIENCY

ADDISON'S DISEASE	Progressive destruction of adrenal cortex

SECONDARY ADRENOCORTICAL INSUFFICIENCY

- Most common, resulting from administration of exogenous corticosteroids and inhibits ACTH production, resulting in partial adrenal insufficiency
- Dependant on dose and duration of administration

DENTAL TREATMENT CONCERNS

- Inability to tolerate stress
- Delayed healing
- Susceptibility to infection
- Hypertension

DENTAL MANAGEMENT

Rule of Twos
Adrenal suppression should be suspected if a patient has received a glucocorticosteroid therapy:
1. In a dose of 20 mg or more of cortisone or its equivalent daily
2. For a continuous period of 2 weeks or longer
3. Within 2 years of dental therapy

Administer exogenous glucocorticosteroids before, during, and possibly after the stressful situation, dependant upon physician evaluation
⚷ Stress reduction protocol

Patients with Thyroid Disease

HYPOTHYROIDISM

Thyroid failure usually caused by disease of the thyroid gland

PRIMARY CAUSES OF HYPOTHYROIDISM	• Autoimmune hypothyroidism • External radiation therapy • Iodine deficiency • Antithyroid drugs • Idiopathic
SECONDARY CAUSES	• Pituitary tumor • Infiltrative disease (sarcoid) of pituitary
DENTAL MANAGEMENT	• Hypothyroid coma may develop if exposed to stressful situations • Untreated patients may be sensitive to narcotics, barbiturates, and tranquilizers
ORAL COMPLICATIONS	• Increased tongue size • Delayed eruption of teeth and malocclusion

HYPERTHYROIDISM

Also called thyrotoxicosis and may progress into thyroid storm

CAUSES	• Graves' disease—toxic diffuse goiter • Toxic multinodular goiter • Toxic uninodular goiter
DENTAL MANAGEMENT	• Thyroid storm in untreated patients may be caused by infection, trauma, stress • Untreated patients are sensitive to epinephrine and other pressor amines and are an absolute contraindication • Hypertension risks in untreated patient • ⚷ Emergency protocol 　Call EMS 　Hydrocortisone (100 to 300 mg) 　CPR if needed
ORAL COMPLICATIONS	• Progressive periodontal disease • Extensive dental caries • Tumors on posterior tongue

Patients with Cancer

DENTAL MANAGEMENT

PREVENTION PROGRAM PRIOR TO CANCER THERAPY	• Plaque control • Daily fluoride therapy • Dietary instructions • Eliminate gross infection • Treat carious lesions

RADIATION TREATMENT

EFFECTS OF RADIATION ON ORAL CAVITY	• Mucositis • Candidiasis • Xerostomia • Loss of taste • Trismus • Cervical caries • Sensitivity to teeth

ORAL MANAGEMENT	<ul><li>Brushing with very soft toothbrush</li><li>Baking soda/saline rinses</li><li>Chlorhexidine rinses to reduce inflammation</li><li>Topical anesthetics rinses or ointments prior to eating for pain</li><li>Xerostomia management</li><li>Management of radiation caries that are predisposed from xerostomia (intensify prevention procedures with daily fluoride therapy)</li><li>Management of fungal infections—candidiasis is most common (treat with antifungal agent that does not contain sugar)</li></ul>

CHEMOTHERAPY

ORAL EFFECTS OF CHEMOTHERAPY	<ul><li>Mucositis</li><li>Excessive bleeding and spontaneous gingival bleeding</li><li>Xerostomia</li><li>Infection</li><li>Poor healing</li></ul>
DENTAL MANAGEMENT	<ul><li>Determine need for antibiotic coverage if granulocyte count is less than $2000/mm^3$</li><li>Control spontaneous bleeding with gauze, periodontal dressing</li><li>Topical fluoride for caries prevention</li><li>Xerostomia management</li></ul>

XEROSTOMIA MANAGEMENT

- Pilocarpine therapy, 5–10 mg
- Saliva substitutes
- Water and ice chips
- Moist food and sugarless gum
- Humidifier

Patient with HIV/AIDS

HIV

Client with HIV has a CD4+ cell count of less than 200/mm^3 or with CD4 percentage less than 14 percent of total CD4+ cell count regardless of opportunistic diseases

VIRAL DISEASE	• Virus infects host cell → replicates self → destroys cell functioning → results in cell death • New viruses released into body → process repeated → CD4+ cells destroyed → immune system malfunctions → death occurs • ☞ Review human physiology
BLOOD ASSAYS	• Evaluate various cells in the blood • Lymphocyte subset detects degree to which CD4+ T lymphocyetes are destroyed and identifies vulnerability of person developing AIDS; must examine CD4+ cell counts over time to determine immune system dysfunction

CD4+ CELL COUNTS AND MEDICAL CONDITIONS

- Healthy—CD4+ counts between 500/mm^3 to 1,500/mm^3 with average around 1000/mm^3
- Opportunistic infections like herpes simplex, herpes zoster, and candidiasis—CD4+ cell counts between 500/mm^3 to 800/mm^3
- Significant immunodeficiency like toxoplasmosis, PCP, and cryptococcal meningitis—CD4+ cell counts less than 200/mm^3
- CD4+ cell counts less than 100/mm^3 at risk of developing lymphoma, cytomegalovirus, and mycobacterium avium complex

☞ Examining CD4+ cell counts only is not an accurate method for determining disease progression; must consider CD4+ cell counts and viral loads over a period of time

VIRAL LOADS AND MEDICAL INTERVENTIONS

- Viral loads measure amount of HIV/RNA found in the blood and are good predictors of virus activity/disease progression
- Viral load—5,000 copies/mL or less; low level of viral replication; no medical intervention needed unless CD4+ count is less than 350
- Viral load—10,000 to 50,000 copies/mL; significant replication; start medical intervention regardless of CD4+ count
- ☞ Viral load—over 100,000 copies/mL; rapid deterioration; therapy needs to be initiated or changed immediately

CD4+ CELL COUNTS AND VIRAL LOAD

- Synergistic relationship between CD4+ cell counts and viral load
- High viral load correlates with low CD4+ cell counts and visa versa

Common HIV+/AIDS-Related Illnesses

MYCOBACTERIUM AVIUM COMPLEX (MAC)

Bacterial infection caused by organisms found in food, water, or dust; this infection can be life-threatening in persons with AIDS

SYMPTOMS	Fever, night sweats, abdominal pain
TREATMENT	Clarithromycin or azithromycin and ethambuto

CANDIDIASIS

Fungal infection commonly identified in the oral cavity but can spread to esophagus and sometimes stomach

SYMPTOMS	Scrapable white or red patches on tongue, palate, gingiva, difficulty swallowing and loss of appetite
TREATMENT	Fluconazole, nystatin, clotrimazole

PNEUMOCYSTIS CARNII PNEUMONIA (PCP)

Pneumonia commonly found in persons with AIDS; caused by a protozoal infection

SYMPTOMS	Fever, dry cough, weight loss, difficulty breathing
TREATMENT	Systemic Bactrim, Septra, Dapsone, or Clindamycin

CYTOMEGALOVIRUS (CMV)

This viral infection can spread to various parts of the body, i.e., eyes, stomach, lungs; CMV is a member of the herpes viruses and only becomes active once the immune system is weakened

SYMPTOMS	In the eyes—blurry vision; in the esophagus—pain, ulcers, difficulty swallowing; in the lungs—pneumonia
TREATMENT	IV or intraocular implants of ganciclovir or foscarnet; some other experimental drugs are also used

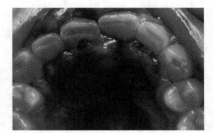

KAPOSI'S SARCOMA

This is a fatal, metastasizing, malignant vascular cancer found in 90% of all patients with AIDS

Figure 9-34

FIGURE 9-34 Kaposi's Sarcoma

SYMPTOMS	Purplish lesions found all over the body and often orally
TREATMENT	Vinblastine, chemotherapy, conventional surgery, laser surgery, or radiation

NEUROPATHY

Pathological changes in the peripheral nervous system

Nerve damage that occurs and is possibly a side effect of drugs or HIV infection

SYMPTOMS	Tingling "pins and needles" feeling in the extremities

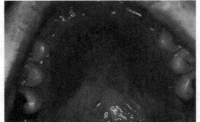

FIGURE 9-35 Candidiasis

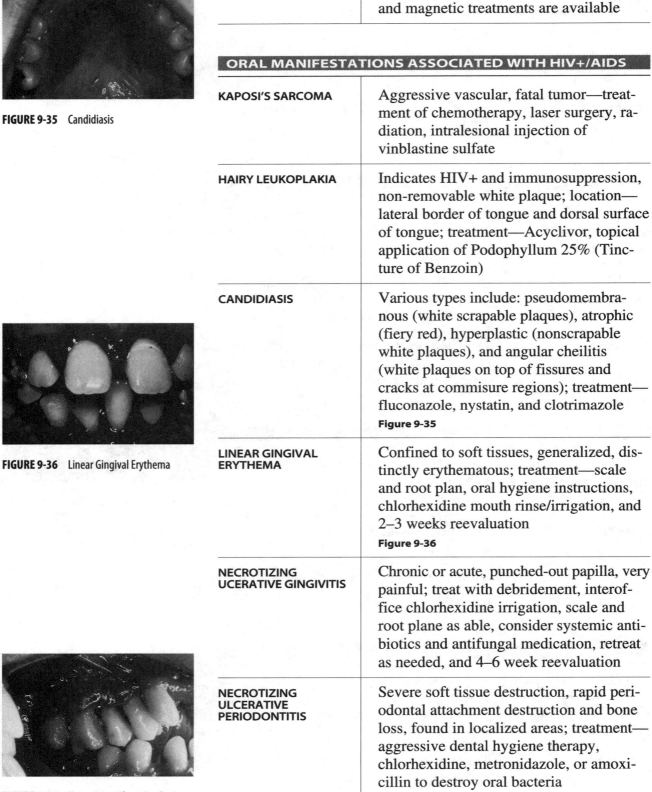

FIGURE 9-36 Linear Gingival Erythema

FIGURE 9-37 Necrotizing Ulcerative Periodontitis

TREATMENT	Currently only experimental medications and magnetic treatments are available

ORAL MANIFESTATIONS ASSOCIATED WITH HIV+/AIDS

KAPOSI'S SARCOMA	Aggressive vascular, fatal tumor—treatment of chemotherapy, laser surgery, radiation, intralesional injection of vinblastine sulfate
HAIRY LEUKOPLAKIA	Indicates HIV+ and immunosuppression, non-removable white plaque; location—lateral border of tongue and dorsal surface of tongue; treatment—Acyclivor, topical application of Podophyllum 25% (Tincture of Benzoin)
CANDIDIASIS	Various types include: pseudomembranous (white scrapable plaques), atrophic (fiery red), hyperplastic (nonscrapable white plaques), and angular cheilitis (white plaques on top of fissures and cracks at commisure regions); treatment—fluconazole, nystatin, and clotrimazole **Figure 9-35**
LINEAR GINGIVAL ERYTHEMA	Confined to soft tissues, generalized, distinctly erythematous; treatment—scale and root plan, oral hygiene instructions, chlorhexidine mouth rinse/irrigation, and 2–3 weeks reevaluation **Figure 9-36**
NECROTIZING UCERATIVE GINGIVITIS	Chronic or acute, punched-out papilla, very painful; treat with debridement, interoffice chlorhexidine irrigation, scale and root plane as able, consider systemic antibiotics and antifungal medication, retreat as needed, and 4–6 week reevaluation
NECROTIZING ULCERATIVE PERIODONTITIS	Severe soft tissue destruction, rapid periodontal attachment destruction and bone loss, found in localized areas; treatment—aggressive dental hygiene therapy, chlorhexidine, metronidazole, or amoxicillin to destroy oral bacteria **Figure 9-37**

Side Effects of Commonly Prescribed Antiretroviral Medications

NUCLEOSIDE ANALOGUE REVERSE TRANSCRIPTASE INHIBITORS	
VIDEX (ddI)	Xerostomia, candidiasis, peripheral neuropathy
ZERIT (d4T)	Peripheral neuropathy, neutropenia, and thrombocytopenia
COMBIVIR (AZT AND 3TC)	GI upset and peripheral neuropathy
EPIVIR (3TC)	GI upset and peripheral neuropathy
HIVID (ddC)	Hypertension, renal failure, GI upset, and peripheral neuropathy
RETONIVIR (AZT, ZDV)	Granulocytopenia, anemia, and GI upset
ZIAGEN (ABCAVIR SULFATE)	Renal failure and GI upset

PROTEASE INHIBITORS	
AGENERASE (AMPRENAVIR)	Anemia, parasthesia, GI upset, diabetes mellitus, and several drug interactions, specifically with Abacavir
CRIXIVAN (INDINAVIR SULFATE)	Anemia, GI upset, diabetes mellitus, renal insufficiency; patients should avoid nonsteroidal anti-inflammatory drugs
FORTOVASE (SAQUINAVIR)	Cardiovascular problems, thrombocytopenia, pancytopenia, anemia, GI upset, peripheral neuropathy, diabetes mellitus, and several drug interactions, specifically with clindamycin
INVIRASE (SAQUINAVIR MESYLATE)	Thrombocytopenia, pancytopenia, and GI upset
NORVIR (RITONAVIR)	Cardiovascular problems, thrombocytopenia, leukopenia, peripheral neuropathy, increased bleeding problems, and parasthesias
VIRACEPT (NELFINAVIR MESYLATE)	Anemia, GI upset, peripheral neuropathy, neutropenia, leukopenia, and increased bleeding

NON-NUCLEOSIDE REVERSE TRANSCRIPTASE INHIBITORS	
RESCRIPTOR (DELVIRDINE MESYLATE)	Anemia, GI upset, thrombocytopenia, neutropenia, skin rashes, drug interactions with Amprenavir, Fluconazole, and Indinavir
SUSTIVA (EFAVINEZ)	Cardiovascular problems, GI upset, skin rashes, drug interactions with Amprenavir, Azithromycin, Fluconazole, Indinavir, Nelfinavir, Ritonavir, Saqunavir, and Zidovudine
VIRAMUNE (NEVIRAPINE)	Decreased hemoglobin, platelets, neutrophils, life-threatening hepatotoxicity, toxic epidermal necrolysis, fever, drug interactions with Amprenavir, Erythromycin, Indinavir, Nelfinavir, Ritonavir, Saqunavir, and Zidovudine

Reviewing a Patient's CBC Results

IMPORTANT BLOOD COMPONENTS	
PLATELETS	These cells initiate blood clotting ☛ Low reading indicates increased risk of bleeding ☛ A count of less than 50,000/mcl requires information on partial thromboplastin time (PTT) and prothrombin time (PT)
HEMOGLOBIN (Hb OR Hgb)	These are red blood cells carrying oxygen ☛ Low reading indicates anemia
HEMATOCRIT (HCT)	Another way of measuring hemoglobin in blood ☛ Low reading indicates anemia
WHITE BLOOD CELL COUNT (WBC)	These cells fight off infection ☛ High reading indicates infection
RED BLOOD CELL COUNT (RBC)	These cells carry oxygen to body organs ☛ Low reading indicates anemia
ABSOLUTE NEUTROPHILS (AB NTS)	• White blood cells • Increased neutrophil reading indicates bacterial infections, haemorrhagia, inflammation, and leukemia

	• Low neutrophils reading indicate viral infections, TB, and typhoid; medications like Carbimazole and Sulphonamides can cause lower than normal reading in neutrophils ☞ If this reading is below 500, the patient will need to be premedicated with antibiotics
ABSOLUTE LYMPHOCYTES	• These cells fight off infection and destroy microorganisms • Increased lymphocyte reading indicates viral infections • Low lymphocyte reading seen in AIDS, steroid therapy, post-chemotherapy, or radiotherapy
ABSOLUTE EOSINOPHILS	Another type of white blood cells; increased reading indicates asthma, parasitic infections, allergic disorders, restrictive cardiomyopathy, and neuropathy
ABSOLUTE MONOCYTES	Part of white blood cells; increased reading indicates acute and chronic infections like TB and protozoa
ABSOLUTE BASOPHILS	Part of white blood cells; increased reading indicates viral infections
CD4+ T LYMPHOCYTES AND VIRAL LOAD	Should also be examined and included as part of the CBC results; most effective way to determine health of person with HIV/AIDS is to examine a trend in CD4+ cell counts and viral loads over time

10 Performing Periodontal Procedures

Demetra Daskalos Logothetis, RDH, MS

Christine Nathe, RDH, MS

Tammy Teague, RDH, BS

➤ ETIOLOGY AND PATHOGENESIS OF PERIODONTAL DISEASES

Periodontology

DEFINITIONS	
SCALING	Instrumentation of the crown and root surfaces of the teeth to remove plaque and calculus
ORAL PROPHYLAXIS	Supra and subgingival scaling and selective polishing combined to remove plaque, calculus, and stain from teeth
ROOT PLANING	Definitive procedure designed for the removal of cementum and dentin that is rough and/or permeated by calculus, or contaminated by toxins and microorganisms
DEPLAQUING	Removal or disruption of bacterial plaque and its toxins subgingivally after debridement has been completed ☛ New concept; it is performed using curet or ultrasonic; not polishing

PERIODONTAL DEBRIDEMENT	Removal of all subgingival plaque and its by-products, clinically detectable plaque retentive factors (calculus and overhangs), detectable calculus-embedded cementum to finish the root surface during periodontal instrumentation while preserving as much of the tooth surface as possible
PERIODONTAL MAINTENANCE PROCEDURES (PMP)	An extension of periodontal therapy that involves continuing periodic assessment and preventive treatment of the periodontal structures to allow for early detection and treatment of new or recurring periodontal disease ☞ AKA maintenance therapy or supportive periodontal therapy (SPT)
ACTIVE THERAPY	Nonsurgical and/or surgical therapy
INITIAL THERAPY	First phase of treatment performed to eliminate or suppress infectious microorganisms and to establish an environment which promotes health of the periodontal tissues

PERIODONTIUM Tissues that attach the tooth to the alveolar process	
GINGIVA	Oral masticatory mucosa that covers the cervical and root portions of the teeth and alveolar process; includes marginal and attached gingiva
MARGINAL GINGIVA	Surrounds the tooth on all surfaces, forming a cuff-like band of tissue; includes the interdental gingiva (facial and lingual papilla connected between the teeth by the col)
ATTACHED GINGIVA	Gingiva that is attached to the cementum of the tooth and to the underlying periosteum of the alveolar processes; it extends from the base of the gingival sulcus to the mucogingival junction ☞ Generally it is widest at the maxillary premolar area and narrowest in mandibular premolar area
LAMINA PROPRIA	The connective tissue of the gingiva composed of gingival connective tissue fibers and intercellular ground substance

GINGIVAL FIBERS

Provide support for the junctional epithelium by providing reinforcement of the gingiva to the tooth

CIRCULAR OR CIRCUMFERENTIAL FIBERS	Encircle each tooth in a cuff within the marginal gingival
DENTOGINGIVAL FIBERS	Embed into the cementum apical to the junctional epithelium and fan out into the marginal and attached gingiva
DENTOPERIOSTIAL FIBERS	Embed into the cementum apical to the junctional epithelium and extend apically over the alveolar crest, pass through the periosteum, and terminate in alveolar bone
TRANSEPTAL FIBERS	Embed in cementum apical to the junctional epithelium and run horizontally between the roots of adjacent teeth
ALVEOLOGINGIVAL FIBERS	Insert in the alveolar crest and splay out onto the free gingival

PERIODONTAL LIGAMENT FIBERS

Collagen fibers that embed into the cementum of the root on one side and the alveolar bone on the other; has physical, formative, nutritive, and sensory functions

SHARPEY'S FIBERS	Terminal end of periodontal ligament fibers
PRINCIPAL FIBER GROUPS	Bundles of periodontal ligament fibers, including oblique, alveolar crest, horizontal, apical, and interradicular
OBLIQUE GROUP	Extends from the alveolar bone to the cementum in an oblique direction; allows the tooth to withstand vertical masticatory stresses ☛ Largest fiber group
ALVEOLAR CREST FIBER GROUP	Extends from cementum obliquely to the alveolar crest
HORIZONTAL FIBER GROUP	Extend from cementum to bone at a right angle to the long axis on the tooth

522 ■ PROVISION OF CLINICAL DENTAL HYGIENE SERVICES

APICAL FIBER GROUP	Forms at the apex of the tooth after the complete formation of the root
INTERRADICULAR FIBER GROUP	Extends from the alveolar bone to the cementum in the furcation area of multi-rooted teeth

CEMENTUM

Calcified connective tissue that covers the root of the tooth and connects the tooth to periodontal ligament fibers

ALVEOLAR PROCESS
Bone that supports the tooth in its socket (alveoli)

ALVEOLAR BONE PROPER	Inner socket wall of compact bone; contains Sharpe's fibers of the periodontal ligament; thicker in the posterior regions; least stable of all the periodontal tissues ☞ Cribriform plate; appears radiographically as the lamina dura
ALVEOLAR CREST	The coronal rim of the alveolar bone proper; normally located 1.5–2mm apical to the CEJ
SUPPORTING ALVEOLAR BONE	Cortical plate and cancellous bone

Etiology Periodontal Disease

BACTERIAL PLAQUE FORMATION

Three stages (pellicle formation, bacterial colonization, and maturation) that forms the dense, nonmineralized, complex mass of colonies called plaque; composition of plaque differs among individuals, differs between various tooth surfaces in the same individual, and changes with age; microorganisms account for 70 to 80% of solid components of plaque; the causative factor in periodontal disease

CALCULUS FORMATION

Mineralization (crystal formation) that occurs in the inner surfaces of the supragingival bacterial plaque and in the attached component of the subgingival plaque; time interval averages 12 days for an undisturbed soft deposit to change to a mineralized form that grows by apposition of new layers; calculus deposits have an irregular surface that acts to retain bacterial plaque

Pathogenesis of Periodontal Disease

ROLE OF BACTERIAL PATHOGEN IN PERIODONTAL DISEASE

- Periodontal pathogen must be present in a virulent form to produce disease
- Periodontal disease is a mixed infection and pathogens must be present in the right combination with sufficient numbers to produce disease
- The host must be susceptible to the pathogen and the numbers of pathogens must exceed the threshold of the host
- The pathogen must be located in a site that is conducive to the virulence of the pathogen

DENTALLY RELATED RISK FACTORS FOR PERIODONTAL DISEASE

- Presence of established periodontal disease
- Missing teeth
- Mouth breathing
- Mobile teeth
- Areas of food impaction
- Poor oral hygiene

☞ Presence of established periodontal disease (2 mm or greater LOA) is the most important risk factor

SUBJECT-RELATED RISK FACTORS FOR PERIODONTAL DISEASE

- Genetics
- Gender (male)
- Race
- Tobacco use
- Chronic alcoholism
- Age
- Stress
- Diet and nutrition
- Drugs
- Systemic disease

BACTERIA ASSOCIATED WITH PERIODONTAL DISEASES

Most periodontopathogenic bacteria are gram-negative, non-motile, and anaerobic

THREE MAJOR MICROORGANISMS ASSOCIATED WITH 98% OF PERIODONTAL DISEASES	• Actinobacillus actinomycetemcomitans (Aa) • Porphyromanas gingivalis (Pg) • Prevotella intermedia (Pi)
MINOR ORGANISMS ASSOCIATED WITH PERIODONTAL DISEASE	• Camplylobacter (Wolinella) recta • Eikenella corrodens • Fusobacterium nucleatum • Spirochetes • Bacteroikes forsynthus
PERIODONTAL PATHOGEN THAT IS GRAM-POSITIVE	Eubacterium

Diseases of the Periodontium

Diagnosis and classification are based on clinical assessments

DISEASES AFFECTING THE GINGIVA (NOT INCLUDING THE SUPPORTING STRUCTURES)

GINGIVITIS	Inflammatory gingival lesion caused by bacterial plaque
CHRONIC GINGIVITIS	Inflammation and tissue destruction confined to the gingival; characterized by redness, gingival bleeding, changes in contour, edema, enlargement, loss of tissue tone, and increase in gingival crevicular fluid; plaque is etiologic factor ☛ Most common form of all periodontal diseases; often asymptomatic
NECROTIZING ULCERATIVE GINGIVITIS (NUG)	Condition characterized by craterlike depressions at the crest of the interdental papilla; severe inflammation usually confined to the marginal gingival; gingival bleeding, necrosis and pain in the papilla; may also include fever, gray-yellow pseudomembrane, malaise, and foul breath; etiology is unknown but poor oral hygiene and a systemically compromised

	host are present; risk factors include stress, poor diet, and smoking
	☛ Provotella intermedia and spirochetes are bacteria commonly associated with NUG
GINGIVITIS ASSOCIATED WITH SYSTEMIC DISEASE	Gingivitis associated with systemic diseases that affect the host response and/or immunosuppressive conditions; examples include leukemia, Addison's disease, diabetes, hemophilia, thrombocytopenia, and Sturge-Weber syndrome
SCORBUTIC GINGIVITIS	Gingivitis associated with severe ascorbic acid deficiencies in patients with scurvy
GINGIVITIS ASSOCIATED WITH HORMONAL CHANGES	Redness, gingival inflammation, edema, and bleeding that results from an exaggerated response to bacterial plaque; may occur due to pregnancy, puberty, menstruation, steroid therapy, or birth control medication

DISEASES OF THE PERIODONTIUM (GINGIVAL AND SUPPORTING STRUCTURES)

All periodontitis is preceded by gingivitis, but not all gingivitis becomes periodontitis

PERIODONTITIS

Diseases of the periodontium characterized by a loss of the connective tissue and alveolar structures (loss of attachment) with the apical migration of the junctional epithelium; results from a host response to microbial plaque
☛ 98% have Aa, Pg, and Pi bacteria

CHRONIC PERIODONTITIS

Most common form of periodontitis, characterized by periodontal pockets, bone loss, and eventually tooth mobility; bone loss is usually bilateral with the interdental bone affected more than buccal and lingual; progression is slow and host response is normal; usually not clinically evident until mid-30s; characterized as early, moderate, or advanced
☛ 90% of patients have Pg bacteria present
☛ 95% of patients have Pi bacteria present

AGGRESSIVE PERIODONTITIS

Aggressive forms of periodontitis associated with rapid progression and abnormalities is neutrophil function, early age of onset; includes prepubertal, juvenile, and rapidly progressive

PREPUBERTAL PERIODONTITIS	Severe gingival inflammation, rapid loss of alveolar bone, mobility, and tooth loss that affects the primary or mixed dentition soon after the eruption of the primary teeth; may be localized or generalized ☛ Associated with leukocyte adherence deficiency and immune diseases
JUVENILE PERIODONTITIS	Severe rapid bone loss that begins in the first molars and incisors that affects the permanent dentition in otherwise healthy adolescents, often as a depressed neutrophil chemotaxis; little or no plaque, calculus, and inflammation present; may be localized to incisors and molars or include the entire dentition ☛ 98% of patients have Aa bacteria present; Pg, Pi, and Capnocytophagia sp. also present; Eikenella corrodens is present in generalized juvenile periodontitis
RAPIDLY PROGRESSIVE PERIODONTITIS (RPP)	Severe rapid bone loss that begins as a young adult; patient may have a neutrophil defect, very similar to localized juvenile periodontitis ☛ Aa, Pg, Pi, E. corrodens, and Campylobacter rectus are associated with RPP
REFRACTORY PERIODONTITIS	Aggressive form of periodontitis that occurs in multiple sites in patients who continue to demonstrate loss of attachment despite apparently appropriate treatment ☛ Aa, Pg, Pi, E. corrodens, Peptostreptococcus, and F. nucleatum may be present

PERIODONTITIS ASSOCIATED WITH SYSTEMIC DISEASES

Loss of clinical attachment associated with systemic conditions such as neutrophil disorders, immunodeficiencies, and blood dyscrasias
☛ Type I diabetes has Capnocytophagia; Type II diabetes has Camplobacter recta associated with it

NECROTIZING PERIODONTAL DISEASES

Ulceration and necrosis and ulceration of the gingival that results in necrosis and exposure of the alveolar bone; very painful
☛ AKA Vincent's infection; Pi and intermediate spirochetes are associated with NUP

➤ PERIODONTAL DEBRIDEMENT

Periodontal Instruments and Instrumentation

A variety of instruments can be used for scaling and root planing including curets, sickles, hoes, files, chisels, and ultrasonic

CURETS

- Blade has two cutting edges, a face, a back, a toe or tip, and two lateral surfaces
- Curets may vary in handle size, shank length, angulation, strength, and blade angulation and size; two types are universal and area specific
- Scaling should be done by adapting the lower 1/3 of the instrument, inserted subgingivally by closing the blade (face toward the tooth at 0 degree), and the angle between the face of the blade and the tooth surface should be between 45 and 90 degrees

Figures 10-1 and 10-2

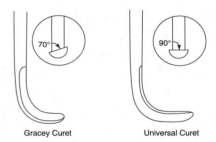
Gracey Curet   Universal Curet

FIGURE 10-1 Blade Angulation of Gracey and Universal Curets

UNIVERSAL CURETS	• One instrument is designed to adapt to all tooth surfaces • Both cutting edges of the blade are used • Blade is angulated so that the face of the blade is 90 degrees to lower shank of the instrument • Blade is curved only in one plane
AREA-SPECIFIC CURETS (GRACEY)	• Only one cutting edge on each blade is used • The blade is "offset" at 70 degrees • Blade is curved in two planes (toe curves up and to side) • When looking down at the face of the blade the larger outer curve is the correct cutting edge (the lower shank should be parallel to the surface to be scaled with the toe pointing in the mesial direction)

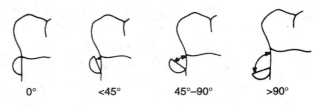

0°   <45°   45°–90°   >90°

FIGURE 10-2

GRACEY 1–2 GRACEY 3–4	Area-specific for the anterior teeth
GRACEY 5–6	Area-specific for anterior and bicuspid teeth
GRACEY 7–8 GRACEY 9–10	Area-specific for posterior buccal and lingual surfaces
GRACEY 11–12	Area-specific for posterior mesial surfaces
GRACEY 13–14	Area-specific for posterior distal surfaces

INSTRUMENTS MODIFIED FOR PERIODONTAL PATIENTS

AFTER FIVE CURETS	Modified Gracey curets that have a 3mm longer terminal shank and thinner blade—they allow extension into deeper pockets
MINI FIVE CURETS	Modified Gracey after five curets that features half the blade length of the after five or standard Gracey—they allow for easier insertion and adaptation in deep, narrow areas
LANGER CURETS	Combination of the shank design of the Gracey's with the 90-degree blade angulation of the universal—a set of three curets, which allows adaptation to the mesial and distal surfaces of the tooth without changing instruments

SICKLES

Two straight cutting edges, formed by the junction of the face and a flat side; sides join to form the sharp, pointed back of the instrument; not good for subgingival calculus removal, used only for supragingival calculus

Principles of Instrumentation

- Pressure on the fulcrum finger and pressure on the instrument blade are the same.
- Keep the fulcrum finger and middle finger together.
- Fulcrum must be close to the working area so lower shank is parallel to surface.
- Handle and shank of instrument should rest on side of middle finger for lateral pressure.
- Thumb should be parallel with curet blade to give direct pressure.
- Index finger should be bent at first knuckle and cocked back on handle of instrument for better pressure.
- Middle finger should be slightly bent at the first knuckle.
- Keep middle and index finger together.
- Handle on instrument should be parallel to the long axis of the tooth.
- Most effective strokes combine wrist motion and finger-flexing motion.
- Wrist motion should be combined with lateral pressure.
- Handle should be positioned on the middle of the thumb pad.
- Readjust the pressure on index finger when rolling instrument
- Pivot on fulcrum while rotating the instrument in your finger when scaling line angles.
- Grasp should be spread out on instrument.

ANTERIOR SICKLE	Two types of sickles—straight and curved; the blade, shank, and handle are in the same plane; a pull stroke is used with a blade angulation of less than 90 but more than 45 degree
POSTERIOR SICKLE	The shank has a contra-angle bend so the blade, shank, and handle are not in the same plane and the instrument can be adapted to posterior teeth, pull stroke is used with a blade angulation less than 90 but more than 45 degrees

HOES
Figure 10-3

- The junction of the face and the beveled toe forms bulky scaler with a single straight cutting edge that can break up large calculus pieces
- Paired instruments that have specific working ends for the buccal, lingual, mesial, and distal
- The blade is thick and lacks adaptability and tactile sensitivity, which limits its use subgingivally; use with a vertical pull stroke

FIGURE 10-3 Hoe

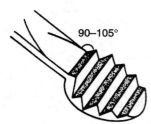

90–105°

FIGURE 10-4   File

- Instrument with multiple cutting edges on a base used to crush or fracture very heavy, tenacious calculus
- Lacks adaptability and tactile sensitivity, thus limiting its subgingival usefulness
- A set of four working ends (one for each area of the tooth) and a pull stroke with a stabilized instrument should be used

Instruments for Periodontal Assessment

PROBE

Only consistently reliable means of detecting pockets, measuring their depth, and determining their shape; vary in design may be flat, round, or oval and also in markings

MARQUIS PROBE	Color-coded by alternating bands that mark 3, 6, 9, and 12 mm; good working end but care must be taken when estimating the mm readings between the markings
WILLIAMS PROBE	Markings are at 1, 2, 3, 5, 7, 8, 9, and 10; working end is sometimes too thick to allow easy insertion
MICHIGAN-O PROBE	Markings are at 3, 6, and 8 mm or may be obtained with Williams's markings; working end is very thin
#2 NABERS PROBE	Has curved, noncalibrated-working ends designed for examination of furcations

EXPLORERS (USED FOR CALCULUS DETECTION) Figure 10-5

Most sensitive instrument, used for detection calculus before, during, and after instrumentation; they come in a variety of shapes and sizes

HU-FRIEDY #3-A	Used for detection of calculus and caries; has a long, curved working end that allows for detection in deep pockets and furcations Figure 10-5 A

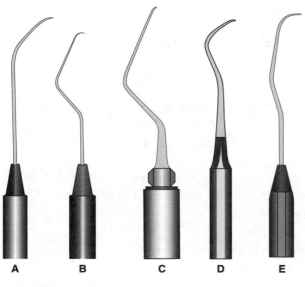

FIGURE 10-5   Explorers

#17 EXPLORER	Used for calculus; has a fine 2-mm tip that is at right angle to the shank; good adaptation is very important **Figure 10-5 B**
PIG-TAILED OR COW-HORN EXPLORERS	Pair and always double ended, the curved, thin tip is easily adapted to most surfaces, but does not extend into deep area; good for children and adults with minimal sulcus depth **Figure 10-5 D**
O.D.U. #11/12	• Paired, double-ended explorer with the shank design adapted from the Gracey 11/12 • Excellent for posterior mesial, buccal, and lingual surfaces and anteriors • Limitations when used in pockets deeper than 4 or 5 mm and on posterior distal line angles **Figure 10-5 E**

Instrument Sharpening

Objective is to produce a sharp cutting edge without changing the original design of the instrument

PRINCIPLES OF SHARPENING

1. Choose an appropriate stone (shape and abrasiveness)
2. Sterilize stone
3. Establish proper angulation between the stone and instrument
4. Maintain a stable, firm grasp of stone and instrument
5. Avoid excessive pressure
6. Avoid formation of a wire edge
7. Lubricate stone during sharpening
8. Sharpen at first sign of dullness

SHARP INSTRUMENTS	The junction of the lateral surface and the face of the blade is a fine line running the length of the instrument that will not reflect light; it will cleanly shave off deposits with less pressure
DULL INSTRUMENTS	Has a rounded surface on the cutting edge, which will reflect light; appears as a white line running the length of the cutting edge; tactile sensitivity is decreased, calculus is burnished, and operator fatigue and heavy handedness result
LUBRICATION OF STONES	Minimizes clogging of the abrasive surface with metal particles ⚷ Examples: oil or water
WIRE EDGE	Small, thin, roughened filaments of metal projecting from the cutting edge, which occurs during sharpening; avoided by finishing sharpening on a down stroke

TYPES OF STONES

May or may not be natural but the surface of the stone is made up of abrasive particles that are harder than the metal of the instrument

UNMOUNTED STONES

Come in a variety of sizes and shapes; instrument is held stabilized and the stone is drawn across it or stone is stabilized and the instrument is drawn across it

CARBORANDUM AND RUBY STONE	Course, artificial stone; lubricate with water
INDIA STONE	Fine artificial stone found in fine or medium abrasiveness; lubricate with oil
ARKANSAS OILSTONE	Natural stone with fine abrasiveness; lubricate with oil

MOUNTED ROTARY STONES

Stones mounted on a metal mandrel and used in a motor-driven handpiece; cylindrical, cone, or disc shaped; they tend to wear down the instrument very quickly and generate frictional heat that may damage the instrument

SHARPENING UNIVERSAL CURETS

- Angle between the face of the blade and the lateral surface is 70 to 80 degrees
- Angle between the face of the blade and surface of the stone should be at 100 to 110 degrees
- Start at shank end of the cutting edge and work toward the toe using consistent, light pressure
- Maintain 100- to 110-degree angulation and keep instrument in continuous contact with stone; sharpen both cutting edges

SHARPENING GRACEY CURETS

- Angle between the face and the lateral surface of the blade is 70 to 80 degrees
- Angle between the face of the blade and the stone will be 100 to 110 degrees
- Identify the correct cutting edge; sharpen with short up and down strokes from the shank end of the blade to the toe ending on a down stroke, to prevent wire edge; preserve the curvature of the blade of the cutting edge

SHARPENING SICKLES

- Angle between the face of the blade and the lateral surface is 70 to 80 degrees
- Angle between the face of the blade and stone will be 100 to 110 degrees
- The lateral surface is usually flat and the entire cutting edge will contact the stone; use consistent, light pressure and keep the stone in continuous contact with the instrument

Powered Instruments

MECHANISMS

ULTRASONIC AND SONIC INSTRUMENTS	Work by converting high frequency electrical current into mechanical vibrations ☞ Ultrasonic instruments work at 20,000 to 50,000 Hz (cycles per second) and not audible, while sonic instruments are audible and are usually at ranges close to 7,000 Hz (cycles per second) **Figure 10-6**

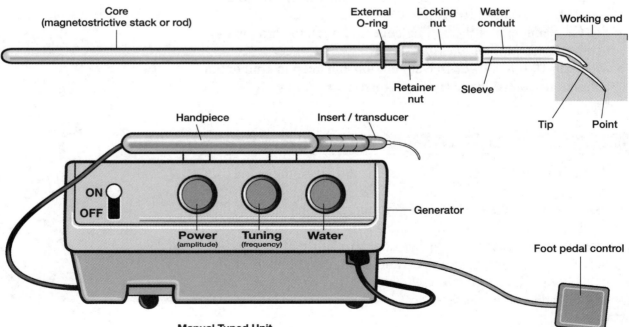

Manual Tuned Unit

FIGURE 10-6 Parts of Ultrasonic Unit

CAVITATION	• Created by vibrations and water ☞ Water helps cool handpiece • Works by removing plaque, LPS, and calculus and removes pathogenic materials without excessive removal of cementum • Gram – bacteria are most sensitive to cavitation and gram + bacteria are more resistant to cavitation ☞ Bacterial endotoxins are removed • Cavitation reaches the base of the pocket much easier than hand instruments

Types of Ultrasonics

MAGNETOSTRICTIVE Figure 10-7

- Flat metal strips or ferromagnetic rod, transducer connect to tip, coil contained within handpiece, which becomes magnetized, causing expanding and contracting currents
- Elliptical/orbital vibrations
☞ All sides work in magnetostrictive ultrasonic tips
- Power dial controls amplitude
☞ Amplitude is the area (range) of the vibration; high power would result in large elliptical movements, whereas low power would result in smaller elliptical movements; when using subgingivally, low power would be preferred
- Tuning dial controls frequency
☞ Some units are auto-tuned; tuning gives you the option to increase the vibrations even when utilizing low power

PIEZOELECTRIC

- Contained within handpiece, alternating electrical current applied to reactive crystals, dimensional change transmitted to tip
- Linear vibrations
☞ Not recommended for use subgingivally

SONIC

Vibrated at a lower frequency, and powered by air
☞ Not recommended for use subgingivally

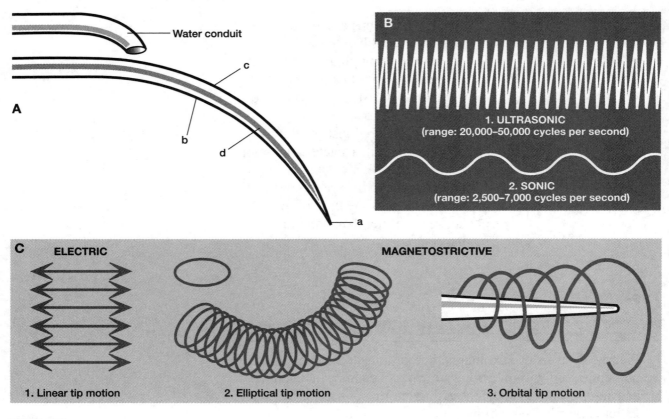

FIGURE 10-7

ULTRASONIC USE	
ADVANTAGES	• Patient comfort ☛ No anesthesia is usually needed • Less bleeding ☛ Visibility is improved • Able to debride in deep pockets and furcations **Figure 10-8** • Removal of less cementum than hand instruments ☛ Promotes healing • Smoother finish than hand instruments • More time efficient ☛ Less fatiguing to hygienist • Increased tactile sense of pocket topography ☛ Amalgam overhang removal
DISADVANTAGES	• Not able to be used with noncontained pacemakers • More difficult to master than hand instruments

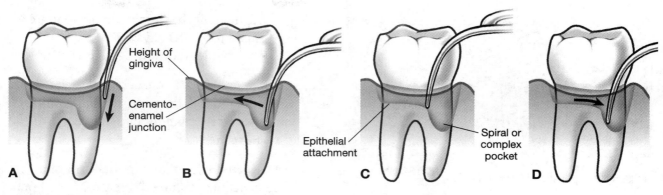

FIGURE 10-8   Using Ultrasonic Tip to Debride in Deep Pocket

☛ Increased risk of damage to patient
• Suction is mandatory

Supportive Treatment Procedures

Therapeutic intervention that augment debridement for the control of periodontal diseases and maintenance of periodontal health including the use of chemical agents and different methods of delivery, desensitization, overhang removal, care of dental implants

ANTIMICROBIAL THERAPY

Use of specific agents for the control or destruction of microorganisms, either systemically or at specific sites

SYSTEMIC ADMINISTRATION

Administration of antibiotics to control infection

LOCAL DELIVERY

Medication is concentrated at site of infection

TETRACYCLINE FIBER	• 12.7 mg tetracycline hydrochloride maintained over 10-day period • Controlled delivery • Contraindications—pregnant or breast-feeding women, allergic to tetracycline, immunocompromised patient (infection related to overgrowth of candida) Figure 10-9

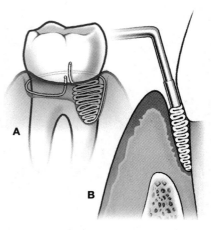

FIGURE 10-9   Application of Tetracycline Fiber

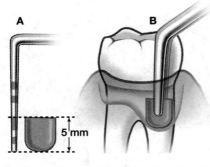

FIGURE 10-10 Application of Chlorhexidine Chip

CHLORHEXIDINE CHIP	• 2.5 mg chlorhexidine gluconate maintained for 7–10 days • Chip biodegrades in 7–10 days **Figure 10-10**
DOXYCYCLINIC POLYMER	Biodegradable liquid form that solidifies; delivered by cannula into pocket **Figure 10-11**
METRONIDAZOLE GEL	Delivered by cannula in the form of a suspension; sustained release 24–36 hours

DESENSITIZATION

TOOTH DESENSITIZATION	Sensitivity to cold, hot, or sweets may follow scaling and root planing, especially if dentin is exposed ☞ Most important factor in hypersensitivity control is plaque control
DESENSITIZING AGENTS	Mechanism of action is unknown but probably results due to: • Denaturing of organic material at the exposed end of the odontoblastic processes

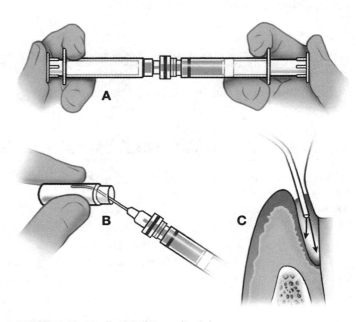

FIGURE 10-11 Applicatino of Doxycycline Polymer

- Deposition of an inorganic salt at the exposed end of the dentinal tubules
- Stimulation of secondary dentin formation within the pulp
- Suppression of inflammation within the pulp

PATIENT-APPLIED DESENSITIZING AGENTS	Patients may use a dentifrice (containing potassium nitrate, strontium chloride, or sodium citrate) or a prescription fluoride dentifrice, rinse, or gel at home; results are acquired after repeated use ⚷ Examples: Denquel and Sensodyne; advise patients not to eat, drink, or rinse for 30 minutes after use
PROFESSIONALLY APPLIED AGENTS	Most common agent is fluoride ⚷ Examples: 2 to 4% sodium fluoride, 0.9% saturated silicofluoride, and 8% stannous fluoride

PERIODONTAL DRESSINGS

Substance applied to cover gingival wounds during healing, which provides patient comfort by protecting the healing wound
⚷ Example: Coe Pak

PERIODONTAL DRESSING PLACEMENT	• Most dressings are activated by mixing two equal amounts of material (zinc oxide and resins with fatty acids) • Lubricate fingers and roll mixture into the length needed to cover the surgical site, dry the site, and place dressing at the gingival margin over the surgical site; use finger pressure to adapt the material and press it interproximally, trim the dressing around each tooth so it follows the CEJ and does not interfere with occlusion; advise patients to not brush the dressing or eat course foods that may dislodge it; they should rinse with salt water to remove debris; patient should not worry if small parts of the dressing come off but should return if all of the dressing comes off in the first day or two or if they are having discomfort **Figure 10-12**

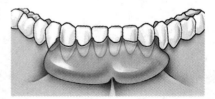

FIGURE 10-12 Placement of Periodontal Dressing

PERIODONTAL DRESSING REMOVAL	Gently insert a curet or cotton pliers under the border of dressing and pry it away from the teeth (watch for sutures) and use a curet to remove any attached pieces of dressing, debride soft tissue with a cotton swab soaked in hydrogen peroxide, and have patient rinse with warm water

SUTURE REMOVAL

Periodontal dressings should be removed and the teeth, tissue, and sutures cleansed before removing the sutures; there are two types: interrupted and continuous

REMOVAL OF INTERRUPTED SUTURES	• Placement is from facial to lingual in a single interproximal space • Removal is done by locating the knot with cotton pliers and the suture is cut between the knot and the tissue • Grasp the knot with cotton pliers and gently pull the suture out of the tissue
REMOVAL OF CONTINUOUS SUTURES	• Continuous sutures are placed from facial to lingual in an interproximal space and continued around the adjacent tooth to the next interproximal space • Removal is accomplished by cutting the suture between the knot and the tissue and the vertical loops of suture material, where it enters the tissue in each interproximal space, facial and lingual • Using cotton pliers, withdraw each strand by pulling on the portion that is wrapped around the buccal and lingual surface of each tooth

➤ REASSESSMENT AND MAINTENANCE

PERIODONTAL TREATMENT

4–6 weeks following the therapeutic appointment

STEPS FOR REEVALUATION	• Visually examine the gingiva • Remeasure pocket depths and compute loss of attachment, reevaluate bleeding points, compare pre-op and post-op scores

	• Evaluate patient's home care • Check for retained calculus
APPROPRIATE RETREATMENT OPTIONS	• Consider chemotherapeutic agents • Consider curettage • Consider refractory periodontitis • Consider referral for periodontal surgery

IMPLANT CARE

IMPLANT PLAQUE	Same as natural teeth, and must be cleaned around posts and surrounding tissues
CLEANING DEVICES	Floss threaders, gauze strips, yarn, tuffed floss
RINSING AND IRRIGATION	Irrigation with an approved antimicrobial before brushing ☛ Chlorhexidine 0.12% has been shown to be effective
FREQUENCY OF APPOINTMENTS	1–2 month intervals during the first year
DENTAL HYGIENE INSTRUMENTATION	• Calculus removal—plastic instruments are indicated for titanium • Do not use ultrasonic scaler • Professional subgingival irrigation is indicated
PATIENT EDUCATION	• Importance for daily home care • Cleaning time takes longer

CHAPTER

11

Using Preventive Agents

Christine Nathe, RDH, MS

➤ FLUORIDES

Mechanisms of Action

Fluoride is an essential nutrient in the formation of teeth and bones
🔑 Fluoride is stored in the crystal lattice of fluorapatite

FLUORIDE ACQUISITION	
TOPICAL	Fluoride exposure inhibits demineralization and enhances remineralization
SYSTEMIC	Fluoride is taken in by drinking and eating food with fluoride and is made available to the developing teeth by way of the blood plasma to the tissues surrounding the tooth bud; after tooth mineralization, but before tooth eruption, fluoride deposition continues in the surface of the enamel

Toxicology

ACUTE TOXICITY

Acute refers to the rapid intake of an excess dose over a short time, such as a child eating a large quantity of toothpaste
Table 11-1

543

Table 11-1

Lethal and Safe Doses of Fluoride

A. Lethal and safe dosages of fluoride for a 70-kg adult.

Certainly Lethal Dose (CLD)

5–10 g NaF

or

32–64 mg F/kg

Safely Tolerated Dose (STD) = ¼ CLD

1.25–2.5 g NaF

or

8–16 mg F/kg

B. CLDs and STDs of fluoride for selected ages

Age (years)	Weight (lbs)	CLD (mg)	STD (mg)
2	22	320	80
4	29	422	106
6	37	538	135
8	45	655	164
10	53	771	193
12	64	931	233
14	83	1,206	301
16	92	1,338	334
18	95	1,382	346

From Heifetz, S.B. and Horowitz, H.S. The Amounts of Fluoride in Current Fluoride Therapies: Safety Considerations for Children, *ASDC J. Dent. Child.*, 51, 257. July–August, 1984.

TREATMENT OF ACUTE TOXICITY	• Call 911 • Induce vomiting • Administer milk or lime water
SYMPTOMS MAY INCLUDE	• Nausea, vomiting, diarrhea • Abdominal pain • Increased salivation, thirst

CHRONIC TOXICITY

- Dental fluorosis can occur from too much systemic fluoride
- Patients with dental fluorosis generally have a low risk of dental caries
- ☞ It is the form of enamel hypomineralization due to excessive ingestion of fluoride during the development of the teeth; may appear as a white spot or as severe browning of tooth and may include pitting of the surface; skeletal fluorosis may include isolated instance of osteosclerosis

DEFLUORIDATION

- The process of removing naturally occurring fluoride from water supplies
- This is done when the fluoride content is well over 1 ppm
- Some fluoride will be left in water for the prevention of dental caries

Methods of Administration

WATER FLUORIDATION

The addition of fluoride in public drinking supplies

Figure 11-1

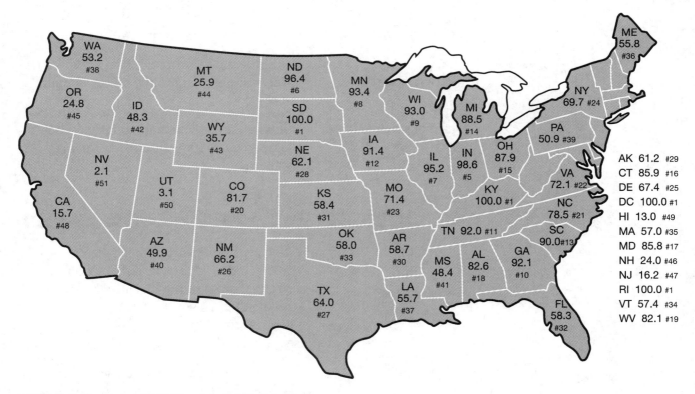

FIGURE 11-1 Fluoridation of Public Water Systems in the United States

Water fluoridation can result in as many as 40–65% fewer carious lesions

SCHOOL FLUORIDATION	• Adding fluoride to a school's water supply to decrease dental caries in the student population; data suggests 40–50% less dental caries in this population • Certain foods naturally contain fluoride, whereas some food sources contain fluoride because of the inclusion of fluoridated water; fluoridated salt has also been used

PROFESSIONALLY ADMINISTERED

FLUORIDE GELS, FOAMS	Delivered by trays or the swabbing method and mouth rinses may be administered by the dental hygienist **Table 11-2**
FLUORIDE VARNISH	Can be used to prevent caries or treat tooth sensitivity
PROPHY PASTES	Most commercial prophy pastes contain fluoride
RESTORATIVE MATERIALS	Glass ionomer cement restoratives and some sealants have fluoride-releasing properties

SELF-ADMINISTERED

FLUORIDE SUPPLEMENTS	Dietary fluoride supplements can be administered as a pill, chewable tablet, lozenge, drop, or mouth rinse for swallowing after rinsing ☛ Prescribed by the dentist **Table 11-3**
VITAMINS	Vitamins may include fluoride ☛ Prescribed by the dentist
PRESCRIPTION FLUORIDE GELS	Prescription fluoride gels can be used at home for patients at risk; patients either brush them on the teeth or place in a fluoride custom tray **Table 11-4**

Table 11-2

Professionally Applied Topical Fluorides

Agent	Form	Concentration	Mode Application	Special Notes
Sodium fluoride (NaF)	Solution 2%	9,040 ppm 090% F ion	Paint on	Cotton-roll isolation absorbs excess solution
pH = neutral	Gel 2%	9,040 ppm 0.90% F ion	Paint on or Tray	Take care not to overfill tray Request patient not to swallow
	Foam 2%	9,040 ppm 0.90% F ion	Tray	Less amount needed to fill tray Less risk of swallowing because of consistency
	Varnish 5%	22,600 ppm 2.3% F ion	Paint on	Sets promptly No risk of swallowing excess F
Acidulated phosphate fluoride (APF)	Solution 1.23%	12,300 ppm	Paint on	Cotton-roll isolation absorbs excess solution Avoid ceramic and composite resin restorations
pH = 3.0 to 3.5	Gel 1.23%	12,300 ppm	Paint on or Tray	Take care not to overfill tray Avoid ceramic and composite resin restorations
	Foam 1.23%	12,300 ppm	Tray	Smaller amount needed to fill tray; less F Avoid ceramic and composite resin restorations

Source: Wilkins, E. *Clinical Practice of the Dental Hygienist* (8th Edition). Philadelphia: Lippincott, Williams & Wilkins, 1999.

Table 11-3

Fluoride Supplements Dosage Schedule (mg F/day)*

Age of Child (years)	Water Fluoride Concentration (ppm)		
	Less than 0.3	Between 0.3 and 6	Greater than 0.6
Birth–6 mo	0	0	0
6 mo–3 yr	0.25 mg	0[†]	0[†]
3–6 yr	0.50 mg	0.25 mg	0
6–16 yr	1.0 mg	0.5 mg	0

*2.2 mg sodium fluoride provides 1 mg fluoride ions.
[†]Infants receiving their total diet from breast-feeding need a 0.25-mg supplement.
(Recommendations from the American Dental Association, Chicago, IL)

Table 11-4	
Procedures to Reduce Fluoride Ingestion during Topical Gel-Tray Application	
Patient	Seat upright
	Instruct not to swallow
	Tilt head forward with trays; tilt away from side with cotton-roll holder
Trays	Custom-made or appropriate size with absorptive liners; post-dam; border rim
	Use minimum amount of gel: 2 mL per tray, less for small tray; no more than total of 5 mL for large trays
Isolation	Use saliva ejector with maximum efficiency suction
	Cotton-roll holder technique: position for security, stability; place saliva absorber in cheek
Attention	Do not leave patient unattended
Timing	Use a timer; do not estimate
Completion	Tilt head forward for removal of tray or cotton-roll holder
	Request patient to expectorate for several minutes; do not allow swallowing
	Wipe excess gel from teeth with gauze sponge
	Use high-power suction to draw out saliva and gel
	Instruct patient not to rinse, eat, drink, or brush teeth for at least 30 minutes

Recommendations based on *Oral Health Policies for Children: Protocol for Fluoride Therapy,* American Academy of Pediatric Dentistry, 211 E. Chicago Avenue, Chicago, IL 60611.

OVER-THE-COUNTER FLUORIDE	Over-the-counter fluoride products include: • Toothpastes • Mouth rinses ☞ Most toothpaste in America contains fluoride **Figure 11-2**

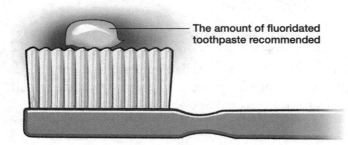

The amount of fluoridated toothpaste recommended

FIGURE 11-2 The Correct Amount of Fluoridated Toothpaste

➤ PIT AND FISSURE SEALANTS

Mechanisms of Action

DEFINITION

Dental sealant is an organic polymer that bonds to the enamel surfaces of the pit and fissures by mechanical retention
• Sealants are 100% effective in preventing pit and fissure caries when retained and remain retained in about 85% of the cases

GOALS OF SEALANT APPLICATION

- Seal off the pit or fissure surfaces
- Fill the pit and fissure as deeply as possible
- Prevent bacteria from collecting in the pit and fissure

MATERIAL

Sealant material is a polymer resin (BisGMA) that may be:
- Filled (glass or quartz particles)
- Unfilled
- Fluoride-releasing filled
• Polymerization may occur with the use of an external light source (autopolymerized) or by the inclusion of a catalyst mixed with the sealant (self-curing)

BONDING

- The etching of the surface, which produces irregularities or micropores in the enamel, completes bonding of the polymer material
- The sealant then becomes mechanically locked in the micropores, sometimes referred to as tissue tags

Techniques for Application

ASSESSMENT OF TOOTH

Teeth with no interproximal decay and deep pit and fissures
☛ Do not apply fluoride (prophy paste may contain fluoride) to pit and fissure surfaces prior to sealant application

APPLICATION PROCEDURE

POLISH	Clean occlusal surface with pumice, air polisher, or toothbrush
RINSE AND DRY	Rinse and dry tooth surface and isolate tooth by the use of cotton rolls, triangles, and/or gauze
ACID ETCH	Apply acid etch (phosphoric acid) to create micropores according to manufacturer's directions ☛ Acid etch may come in a variety of forms • Liquid, use cotton pellets to apply • Gel • Semi-gel
RINSE AND DRY	Rinse and dry tooth; isolate tooth
APPLICATION OF MATERIAL	Apply sealant by covering pits and fissures but not overfilling the surface ☛ Self-cured sealant will need to be applied after mixing sealant and catalyst; light-cured sealant will need to be applied and a light source will need to be placed on top of surface for the manufacturer's recommended time
EXAMINE SEALANT	Check sealant adhesion and occlusion adjust if necessary ☛ If sealant is placed incorrectly in the interproximal area, acid etch can be used to remove it so flossing may be accomplished
SEALANT FAILURE	If sealant has not adhered to the tooth surface, rinse and dry tooth and repeat the etching and sealant placement procedures

➤ OTHER PREVENTIVE AGENTS

ORAL APPLIANCES

ATHLETIC MOUTHGUARDS	Athletic mouthguards are utilized to prevent ora-facial trauma and concussions during athletics ⚷ Athletic mouthguards are made of thermoplastic material; can be fabricated by the dental hygienist or purchased in the sporting goods section of a store as stock guard (small, medium, and large) or boil-n-bite guard (which the patient bites while softened to indent with his/her dentition)

CUSTOM FLUORIDE TRAYS

Custom fluoride trays are made by the dental hygienist to hold fluoride for patients at high risk for dental caries
⚷ Fluoride custom trays are made of thermoplastic material

12 Providing Supportive Treatment Services

Christine Nathe, RDH, MS

➤ PROPERTIES AND MANIPULATION OF MATERIALS

DIMENSIONAL CHANGE

Change occurring in dimension of materials
☛ Sometimes refered to as microleakage or percolation

THERMAL CONDUCTIVITY

Rate of heat flow of the material
☛ Amalgam has high heat flow, whereas composites have a low rate of heat

ELECTRICAL PROPERTIES

☛ Corrosion is irreversible

CORROSION	Dissolution of metal
TARNISH	Surface discoloration ☛ Tarnish is reversible and can be removed with a finishing and polishing procedure
GALVANISM	The generation of electrical currents the patient can feel; saliva acts as an electrolyte conductor **Figure 12-1**

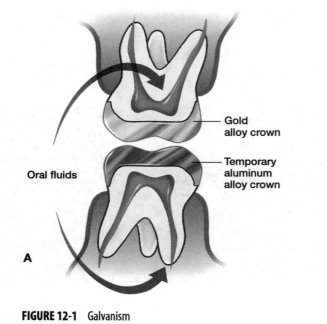

Gold
alloy crown

Temporary
aluminum
alloy crown

Oral fluids

A

Aluminum
crown

B

FIGURE 12-1 Galvanism

ADHESION

Forces of attraction between two different objects
☞ One example would be a cemented orthodontic band that falls off once the patient is at home; the cement is still attached to the band; the problem was adhesion, probably due to saliva contamination

COHESION

The forces of attraction within an object
☞ Utilizing the same scenario as above, the patient returns with cement on the band and the tooth; the problem was cohesion, probably due to the mixing of the cement

WETTABILITY

The spreading of a drop of liquid sometimes referred to as the contact angle
☞ A material that has good wettability would remain in close contact, such as sealant materials, fluoride, etc

Figure 12-2

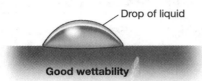

FIGURE 12-2 Wettability

STRESS

Materials' response to force

Figure 12-3

STRAIN

The change in length produced by stress
🔑 Try bending a paper clip back and forth; the permanent change caused by the constant stress is called strain

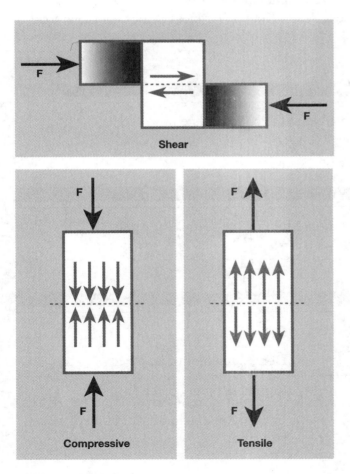

FIGURE 12-3 Types of Stress

ELASTIC MODULUS

The measure of stiffness of a material
⚷ Resistance to deformation under force

FATIGUE

Weakening of a material caused by repeated loading at a stress level below the fracture strength

CREEP

The time-dependent deformation of an object subjected to constant stress or the flow of that material

HARDNESS

Materials' resistance to indentation
⚷ Mohs Hardness Scale, Knoop Hardness Scales, and Diamond Pyramid

IMBIBITION

The taking up of fluid in the colloid system
⚷ "Swelling"

SYNERESIS

The exudation of liquid film on the surface of a gel
⚷ "Evaporation"

COLOR

⚷ Such as red, yellow, blue

HUE	Dominant color of an object
VALUE	Lightness of an object
CHROMA	Intensity or extent of saturation of a certain color

DYNAMIC PROPERTIES

- The property at extremely high rates of loading, such as an impact
- The amount of energy the materials are able to absorb
- ☛ Seen in the effects of the prevention of concussions and oral trauma due to wearing an athletic mouthguard

Manipulation of Materials

STAGES OF MANIPULATION

MIXING TIME	The time from the onset of the procedure to the completion of mixing
WORKING TIME	The time from the onset of mixing until the onset of the initial setting time
INITIAL SETTING TIME	Time at which the material is resistant to further manipulation
FINAL SETTING TIME	Time at which the material is practically set as defined by its resistance to indentation

REACTIONS

PHYSICAL	Solidifies by drying or cooling ☛ Exothermic reaction, such as the heat felt on the base when a study model is setting
CHEMICAL	Solidifies by the bonding process ☛ Polymerization reaction, such as that seen when a sealant is being polymerized by light

MATERIAL SYSTEMS

Systems by which dental materials are commonly dispensed (i.e., glass ionomer cement is prepared by mixing a powder material with a liquid material)

- Powder/liquid
- Powder/water
- Paste/paste
- Paste/light

Three different stages occur during the manipulation of dental materials

MIXING	Length of time of the mixing stage
WORKING	Length of time of the working stage
SETTING	Length of time of the setting stage

➤ POLISHING NATURAL AND RESTORED TEETH

GOALS

- Reduce chance of decay
- Easier to keep clean
- Esthetics
- Less irritation to tissues

PRINCIPLES

ABRASION	Wearing away or removal of material by the act of rubbing, cutting, or scraping
CUTTING	Removing of material by a shearing-off process
FINISHING	The process by which a restoration or appliance is contoured to remove excess material and produce a reasonably smooth surface
POLISHING	Refers to the final removal of material from a restoration or appliance to result in a smooth surface ⚷ Polishing always follows finishing

FACTORS THAT AFFECT CUTTING, FINISHING, POLISHING

HARDNESS	The hardness of abrasive as well as the hardness of the material to be abraded ⚷ Review Moh's scale: Diamond is the hardest abrasive
SHAPE	A spherical particle will be less abrasive than an irregularly cut particle **Figure 12-4**

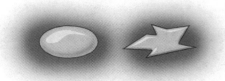

FIGURE 12-4 The Shape of Particles Affects Their Abrasiveness

SIZE	Larger particles abrade more rapidly than smaller particles ☞ Grit size of prophy paste determines coarse, medium, fine, and extra fine grit
PRESSURE	The more pressure applied, the more abrasion accomplished
SPEED	The faster the abrasive is applied, the more abrasion accomplished
LUBRICATION	Adding lubricators such as water will decrease the abrasive effect
INSTRUMENTS	Instruments with cutting edges and abrasive particles impregnated will result in abrasion

POLISHING AGENTS

PUMICE	A natural glass that is rich in silica; produced from volcanoes
POLISHING PASTE	May contain pumice, silicon dioxide or zirconium silicate and usually contains fluoride

SELECTIVE POLISHING

Selective polishing refers to the polishing of teeth only when stain cannot be removed by hand or ultrasonic instruments; only the enamel part of the tooth can be polished
☞ Evidence-based practice dictates the use of selective polishing

Polishing Restored Teeth

POLISHING AGENTS	
ALUMINUM OXIDE	Used to *smooth* enamel (after a slight fracture or chip) or finish metal alloys and ceramic materials
CARBIDES	Used to cut cavity preparations or finish composite restorations: • Silicon carbide • Boron carbide • Tungsten carbide
CHALK	Used to polish teeth, gold and amalgam restorations, and plastic materials; sometimes it is referred to as whiting or calcium carbonate
CUTTLE	A fine grade of quartz, although it was historically derived from fish bones; it is used to finish gold alloys, acrylics, and composites
DIAMOND	Used to finish and polish composite restorations, and to cut crown and bridge preparations
EMERY	Used to grind off rough areas and contour acrylic appliances and custom trays
GARNET	Used for grinding plastics and metal alloys
PUMICE	A silicate that is used to polish enamel, gold foil, and dental amalgam and to finish acrylic denture bases
ROUGE	Is red in color and is used on a rag wheel to polish gold alloys
SAND	Used to grind metals and plastics
TIN OXIDE	Used as a final polishing paste for enamel and metallic restorations
TRIPOLI	Used to polish gold alloys
ZIRCONIUM SILICATE	Used to polish enamel

Dental Restorative Materials

RESTORATIVE MATERIALS	
AMALGAM	A metal alloy with one of its elements consisting of mercury; utilized to fill cavity preparations
COMPOSITE	An esthetic restoration composed of polymers (resin) and glass particles (fillers) ☞ Composite materials can be used as: • Anterior and posterior restorations • Bonding • Veneers • Inlays
GLASS IONOMER	Dental cement utilized for class V cavity preparations; newer glass ionomer restorations release fluoride
PORCELAIN (CERAMICS)	An esthetic restoration ☞ Porcelain may be used for: • Jacket crowns • Porcelain fused to metal crowns and bridges • Veneers • Inlays and onlays • Denture teeth
GOLD	An alloy of gold and other noble (precious) metals ☞ Types of gold restorations: • Gold foil • Gold crowns and bridges
ACRYLICS	Acrylic plastics may be soft and flexible or rigid and brittle and can be used for a wide variety of applications ☞ Acrylic plastics can be used for: • Dentures and denture teeth • Denture liners • Oral appliances

Instruments and Materials Used to Polish Restorations

INSTRUMENTS	
BURS	Attached to a handpiece and can either be instruments with cutting edges or impregnated with abrasive particles
DISKS	Attached to a handpiece and impregnated with abrasive particles
POWDERS	Utilized during the polishing sequence in conjunction with a rag wheel
RAG WHEELS	Wheel with a cloth rag that is attached to the dental lathe
RUBBER CUPS, POINTS, BRUSHES	Can be attached to a prophy angle or contra angle for the purpose of polishing
STONES	Can be used to impregnate burs, disks, and strips and as an ingredient in paste
STRIPS	Impregnated strips used to finish and polish

➤ MAKING IMPRESSIONS AND PREPARING STUDY CASTS

Impression Materials

PRINCIPLES

Impressions are negative replications of the oral cavity, whether dentition or edentulous; impressions accurately record the oral cavity
- ⚷ Uses include:
  - Study models
  - Patient education
  - Baseline
  - Appliance fabrication
  - Restoration fabrication

REQUIREMENTS OF IMPRESSION MATERIAL

- Fluid enough to flow into or around area
- Must harden once positioned in the mouth

- Biocompatible
- Dimensionally stable
- Easy to handle
- Able to disinfect material

INELASTIC (RIGID)

Exhibits little or no spring-like quality when deformed; basically any significant deformation produces a permanent change in the shape; cannot be used in undercut areas

- Plaster
- Compound
- Zinc oxide eugenol—a phenol that is derived from oil of cloves

⚷ Undercut—an area that has enough of a curve (e.g., a tooth) to make it difficult for a more rigid material to not tear upon removal

Figure 12-5

ELASTIC MATERIALS

Can be removed from undercuts without undergoing any permanent distortion in shape; can be used for both dentulous and edentulous procedures

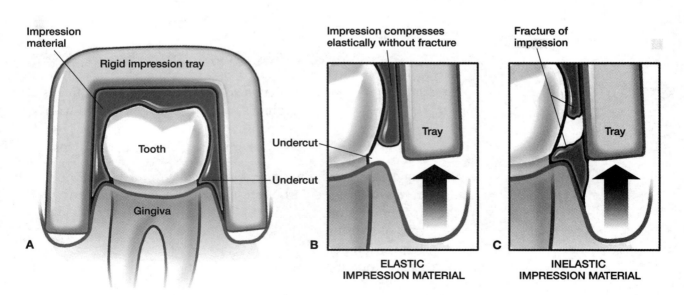

FIGURE 12-5 A) Making an Impression; B) Removing Elastic Impression Material; C) Removing Inelastic Impression Material

FLEXIBLE HYDROCOLLOIDS	• Hydrocolloids contain large amounts of water and have limited stability once they are removed from the mouth • Agar-Agar—reversible and transforms from a fluid paste to a rubber-like solid by a physical process that can be reversed simply by altering its temperature • Alginate—irreversible and supplied as a powder/water system; not as dimensionally accurate as agar, but easier to use
FLEXIBLE, ELASTOMERIC, OR RUBBER	• Polysulfide rubber • Silicone rubber (☛ sometimes referred to as condensation silicone) • Polyether rubber • Polyvinyl siloxane (☛ sometimes referred to as addition silicone)

Model and Die Material

DEFINITIONS

Models, casts, and dies are positive replications of the oral cavity

MODEL	Used for observation
CAST	Used for fabrication
DIE	A cast used for a single tooth or a few teeth

TYPES

GYPSUM	Calcium sulfate dihydrate, a rock that is ground to a powder and the mixed with water ☛ Plaster statues are made from gypsum

Gypsum can be ground into irregularly shaped, fluffy plaster or denser, regular-shaped particles for stone; the denser the particles, the stronger the stone
☛ Types of gypsum products:
• Impression plaster
• Laboratory or model stone

- Die stone
- High strength stone

ELECTROPLATING	Casts that are plated with metal to make them harder and more stable
EPOXY DIES	Epoxy resins that are toxic and not regularly used

➤ OTHER SUPPORTIVE SERVICES

Temporary Restorations

DEFINITION

Temporary restorative may be in the form of a tooth filling or a crown

🔑 Temporary restoratives are utilized to:
- Provide protection to the pulp
- Provide a palliative effect on the pulp; to be obtudant to the pulp
- Maintain tooth position
- Provide esthetic properties

MATERIALS

- Zinc oxide eugenol (ZOE)—has a palliative effect on the pulp
- MMA/PMMA filling materials
- Bisacrylic filling materials

Rubber Dams and Matrices

PRINCIPLE FOR USE

Rubber dams provide an isolated working area for restorative procedures

MATERIALS

RUBBER DAM	Rubber sheets that provide isolation; holes are cut to allow for tooth position above the rubber dam field

CLAMPS	Used to provide stability and further isolation of materials
LUBRICANT	Allows easier work with the rubber dam isolation
NAPKINS	Used occasionally for the comfort of the patient's face
RUBBER DAM HOLDERS	Used for stabilization of the rubber dam and to stretch the rubber material
MATRIX BAND	Utilized during a filling procedure to provide effective margination of the restoration

Margination

PRINCIPLES

MARGINATION	The process by which restorations are made flush with the enamel or cement surface ☞ When a gap exists between these surfaces, plaque, food debris, and saliva can pass in and out of the gap; this is referred to as percolation or micro-leakage **Figure 12-6**
OVERHANG REMOVAL	Performed when the restoration is overhanging in the interproximal area Contraindications include: • Tooth sensitivity • Recurrent decay • Defective restoration ☞ Performing margination on a restoration will: • Decrease tarnish • Decrease corrosion • Increase integrity of the junction of the tooth • Decrease recurrent decay • Improve gingival health • Improve maintenance by the patient • Increase patient comfort • Improve appearance of restoration • Maintains oral health tooth and function **Figure 12-7**

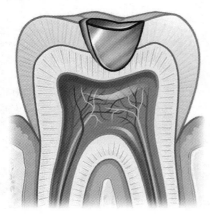

FIGURE 12-6 Gap between Tooth and Restoration

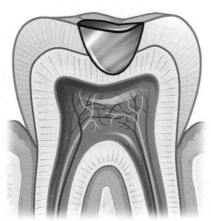

FIGURE 12-7 Margination

PROCEDURE

- A bur may be used when the restoration is grossly overhanging
- Gold knife instrument may be used
- A prophen or EVA system is a handpiece that rotates and is impregnated with diamond chips that help reduce an overhang
- Polishing should then be accomplished to further smooth the restorative material; pumice and tin oxide are generally used to polish

Debonding

PRINCIPLE

Debonding is the removal cements or any luting agent such as composite material; removal is accomplished by mechanical instrumentation and polishing to smooth the area

☛ Dental hygienists often remove excess cement from orthodontic bands upon removal

Community Health and Research Principles

➤ Promoting Health and Preventing Disease within Groups

➤ Participating in Community Programs

➤ Analyzing Scientific Literature, Understanding Statistical Concepts, and Applying Research Results

13 Promoting Health and Preventing Disease within Groups

Christine Nathe, RDH, MS

TARGET POPULATIONS

DEFINITION	A group of people with similar characteristics
CAREGIVERS	Dental hygienists must concentrate on teaching those individuals that provide care to patients ☛ These groups may include teachers, family or home health caregivers, nurses assistants, aides, etc
PERSONAL CONTACT	In order to ensure program effectiveness, it is helpful to have contact with your target population
MINORITY GROUPS	When working with programs targeted at minorities, it is helpful to have minority leaders supporting your program
SCHOOL-AGED CHILDREN	• Second- and sixth-grade classes are targeted for dental sealant programs because of the eruption dates of the first and second molars ☛ Review the eruption pattern of teeth • School fluoridation and school fluoride mouth rinse programs are targeted for children in nonfluoridated localities

SOCIOECONOMIC STATUS (SES)

Includes education, income, occupation, and culture

☞ This is used as it relates to dental health issues, for example, a low SES yields an increased risk of caries

BARRIERS TO CARE

Some populations face many obstacles when trying to access dental hygiene and dental care

Table 13-1

TEACHING STRATEGIES

HEALTH EDUCATION	The education of health behaviors that brings an individual to a state of health awareness
HEALTH PROMOTION	The informing and motivating of people on healthy behaviors
BEHAVIOR CHANGE	• When teaching a target population to adopt positive health behaviors, it is necessary to change the opinions they may have about oral health **Figure 13-1** • Behavior change will not commence until value adoption is complete • Providing dental health education to a target population does not ensure that behavior will change • Without motivation, no learning can take place

Table 13-1

Barriers to Dental Hygiene and Dental Care

Age	Language	Habit
Culture	Limited finances	Lack of faith in treatment
Education	Misunderstanding	Fear
Transportation	Values	Safety of treatment
Illiteracy	Attitudes	Denial of disease
No dental providers	Belief in invulnerability	Convenience
Social issues	Education levels	Provider conflicts

Source: Nathe, C. *Dental Public Health.* Upper Saddle River, NJ: Prentice Hall, 2000.

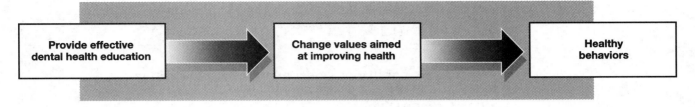

FIGURE 13-1 Goals of Dental Health Education

THEORIES	• Health Belief Model suggests that for an individual to display readiness to take action to avoid disease or to act in a preventive manner, he would need to believe he was susceptible and that the disease has serious consequences and that it is important • Stages of learning depicts an individual's natural progression from knowledge absorption to value adoption • Classical conditioning suggests that individuals become conditioned to specific stimuli to act in a specific way • Operant conditioning is based on the concepts of rewards and punishment • Modeling behavior can facilitate learning through imitation
TEACHING PRINCIPLES	• Utilize the dental hygiene process of care when planning a lesson **Table 13-2** • There are various methods of teaching to utilize when presenting information to a population **Table 13-3**
LEARNING PRINCIPLES	• Involvement of the group is necessary for learning to take place • School teachers should serve as role models during the year on positive dental health values and behaviors

Table 13-2

Lesson Plan Development

Assessment
- Assess target populations' needs, interests, and abilities
- Assess resources

Dental Hygiene Diagnosis
- Formulate findings from assessment
- Prioritize goals

Planning
- Broad goal formulation
- Specific objectives
- Select teaching method(s)

Implementation
- Be prepared
- Effective teacher characteristics

Evaluation
- Qualitative measurement
- Quantitative measurement
- Information provided to appropriate parties

Source: Nathe, C. *Dental Public Health.* Upper Saddle River, NJ: Prentice Hall, 2000.

EDUCATIONAL MATERIALS

TEACHER-PRODUCED MATERIALS	Develop materials that can be utilized for the intended target population
	☞ Types of materials:
	• Slide series
	• Overhead transparencies
	• Flip chart
	• Actual models of interventions (i.e., toothbrushes, floss, instruments, etc.)
	• Books
	• Pamphlets
	• Videotapes

Table 13-3

Teaching Methods

Lecture	Self-study
Discussion	Inquiry
Presentation	Simulation
Interaction Activities	Demonstration

Source: Nathe, C. *Dental Public Health.* Upper Saddle River, NJ: Prentice Hall, 2000.

	• CD interactive games and websites • Worksheets, puzzles, word finds, etc
PROFESSIONALLY PRODUCED MATERIALS	• Materials are developed by dental hygiene and dental organizations • Materials may be developed by dental industry • When distributing education materials, be careful to scrutinize your materials so that you are not blatantly promoting dental care products and the fact that the information is factual

PREVENTIVE MODALITIES

DENTAL HYGIENE CARE	Dental hygiene treatment—oral exam, radiographs, periodontal debridement, selective polishing, application of fluoride and sealants
FLUORIDATION	• Water fluoridation has proven cost effective • See section on Preventive Agents for more information on fluoridation • The only claim made by opponents that cannot be discredited is that fluoridation may violate human rights **Table 13-4** • Advocates of water fluoridation may find it beneficial to develop long-term strategies for adoption

Table 13-4

Water Fluoridation Oppositions

• Violation of personal freedom
• Cause of disease(s) and/or medical conditions: cancer, AIDS, fatigue, etc.
• Forced medication
• Communist plot
• An abuse of police power

Source: Nathe, C. *Dental Public Health.* Upper Saddle River, NJ: Prentice Hall, 2000.

	☞ Methods utilized to implement water fluoridation • Administrative decision, for example, mayor, city council, etc • Initiative petition and/or referendum may be employed • State legislative action
OTHER FLUORIDE MODALITIES	• School water fluoridation • School fluoride mouthrinse programs • Dietary fluoride supplements • Professional fluoride applications • Over-the-counter fluoride dentifrices, mouthrinses, impregnated floss and strips
DENTAL SEALANT	• Proven to be 85% effective in preventing pit and fissure caries • Recommended for children and young adults

Table 13-5

Types of Mouthguards

Type of Mouthguard	Description
Stock	Not custom-made Can be purchased in athletic store or discount department stores Not preferred due to poor fit and excess bulk
Mouth-formed	Referred to as "boil and bite" Comes in stock sizes, but can be heated in water and then placed in the mouth for a more exact fit Can become distorted Not definitive to dentition
Custom-made	Made in the dental office Fabricated from the patient's study model Reduces injuries because it fits better

Source: Nathe, C. Oral Appliances in Gladwin, M. and B. Bagby, *Clinical Applications of Dental Materials.* Philadelphia: Williams and Wilkins, 1999.

ORAL CANCER EXAMINATIONS	Dental hygienist or dentist provide examination to screen for oral cancer • Education targeted at signs and symptoms of oral cancer and lifestyle choices to decrease the chance of oral cancer • The implementation of tobacco cessation programs ☞ Early detection has a tremendous effect on mortality rates
ATHLETIC MOUTHGUARDS	Athletic mouthguards can be made by the dental hygienist or dentist or bought at a sporting supply store **Table 13-5** ☞ Use of athletic mouthguards prevents oral trauma and concussions
MASS EDUCATION	• Dental hygienists present information to a target population to promote dental health • Dental care product advertisements promote preventive dental health care

CHAPTER

14 Participating in Community Programs

Christine Nathe, RDH, MS

COMMUNITY PROGRAMS

COMPARISON	Comparing dental public heath with private dental practice will aid in the understanding of hygienists' roles **Table 14-1**
DENTAL PUBLIC HEALTH PROGRAM	• The dental public health paradigm utilizes the dental hygiene process of care to define program development **Table 14-2** • The dental public health program must reach a significant amount of people to be worthwhile • When initiating a dental public health program, it is necessary to first contact the head administrator for approval and support • Collaborative efforts between administration, dental hygienists, populations, caregivers, and communities are needed to ensure effectiveness

Table 14-1

A comparison of the Provision of Dental Hygiene Care for a Private Patient and for a Community

What the Dental Hygienist Does in Private Practice	What the Dental Hygienist Does in Public Health
Assessment	**Assessment**
Conducts initial health assessment by reviewing health and dental history with patient	Conducts a needs assessment of the target populations
Conducts a comprehensive oral examination	Analyzes needs of the community
Dental Hygiene Diagnosis	**Dental Hygiene Diagnosis**
Provides dental hygiene diagnosis of the patients	Provides dental hygiene diagnosis of the community
Planning	**Planning**
Develops a treatment plan based upon the diagnosis, patient interaction and the priorities and method of payment; utilizes assessment mechanisms that are measurable	Develops a program based not the analysis of needs assessment data, priorities and alternatives, community interaction, and the resources available; utilizes assessment mechanisms that are measurable
Selects appropriate health care workers to provide comprehensive care	Selects appropriate labor to implement program
Implementation	**Implementation**
Implements self-generated treatment plan effectively, changing plan when necessary	Implements self-generated treatment plan effectively, changing the plan when necessary
Evaluation	**Evaluation**
Evaluation of treatment via dental, gingival and periodontal evaluations	Evaluates program via index and community evaluations

Source: Nathe, C. *Dental Public Health.* Upper Saddle River, NJ: Prentice Hall, 2000.

Assessing Populations

NEEDS ASSESSMENT	
INDICES	Assessing the dental needs of the population via dental indexes and/or surveys
COMMUNITY PROFILE	Focus on community organization of power (local politics), leadership, facility, resources, median age, SES, etc
RESOURCES	Assessing resources, which include facilities, funding, personnel, supplies, and equipment

Table 14-2

Dental Hygiene Program Planning Paradigm

ASSESSMENT

Assessment via surveys, existing data, or dental screenings:
- Populations' dental needs
- Demographics
- Facility
- Personnel (manpower)
- Existing resources
- Funding

↓

DENTAL HYGIENE DIAGNOSIS

Prioritization to provide goals and objectives for blueprint

↓

PLANNING

Methods to measure goals should be identified
Blueprint should be developed
Address constraints and possible alternatives

↓

IMPLEMENTATION

Program will begin operation
Revision and changes identified and employed

↓

EVALUATION

Measuring of goals via surveys and dental indices
Ongoing revisions employed

↵

Source: Nathe, C. *Dental Public Health.* Upper Saddle River, NJ: Prentice Hall, 2000.

Program Planning

DENTAL HYGIENE DIAGNOSIS

Formulated after completing a comprehensive assessment

PRIORITIZING

Prioritizing is a necessary component during the planning stage of program development

GOALS AND OBJECTIVES

When planning a program, it is necessary to develop measurable goals and objectives so that the program can be effectively evaluated

LABOR FORCE PLANNING

NEED	Defined as a normative, professional judgment as to the amount and kind of health care services required to attain or maintain health
DEMAND	The particular frequency or desired frequency of dental care from a population
SUPPLY	Quantity of dental care services available
UTILIZATION	The number of dental care services actually consumed, not just desired; this can be of importance when speculating on the available supply of personnel to meet the demand and/or need ☛ A great example of the difference between need and demand can be seen when looking at the fact that although the state projects that 50% of the population needs dental restorative work, the state dental association's report suggests that 30% of a dentist's schedule remains unfilled; these two statements emphasize the difference between need and demand

OPERATION

Planning the activities, promotion of the program, timetables, costs, and possible constraints

Program Implementation

ACTUAL IMPLEMENTATION OF OPERATION

Implementing the activities, promotion of the program, timetables, costs, and possible constraints

| MODIFY TREATMENT PLAN | Implements treatment plan, changing when necessary |
| MANAGEMENT | Important to have management for effective coordination, thus smooth operation |

Evaluation of Programs

MEASURING PROGRAM

Utilize effective dental indexes and surveys to evaluate program
See Dental Indexes section

QUALITATIVE EVALUATION (FORMATIVE)

Evaluation utilizing personal interviews, short item, and fill-in-the-blank answers on surveys; some see this as unscientific, but definitely helpful in evaluation and making useful revisions to a program

QUANTITATIVE EVALUATION (SUMMATIVE)

Evaluative program utilizing dental indexes and numbered questions on surveys

Dental Indexes

CHARACTERISTICS OF A DENTAL INDEX

CLARITY	Criteria are understandable
SIMPLICITY	Easily memorized
OBJECTIVITY	Not subject to individual interpretation
VALIDITY	Measures what is intended
RELIABILITY	Reproducible examiner consistency and calibration
QUANTIFIABLE	Statistics can be applied
SENSITIVITY	Ability to detect small degrees of difference
ACCEPTABILITY	No pain to subjects Minimal expense

PLAQUE, DEBRIS, AND/OR CALCULUS INDEXES

PHP: PATIENT HYGIENE PERFORMANCE	Assesses the extent of plaque and debris over a tooth surface
PHP-M: PATIENT HYGIENE PERFOR-MANCE—MODIFIED	A modification of the PHP index
PLAQUE CONTROL RECORD	Records the presence of bacterial plaque on individual tooth surfaces
PLAQUE-FREE SCORE	Determines the location, number, and percent of plaque-free surfaces of individual motivation and instruction
PL1: PLAQUE INDEX	Assesses the thickness of plaque at the gingival area
OHI: ORAL HYGIENE INDEX	Measures existing plaque and calculus as an indication of oral cleanliness; the OHI has two components, the debris index and the calculus index; the practitioner can evaluate both or just one
OHI-S: SIMPLIFIED ORAL HYGIENE INDEX	The same as the OHI, but only used on 6 specific teeth
VMI: VOPE-MANHOLD INDEX	Assesses the supragingival calculus after a dental cleaning

BLEEDING INDEXES

GBI: GINGIVAL BLEEDING INDEX	Records the presence or absence of gingival inflammation as determined by bleeding from interproximal gingival sulci
SBI: SULCUS BLEEDING INDEX	Locates areas of the gingival sulcus bleeding upon gentle probing
EASTMAN INTER-DENTAL BLEEDING INDEX	Measures papillary bleeding
GI: GINGIVAL INDEX	Assesses the severity of gingivitis based on color, consistency, and bleeding on probing
MGI: MODIFIED GINGIVAL INDEX	A modified GI does not utilize bleeding upon probing

P-M-A: PAPILLARY MARGINAL ATTACHED INDEX	Assesses the extent of gingival changes including papillary, gingival margin, and attached gingiva in large studies

PERIODONTAL DISEASES INDEX

PI: PERIODONTAL INDEX	Assesses and scores the periodontal disease status of populations in large studies
PDI: PERIODONTAL DISEASE INDEX	Assesses the prevalence and severity of gingivitis and periodontitis and to show the periodontal status of an individual or a group
CPITN: COMMUNITY PERIODONTAL INDEX OF TREATMENT NEEDS	Screens and monitors individual or group periodontal treatment needs
PSR: PERIODONTAL SCREENING AND RECORDING	A modified version of the CPITN to screen and monitor individuals or group periodontal needs
LPA: LOSS OF PERIO-DONTAL ATTACHMENT	Assesses the loss of periodontal attachment
ESI: EXTENT AND SEVERITY INDEX	Measures the extent and severity of loss of periodontal attachment
GPI: GINGIVAL PERIO-DONTAL INDEX	Assesses the gingivitis and pocket depth in the dentition

DENTAL CARIES INDEXES

DEFT OR S: DECAYED, EXTRACTED, FILLED PRIMARY TEETH OR TOOTH SURFACES	Calculates the status of decay, extractions, and filled primary teeth or tooth surfaces
DMFT OR S: DECAYED MISSING FILLED PERMANENT TEETH	Calculates the status of decay, missing, and filled teeth or surfaces within the dentition, an indicator of dental caries activity
RI: ROOT CARIES INDEX	Calculates the status of root caries, usually recommended for adult surveys

MALOCCLUSION INDEXES

MALIGNMENT INDEX	Assesses the rotations and tooth displacements
OCCLUSAL FEATURE INDEX	Assesses the crowding and interdigitation and vertical and horizontal overbites
HLD INDEX	Assesses orthodontic treatment needs
TREATMENT PRIORITY INDEX	Assesses orthodontic treatment needs
OCCLUSAL INDEX	Assesses the various characteristics of occlusion including, dental age, molar relation, overbite, overjet, posterior crossbite, posterior open bite, tooth displacement, midline relations, and missing permanent maxillary incisors
DENTAL AESTHETIC INDEX	Assesses esthetics of occlusion based on the impact it has on the social and psychological well-being of the individual

DENTAL FLUOROSIS INDEXES

DEVELOPMENTAL DEFECTS OF DENTAL ENAMEL	Scores enamel opacities, regardless of origin to avoid any bias
FLUOROSIS INDEX	Rate of fluorosis within a population, sensitive to very mild through severe cases
FLUOROSIS RISK INDEX	Assesses fluorosis, particularly the specific time of enamel formation
TOOTH SURFACE INDEX OF FLUOROSIS	Rate of fluorosis within a population; more sensitive than the Fluorosis Index

OTHER INDEXES

CLEFT/LIP PALATE	Calculated as the terms of rate in the number of births in a population
ORAL CANCER	Calculated as the terms of rate in a population, sometimes broken down into strata

15 Analyzing Scientific Literature, Understanding Statistical Concepts, and Applying Research Results

Christine Nathe, RDH, MS

➤ CRITIQUING RESEARCH

EVALUATIONS

PURPOSE	Purpose of study should explain what is to be studied
PROBLEM	Research problem and goal clearly identified
LITERATURE REVIEW	Review of literature included, which is thorough and current
METHODS	Describes methods, research designs, and materials to be used in the study
RESULTS/DISCUSSION	Discussion of results clearly described and conclusions justifiable, recommendations for further research

PEER REVIEWED JOURNAL	Reported in a peer-reviewed journal, ensuring effective critique of research •‣ Peer reviewed is sometimes referred to as blind review or refereed •‣ Primary sources come from an original research study •‣ Secondary sources come from a literature review **Table 15-1**

➤ UNDERSTANDING STATISTICAL CONCEPTS

Descriptive Statistics

MEASURES OF CENTRAL TENDENCY	
MEAN	Mean is the arithmetic average ($x = \Sigma\ x/n$) •‣ A dental hygienist has just probed the facial mesial area of the 6 Ramfjord teeth. The measurements were 5,3,3,4,5,5. What is the mean? Answer = 4.2
MEDIAN	Median is the middle item of the data set (the midpoint) •‣ A dental hygienist has just probed the facial mesial area of the 6 Ramfjord teeth. The measurements were 5,3,3,4,5,5. What is the median? Answer = 4.5

Table 15-1

Criteria for Judging a Research Report

- When was the work published?
- Where was it published?
- Are the qualifications of the authors appropriate?
- Is the purpose clearly stated?
- Is the experimental design clearly described?
- Have the possible influences on the findings been identified and controls instituted?
- Has the sample been appropriately selected?
- Has the reliability of the scoring been assessed?
- Is the experimental therapy compared appropriately to the control therapy?
- Is the investigation of sufficient duration?
- Is the statistical analysis appropriate to answer the research questions or hypotheses?
- Have the research questions or hypotheses been answered?
- Do the interpretations and conclusion logically follow from the experimental findings?

| **MODE** | Mode is the most frequently occurring number in the data set; there can be two modes (bimodal) or three modes (tri-modal), etc
🔑 A dental hygienist has just probed the facial mesial area of the 6 Ramfjord teeth. The measurements were 5,3,3,4,5,5. What is the mode?
Answer = 5 |

MEASURES OF DISPERSION OR SPREAD

RANGE	Range is the measurement of the highest score minus the lowest score (highest score – lowest score = range) 🔑 A dental hygienist has just probed the facial mesial area of the 6 Ramfjord teeth. The measurements were 5,3,3,4,5,5. What is the range? Answer = 2
VARIANCE	Variance is the sum of the square devia-tions about the sample mean divided by one less than the total numbers of items; the larger the variance, the more the data items are spread about the means 🔑 A dental hygienist has just probed the facial mesial area of the 6 Ramfjord teeth. The measurements were 5,3,3,4,5,5. What is the variance? Answer = .66
STANDARD DEVIATION	Standard deviation is the square root of the variance 🔑 A dental hygienist has just probed the facial mesial area of the 6 Ramfjord teeth. The measurements were 5,3,3,4,5,5. What is the standard deviation? Answer = .81

GRAPHING DATA

Data can be depicted on a histogram or bar graph, frequency polygon, scattergram, or pie chart

Figure 15-1

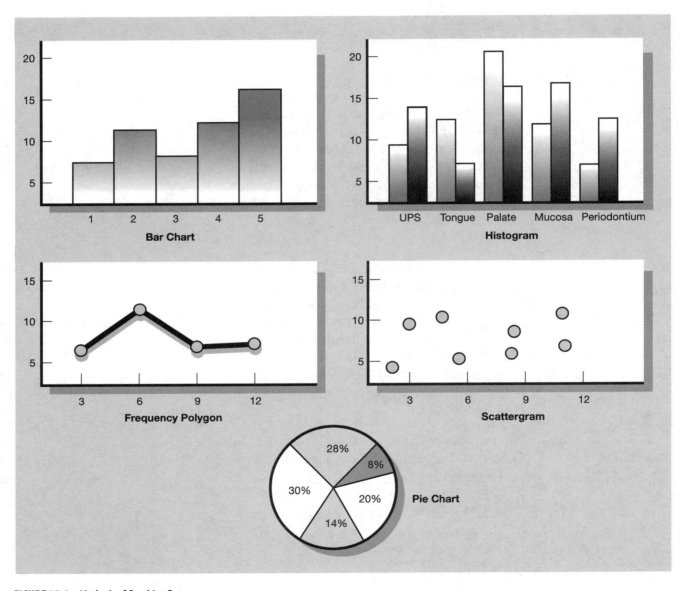

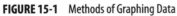

FIGURE 15-1 Methods of Graphing Data

DISTRIBUTION

NORMAL DISTRIBUTION	Normal distribution is sometimes called the bell curve; it is a frequency distribution of scores that when graphed yields a bell-shaped curve **Figure 15-2**
SKEWED	Skew means that extreme scores affect the distribution **Figure 15-3**

CORRELATION

Correlation measures the extent of the linear relationship between two variables

POSITIVE CORRELATION	In a positive linear relationship, the scores being correlated vary together—when one score is high, the other score is high ☛ An increase in sugar uptake may yield an increase in dental caries
NEGATIVE CORRELATION	In a negative relationship, the scores are inverse—when one score is high, the other score is low ☛ An increase in fluoride application may yield a decrease in dental caries

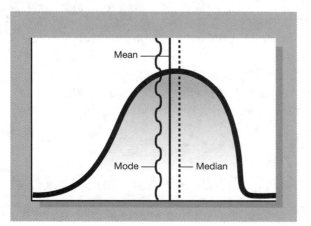

FIGURE 15-2 Normal Distribution (Bell Curve)

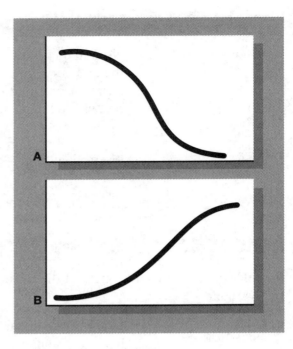

FIGURE 15-3 Skewed Distribution

PERFECT OR STRONG CORRELATION	A perfect correlation relationship would be close to +1 or −1
NO CORRELATION	Coefficients close to 0 would yield little relation, and a 0 would yield no relationship

P VALUES/STATISTICAL SIGNIFICANCE

Significant p-values indicate that the association between the dependent and independent variables was not due to random chance ⚷ Basically, small p-values indicate rare chance occurrences and a statistically significant result (< .05); whereas, large p-values indicate that chance occurrences were likely to have accounted for the results (>.05)

TYPE I ERROR

Type I error is concluding that the null hypothesis is false when it is actually true

HYPOTHESIS

RESEARCH (POSITIVE) HYPOTHESIS	Stated in terms that express the prediction of the investigator 🔑 Brand Y does significantly reduce supragingival calculus formation
NULL HYPOTHESIS	The researcher is attempting to discover a difference by disproving the null 🔑 There is no statistically significant difference between brand Y and a placebo when comparing the formation of supragingival calculus

TYPE II ERROR

A Type II error is concluding that the null hypothesis is true when it is actually false

SAMPLING

To generalize research, it is necessary to utilize a small sample of the population due to time, feasibility, etc

RANDOM SAMPLING	Every possible subject is selected independently and has an equal chance of being selected 🔑 Random sampling is the preferred method; this can be done by lottery for a small sample or by computer selection for a large sample
SYSTEMATIC SAMPLING	Systematic technique samples every nth subject 🔑 This method may be accomplished by choosing every 9th number in a telephone book
CONVENIENCE SAMPLING	Sampling subjects that are readily available 🔑 Using a sample from Dr. Fones' dental practice

STRATIFIED SAMPLING	A researcher has the ability to further stratify the sample during the study by defining information such as age, gender, income level, or educational levels of subjects; the investigator can further generalize results to these strata

Applying Research Results

DEFINITIONS

MORTALITY	The ratio of the number of deaths from a given disease or condition to the total number of cases reported
MORBIDITY	The ratio of sick (affected) individuals to well individuals in a community
PREVALENCE	The number of *all* existing cases of a disease or condition in a population at a given time
INCIDENCE	The number of *new* cases of a disease or condition in a population over a given time
EPIDEMIC	A disease or condition occurring among many individuals in a community or region at the same time, usually spreading rapidly ⚷ Often referred to as an outbreak
PANDEMIC	Widespread outbreak of disease or condition across a region or continent
ENDEMIC	A relatively low but constant level of occurrence of a disease or condition in a population ⚷ The common cold may be an endemic, although during some months it may become an epidemic in a particular locality or region
RISK FACTORS	Characteristics of an individual or population that may increase the likelihood of experience of a given health problem ⚷ Examples may be age, gender, SES, tobacco habits, etc

INDEPENDENT VARIABLE	The condition of the experiment that is manipulated or controlled or the "experimental" variable ☛ In this scenario, Arm & Hammer Dental Care PM® toothpaste is the independent variable. What are the effects of Arm & Hammer Dental Care PM® toothpaste on halitosis?
DEPENDENT VARIABLE	The measure thought to change as a result of the manipulation of the independent variable ☛ In this scenario, halitosis is the dependent variable. What are the effects of Arm & Hammer Dental Care PM® toothpaste on halitosis?
EXTRANEOUS VARIABLE	Uncontrolled variables that are not related to the purpose of the study but may influence the outcome ☛ For example, if you are studying the outcome of dental health education during children's dental health month in February, the results may be affected by the additional promotion of dental health in that month
STATISTICALLY SIGNIFICANT	A term that means the obtained result is likely to be a result of the independent variable
SURVEILLANCE	Methods of systems used to monitor disease in a population periodically or on an ongoing basis
ETIOLOGY	The theory of the causation of disease
VALIDITY	The degree to which the research measured what it was supposed to measure
RELIABILITY	The study was conducted in a controlled manner and if reproduced would yield the same results
PILOT STUDY	Small study that is done prior to a large study to help ensure validity and reliability
PLACEBO	Commonly thought of as "the sugar pill" ☛ A nontreatment

STUDY TYPES

BLIND	When the subject does not know whether or not he/she is receiving actual treatment ⚷ Double blind ensures that both the researcher and the subject do not know whether or not the subject is receiving actual treatment
CROSS-OVER	When the subject is tested on two different treatments at different times
SPLIT-MOUTH	Half of the mouth is used for one treatment and the other half as a control or a different treatment
LONGITUDINAL STUDY	An investigation over a long period of time
PROSPECTIVE STUDY (EXPERIMENTAL)	Clinical trials ⚷ Investigation of tooth-densentizing agents on hypersensitive root surfaces
RETROSPECTIVE (EX POST FACTO)	Looks at a group of people with the disease in the past ⚷ Utilizing past medical records to describe a mother's fluoride uptake during gestation compared to child's current dental health
EPIDEMIOLOGICAL RESEARCH	Study of those factors that influence the occurrence and distribution of health, disease, defect, disability, and death in populations. ⚷ Useful in determining the needs of populations
DESCRIPTIVE RESEARCH	Involves description, documentation, analysis, and interpretation of current conditions
CASE STUDY	Intensive investigation of a person, a family, a group, a social institution, or an entire community in a natural setting

References

➤ Chapter 1

Aquir, A. *Giant's Atlas of Anatomy* (10th ed.). Philadelphia: Lippincott Williams and Wilkins, 1999.

Brand, R. & Isselhard, D. *Anatomy of Orofacial Structures* (6th ed.). St. Louis, MO: Mosby, 1998.

Brand, R. & Isselhard, D. *Study Guide to Accompany the Sixth Edition of Anatomy of Orofacial Structures.* St. Louis, MO: Mosby, 1998.

Fremgen, B. & Frucht, S. *Medical Terminology: An Anatomy and Physiology Systems Approach* (2nd ed.). Upper Saddle River, NJ: Prentice Hall, 2002.

Karst, N. & Smith, S. *Dental Anatomy: A Self-Instructional Program* (10th ed.). Stamford, CT: Appleton and Lange, 1998.

Martinti, H. & Bartholomew, E. *Essentials of Anatomy and Physiology* (2nd ed.). Upper Saddle River, NJ: Prentice Hall, 1999.

Smith, S. & Karst, N. *Head and Neck Histology and Anatomy.* Stamford, CT: Appleton and Lange, 2000.

➤ Chapter 2

Fremgen, B. & Frucht, S. *Medical Terminology: An Anatomy and Physiology Systems Approach* (2nd ed.). Upper Saddle River, NJ: Prentice Hall, 2002.

Martinti, H. & Bartholomew, E. *Essentials of Anatomy and Physiology* (2nd ed.). Upper Saddle River, NJ: Prentice Hall, 1999.

➤ Chapter 3

Insel, P., Turner, E., & Ross, D. *Nutrition.* Jones and Bartlett, 2001.

Recommended Dietary Allowances, 10th ed., Subcommittee on the Tenth Edition of the RDAs, Food and Nutrition Board, Commission of Life Sciences, National Research Council, National Academy Press, Washington, DC, 1989.

Whitney, N. & Rolfes, S: *Understanding Nutrition.* Boulder, CO: Wadsworth, 1999.

Zeman, F. & Ney, D. *Applications in Medical Nutrition Therapy* (2nd ed.). Upper Saddle River, NJ: Prentice Hall, 1996.

➤ Chapter 4

Alcamo, I.E. *Fundamental of Microbiology* (5th ed.). Menlo Park, CA: Addison Wesley Longman, 1997.

Jensen, M., Wright, D., & Robison, R. *Microbiology for the Health Sciences* (4th ed.). Upper Saddle River, NJ: Prentice Hall, 1997.

➤ Chapter 5

Ibsen, O. & Phelan J. *Oral Pathology for the Dental Hygienist* (3rd ed.). Philadelphia: W.B. Saunders, 2000.

Langlais R.P. & Miller C.S. *Color Atlas of Common Oral Conditions.* Philadelphia: Williams and Wilkins, 1998.

Newland, R., Meiller, T., Wynn, R., & Crossley, H. *Oral Soft Tissue Diseases.* Hudson, OH: Lexi-Comp, 2001.

Neville, D. & Allen B. *Oral and Maxillofacial Pathology.* Philadelphia: W.B. Saunders, 1995.

➤ Chapter 6

Christ, D. *High-Yield Pharmacology.* Philadelphia: Lippincott,Williams and Wilkins, 1999.

Haveles, E. *Pharmacology for Dental Hygiene Practice.* Cincinatti, OH: Delmar, 1997.

Requa-Clark. *Applied Pharmacology for the Dental Hygienist* (4th ed.). St. Louis, MO: Mosby, 2000.

Whynn R., Meiller T., & Crossley, H. *Drug Information Handbook for Dentistry* (5th ed.). Hudson, OH: Lexi-Comp, 1999.

➤ Chapter 7

Annals of Periodontology: 1996 World Workshop in Periodontics, Vol. 1. Chicago: American Academy of Periodontology, 1996.

Darby, M.L. & Walsh, M.M. *Dental Hygiene Theory and Practice.* Philadelphia: WB Saunders, 1995.

Tong, D. & Rothwell, B. Antibiotic Prophylaxis in Dentistry: A Review and Practice Recommendations. *JADA,* Vol. 131, March 2000, pp. 368–374.

Wilkins, E.M. *Clinical Practice of the Dental Hygienist* (8th ed.). Philadelphia: Lippincott, Williams and Wilkins, 1999.

Woodall, I.R. *Comprehensive Dental Hygiene Care* (4th ed.). St. Louis, MO: Mosby, 1993.

➤ Chapter 8

Frommer, H. *Radiology for Dental Auxiliaries* (7th ed.). St. Louis, MO: Mosby, 2001.

Haring, J.I. & Lind L. *Dental Radiography: Principles and Techniques.* Philadelphia: WB Saunders, 1996.

Johnson, O., McNally, M., & Essay, C. *Essentials of Dental Radiography for Dental Assistants and Hygienists* (6th ed.). Stamford, CT: Appleton and Lange, 1999.

Thomson-Lakey, E. *Exercises in Oral Radiography Techniques: A Laboratory Manual.* Upper Saddle River, NJ: Prentice Hall, 2000.

White S. & Pharoah, M. *Oral Radiology Principles and Interpretation.* St. Louis, MO: Mosby, 2000.

➤ Chapter 9

Centers for Disease Control. *HIV/AIDS Surveillance Report.* Online. *http://www. cdc.gov/nchstp/hiv_aids/stats/hasr 1001.pdf.* 1998;1:3.37–40.

Darby, M.L. & Walsh, M.M. *Dental Hygiene Theory and Practice.* Philadelphia: WB Saunders, 1995.

Evans, D. *HIV Diagnostic Tests.* Online. *http://www.projinf. org/fs/HIV DiagTest.htm1#CommonLabTests.* 1997:1–14.

Evans, D. *Project Inform Perspective: Number 21-March 1997.* Online. *http:// www.projinf.org/pub/21/ViralLoad.html.* 1997:1–3.

Hughes, M., et al. CD4 cell count as a surrogate endpoint in HIV clinical trials: A metaanalysis of studies of the AIDS Clinical Trials Group. *AIDS* 1998;12: 1823–1832.

Hughes, M., et al. Monitoring plasma HIV-1 RNA levels in addition to CD4+ lymphocyte count improves assessment of antiretroviral therapeutic response. *Annals of Internal Medicine* 1997;126:929–938.

Little, J.W. & Falace, D. *Dental Management of the Medically Compromised Patient.* St. Louis, MO: Mosby, 1997.

Malamed, S. *Handbook of Local Anesthesia* (4th ed.). St. Louis, MO: Mosby, 1997.

Malamed, S. *Medical Emergiencies in the Dental Office.* St. Louis, MO: Mosby, 1993.

Mancano, M. Focus on selected meperidine and codeine drug interactions. *Pharmacy Times* April 2000, pp. 38–22.

Miller-Keane. *Encyclopedia and Dictionary of Medicine, Nursing, & Allied Health.* Philadelphia: WB Saunders, 1996.

Rhoades, R. & Pflanzer, R. *Human Physiology.* Philadelphia: WB Saunders, 1992.

Stein, D.S., Korcik, J.A., & Vermund, S.H. CD4+ lymphocyte cell enumeration for prediction of clinical courses of human immunodeficiency virus disease: A review. *J of Inf Diseases* 1992;165:352–363.

Treatment Strategy. *Project Inform Discussion Paper.* San Francisco, 1996.

UNAIDS Press Release: AIDS moves up to fourth place among would-be killers. Online. *http://www.unaids.org/highband/ press/whr99.html* 1999:1–2.

Whitney, N. & Rolfes, S. *Understanding Nutrition.* Boulder, CO: Wadsworth, 1999.

Wilkins, E.M. *Clinical Practice of the Dental Hygienist* (8th ed.). Philadelphia: Lippincott, Williams and Wilkins, 1999.

Woodall, I.R. *Comprehensive Dental Hygiene Care* (4th ed.). St. Louis, MO: Mosby, 1993.

➤ Chapter 10

Carranza, R.E. *Glickman's Clinical Periodontology* (6th ed.). Philadelphia: WB Saunders, 1995.

Carranza, R.E. & Newman, M.G. *Clinical Periodontology* (8th ed.). Philadelphia: WB Saunders, 1996.

Darby, M.L. & Walsh, M.M. *Dental Hygiene Theory and Practice.* Philadelphia: WB Saunders, 1995.

Hodges, K. *Concepts in Nonsurgical Periodontal Therapy.* Cincinnati, OH: Delmar, 1997.

Pattison, A. & Pattison, G. *Periodontal Instrumentation* (2nd ed.). Stamford, CT: Appleton and Lange, 1992.

Wilkins, E.M. *Clinical Practice of the Dental Hygienist* (8th ed.). Philadelphia: Lippincott, Williams and Wilkins, 1999.

➤ Chapter 11

Darby, M.L. & Walsh, M.M. *Dental Hygiene Theory and Practice.* Philadelphia: WB Saunders, 1995.

Nathe, C. *Dental Public Health: Contemporary Practice for the Dental Hygienist.* Upper Saddle River, NJ: Prentice Hall, 2001.

Wilkins, E.M. *Clinical Practice of the Dental Hygienist* (8th ed.). Philadelphia: Lippincott, Williams and Wilkins, 1999.

➤ Chapter 12

Craig, R., Obrien, W., & Powers, J. *Dental Material: Properties and Manipulation* (5th Edition). St. Louis, MO: Mosby, 1992.

Gladwin, M. & Bagby, M. *Clinical Aspects of Dental Materials.* Philadelphia: Lippincott, Williams and Wilkins, 2000.

Ferrace, J. *Materials in Dentistry: Principles and Applications* (2nd ed.). Philadelphia: Lippincott, Williams and Wilkins, 2000.

➤ Chapter 13

Nathe, C. *Dental Public Health: Contemporary Practice for the Dental Hygienist.* Upper Saddle River, NJ: Prentice Hall, 2001.

US Department of Health and Human Services. *Healthy People 2010.* Hyattsville, MD: US Department of Health and Human Services, National Center for Health Statistics, 2001.

US Department of Health and Human Services. *Oral Health in America: A Report of the Surgeon General.* Rockville, MD: US Department of Health and Human Services, National Institute of Dental and Craniofacial Research, National Institutes of Health, 2000.

➤ Chapter 14

Darby, M. & Bowen, D. *Research Methods for the Oral Health Professionls: An Introduction.* Pocatello, ID: JT McCann, 1986.

DeBiase, C. *Dental Health Education Theory and Practice.* Philadelphia: Lea & Febiger, 1991.